E

EBV	Epstein-Barr virus
ECG, EKG	Electrocardiogram
ECHO	Echocardiography
EEG	Electroencephalogram
EGD	Esophagogastroduodenoscopy
ELISA	Enzyme-linked immunosorbent assay
EMG	Electromyography
ENG	Electroneurography
EP	Evoked potential
EPS	Electrophysiologic study
ERCP	Endoscopic retrograde cholangiopancreatography
ESR	Erythrocyte sedimentation rate
EUG	Excretory urography

F

FBS	Fasting blood sugar
FDPs	Fibrin degradation products
FSH	Follicle-stimulating hormone
FSPs	Fibrin split products
FTA-ABS	Fluorescent treponemal antibody absorption test
FTI	Free thyroxine index
FUT	Fibrinogen uptake test

G

G-6-PD	Glucose-6-phosphate dehydrogenase
Gal-1-PUT	Galactose-1-phosphate uridyl transferase
GB series	Gallbladder series
GE reflux	Gastroesophageal reflux scan
GGT	Gamma-glutamyl transferase
GGTP	Gamma-glutamyl transpeptidase
GHb, GHB	Glycosylated hemoglobin
GI series	Gastrointestinal series
GTT	Glucose tolerance test

H

HAA	Hepatitis-associated antigen
HAV	Hepatitis A virus
Hb, Hgb	Hemoglobin
HBV	Hepatitis B virus
HCG	Human chorionic gonadotropin
HCO$_3^-$	Bicarbonate
HCS	Human chorionic somatomammotropin
Hct	Hematocrit
HDL	High-density lipoprotein
HIV	Human immunodeficiency virus
HPL	Human placental lactogen
HSV 2	Herpes simplex virus, type 2

Mosby's
**Diagnostic and
Laboratory
Test Reference**

Mosby's Diagnostic and Laboratory Test Reference

Kathleen Deska Pagana, PhD, RN

Associate Professor
Department of Nursing
Lycoming College
Williamsport, Pennsylvania

Timothy James Pagana, MD, FACS

Surgical Oncologist
Williamsport, Pennsylvania

Illustrated

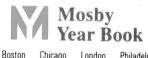

Mosby
Year Book

St. Louis   Baltimore   Boston   Chicago   London   Philadelphia   Sydney   Toronto

Mosby
Year Book

Dedicated to Publishing Excellence

Executive Editor: Don Ladig
Developmental Editor: Robin Carter
Project Supervisor: Barbara Merritt
Copyeditor: Roger McWilliams
Designer: Liz Fett
Design Consultant: Ken Wendling
Illustrator: Mark Swindle

Printed in the United States of America
Mosby–Year Book, Inc. 11830 Westline Industrial Drive,
St. Louis, Missouri 63146

Library of Congress Cataloging-in-Publication Data

Pagana, Kathleen Deska
    Mosby's diagnostic and laboratory test reference / Kathleen Deska
Pagana, Timothy James Pagana.
        p.   cm.
    Includes bibliographical references and index.
    ISBN 0-8016-3756-2
    1. Diagnosis, Laboratory—Handbooks, manuals, etc. 2.   Nursing—
Handbooks, manuals, etc.   I. Pagana, Timothy James
II. Title.
    [DNLM: 1. Diagnosis, Laboratory—handbooks.   QY 39 P128m]
RB37.P24   1992
616.07′5—dc20
DNLM/DLC
for Library of Congress   91-27324
                                                                     CIP

    93   94   95   96   C/D   9   8   7   6   5   4

Consultants

Mary Anthony, MSN, RN
Assistant Professor
MacMurray College
Jacksonville, Illinois

Diane M. Billings, RN, EdD
Professor of Nursing
Indiana University
Indianapolis, Indiana

Barbara Bogdan, MSN, RN
Nursing Instructor
South Suburban College
South Holland, Illinois

Sheila Bollinger, RN, EdD
Instructor
Houston Community College
Houston, Texas

Joyce Engel, RN, MEd
Assistant Professor
University of Lethbridge
Lethbridge, Alberta

Joan S. Grant, RN, DSN, CS
Assistant Professor
University of Alabama
Birmingham, Alabama

Jane Lancour, MSN, RN
Consultant
JML and Associates
Irvine, California

Charlotte Ludwig, MS, ET
Assistant Professor
Erie Community College
Williamsville, New York

Edwina A. McConnell,
PhD, RN
Consultant
Madison, Wisconsin

Andrew McPhee, BS, MA
(candidate)
Staff Nurse
Rushford Treatment Center
Middletown, Connecticut

Tracy A. Riley, BSN, RN
Nursing Instructor
Aultman Hospital School of
    Nursing
Canton, Ohio

Anna Louise Scandiffio,
MS, RN
Nursing Quality Improvement
    Coordinator
Department of Veterans Affairs
Baltimore, Maryland

Brenda Shelton, MS, RN,
CCRN, OCN
Critical Care Clinical Nurse
    Specialist
The Johns Hopkins Oncology
    Center
Baltimore, Maryland

Teresa M. Smiley, PhD, RN
Assistant Professor
University of Wisconsin-
    Oshkosh
Oshkosh, Wisconsin

Sarah Jane Tobiason,
MA, RN
Assistant Professor
Arizona State University
Tempe, Arizona

Marilyn J. Vontz, MA, RN, Doctoral Candidate
Instructor
Bryan Memorial Hospital School
  of Nursing
Lincoln, Nebraska

Mary Wallace, MSN, RNC
Associate Professor
Northern Michigan University
Marquette, Michigan

We lovingly dedicate this book to our daughters

Jocelyn Marie Pagana
Denise Kathleen Pagana
Theresa Noel Pagana

Preface

Mosby's Diagnostic and Laboratory Test Reference provides the user with an essential reference that allows easy access to 564 clinically relevant laboratory and diagnostic tests. A unique feature of this handbook is its consistent format, which allows for quick reference without sacrificing the depth of detail necessary for a thorough understanding of the nurse's important role in diagnostic and laboratory testing. All tests are listed in alphabetical order by their complete name. The alphabetical format is a strong feature of the book; it allows the user to locate tests quickly without having to place tests in an appropriate category or body system. Every feature of this book is geared to provide pertinent information in a sequence that best simulates nursing priorities in the clinical setting.

The following information is provided, whenever possible, for effective diagnostic and laboratory testing:

Name of test. Tests are listed by their complete name. A complete list of abbreviations and alternate test names follows each main entry.

Type of test. This section identifies whether the test is, for example, an x-ray procedure, ultrasound, nuclear scan, blood test, urine test, sputum test, or microscopic examination of tissue. This section helps the reader identify the source of the laboratory specimen or location of the diagnostic procedure.

Normal findings. Normal values are listed, when applicable, for the infant, child, adult, and elderly person. Also, where appropriate, values are separated into male and female. It is important to realize that normal ranges of laboratory tests vary from institution to institution. This variability is even more obvious among the various laboratory textbooks. For this reason, we have deliberately chosen *not* to add a table of normal values as an appendix, and we encourage the user to check the normal values at the institution where the test is performed. This should be relatively easy, since most laboratory reports indicate normal values.

Possible critical values. These values give an indication of results that are well outside the usual range of normal. These results generally require immediate intervention.

Test explanation and related physiology. This section provides a concise, yet comprehensive description of each test. This explanation includes fundamental information about the test itself, specific indications for the test, how the test is performed, what disease or disorder various results may show, how it will affect the patient or client, and relevant pathophysiology that will enhance understanding of the tests.

Contraindications. These data are crucial because they alert the nurse to patients who should not have the test. Patients frequently highlighted in this section include those who are pregnant, who are allergic to iodinated or contrast dyes, and who have bleeding disorders.

Potential complications. This section alerts the nurse to potential problems that will necessitate astute nursing assessments and interventions. For example, if a potential complication is renal failure, the nursing implication may be to hydrate the patient before the test and force fluids after the test. A typical potential complication for many x-ray procedures is allergy to iodinated dye. Patient symptoms and appropriate nursing interventions are described in detail.

Interfering factors. This section contains pertinent information because many factors can invalidate the test or make the test results unreliable. An important feature of this section is the inclusion of drugs that can interfere with test results. Drugs that increase or decrease test values are always listed at the end of this section for consistency and quick access.

Procedure and patient care. This section emphasizes the nurse's role in diagnostic and laboratory testing by addressing psychosocial and physiologic nursing interventions. Patient education and rationale are included. For quick access to essential information, this section is divided into *before, during,* and *after* time sequences.

Before. This section addresses the need to explain the procedure and to allay patient concerns or anxieties. If a consent is usually required, this is always listed as the second bulleted item in this section. Other important features of this section include requirements such as fasting, obtaining baseline values, and performing bowel preparations.

During. This section gives specific directions for clinical specimen studies (e.g., urine and blood studies). An estimate of the approximate amount of a specimen is sometimes given; however, this amount may vary from institution to institution. This section describes pointers that new nurses may not realize or practicing nurses may forget. Diagnostic procedures and their variations sometimes are described in a numbered, usually step-by-step format. Important information, such as who performs the test, where the study is performed, patient sensation, and duration of the procedure, are bulleted for emphasis. The duration of the procedure is very helpful for patient teaching because it indicates the time generally allotted for each study.

After. This section includes vital information that the nurse should perform or convey following the test. Examples include factors such as maintaining bed rest, comparing pulses to baseline values, encouraging fluids, and observing for signs and symptoms of sepsis.

Abnormal findings. As the name implies, this section lists the abnormal findings for each study. Increased or decreased values are listed when appropriate.

The blank space at the end of each test facilitates individualizing the studies according to the institution performing the test. Variations in any area of the test (e.g., patient preparation, test procedure, normal values, postprocedural care) can be noted.

This logical format emphasizes clinically relevant information; the clarity of this format will facilitate a quick understanding of content essential to practicing nurses and student nurses. Color has been used to help locate tests and highlight critical information (e.g., possible critical values). Extensive cross-referencing exists throughout the book. This permits full understanding and helps the reader tie together or locate related studies, such as the cardiac enzymes (CPK, LDH, AST).

For easy access, a listing of abbreviations for test names is included on the book's endpapers. The Appendix provides a list of typical abbreviations and units of measurement. Following the Appendix is a detailed Bibliography. This is followed by an index of studies according to *body systems*. This listing may familiarize the reader with other related studies the patient or client may need or the user may want to review. This should be especially useful for nursing students and for nurses working in specialized areas. A second index provides a listing of studies according to *test type*. This listing may help the user read and learn about similarly performed tests and procedures (e.g., x-rays of the skull, chest, and abdomen). Finally, a comprehensive index includes names of all tests and their synonyms and any other relevant terms found within the tests.

All studies in this book have been extensively critiqued by several reviewers. This has greatly improved the book's accuracy and usefulness. We are most appreciative of the excellent reviewers, and we thank them all. We sincerely thank our nursing editors, Don Ladig and Robin Carter, for helping us to develop the idea and format for this book and for their continual support. We also want to thank Karen Olson and Kathy Weiland of Olson Business Services for the typing of this manuscript. Their pleasant manner and enthusiasm through countless revisions was most appreciated, and we sincerely acknowledge their help.

We invite comments from users of this book so that we may continue to provide useful, relevant diagnostic and laboratory test information to users of future editions.

Kathleen D. Pagana

Timothy J. Pagana

Contents

Diagnostic and laboratory tests, p. 1

Appendix:
  **Typical abbreviations and units of
    measurement, p. 799**
  Bibliography, p. 801

Indexes:
  Tests by body system, p. 803
  Tests by type, p. 809
  Comprehensive index, p. 815

Mosby's
Diagnostic and Laboratory Test Reference

acid-fast bacilli (AFB)

Type of test Sputum

Normal findings No bacilli seen

Test explanation and related physiology

Sputum collection and analysis are usually ordered when tuberculosis is suspected. *Mycobacterium tuberculosis,* after taking up a dye such as fuchsin, is not decolorized by acid alcohol (i.e., it is acid fast) and is seen under the microscope as a red, rod-shaped organism. If this bacillus is seen, the patient has active tuberculosis.

Procedure and patient care

Before

- Explain to the patient the procedure for sputum collection.
- Remind the patient that the sputum must be coughed up from the lungs and that saliva is not sputum.
- Hold antibiotics until after the sputum has been collected.
- Give the patient a sterile sputum container the night before the sputum is to be collected so that the morning specimen may be obtained when the patient awakens.
- Instruct the patient to rinse out his or her mouth with water before the sputum collection to decrease contamination by particles in the oropharynx. Remind the patient not to use mouthwash.

During

- For best results, obtain sputum collection when the patient awakens in the morning.
- Collect at least 1 teaspoon of sputum in a sterile sputum container.
- Obtain sputum usually by having the patient cough after taking several deep breaths.
- If the patient is unable to produce a sputum specimen, stimulate coughing by lowering the head of the patient's bed or by giving an aerosol administration of a warm hypertonic solution.

- Note that other methods to collect sputum, such as endotracheal aspiration, fiberoptic bronchoscopy, and transtracheal aspiration, may be used if necessary.
- Usually, for AFB determinations, collect sputum on three separate occasions.

After

- Avoid personal contamination and wear gloves when handling all patient secretions.
- Inform the patient to notify the nurse as soon as the specimen is collected.
- Label the specimen and send it to the laboratory as soon as possible.

Abnormal finding

Tuberculosis

Notes

acid phosphatase (Prostatic acid phosphatase [PAP])

Type of test Blood

Normal findings

Adult/elderly: 0.11-0.60 U/L (Roy, Brower, Hayden; 37° C) or 0.11-0.60 U/L (SI units)
Child: 8.6-12.6 U/ml (30° C)
Newborn: 10.4-16.4 U/ml (30° C)

Test explanation and related physiology

The enzyme acid phosphatase, often referred to as prostatic acid phosphatase, is found in highest concentrations in the prostate gland. The determination of acid phosphatase level is primarily used to diagnose and stage prostatic carcinoma and to monitor the efficacy of treatment. Elevated levels are seen in patients with prostatic cancer that has metastasized beyond the capsule to other parts of the body, especially the bone. If the tumor is successfully treated by surgery, acid phosphatase levels decrease in several days. If the tumor is treated by estrogen therapy, enzyme levels return to normal in several weeks. Rising levels of acid phosphatase may indicate a poor prognosis.

Acid phosphatase is also found in high concentrations in seminal fluid. For this reason, acid phosphatase tests may be done on vaginal secretions to investigate alleged acts of rape.

Interfering factors

- Falsely high levels of acid phosphatase may occur in males after a rectal examination or after instrumentation of the prostate (e.g., cystoscopy) because of prostatic stimulation.
- Drugs that may cause elevated levels include androgens (in females) and clofibrate (Atromid S).
- Drugs that may cause decreased levels include flourides, phosphates, oxalates, and alcohol.

Procedure and patient care

Before

- Explain the procedure to the patient.
- Tell the patient that no food or drink restrictions are associated with this test.

- Remember that some laboratories request they be notified before the blood sample is drawn so that immediate attention (less than 1 hour) can be given to the sample.

During
- Collect approximately 5 to 10 ml of blood in a red-top tube.
- Avoid hemolysis.
- Note on the laboratory slip if the patient has had a prostatic examination or instrumentation of the prostate within 24 hours.

After
- Apply pressure or a pressure dressing to the venipuncture site.
- Assess the venipuncture site for bleeding.
- Have the test performed without delay, or freeze the specimen.
- Do *not* leave the specimen at room temperature for 1 hour or longer because the enzyme is heat and pH sensitive and its activity will decrease.

Abnormal findings
Increased levels

Prostatic carcinoma
Multiple myeloma
Paget's disease
Sickle cell crisis
Gaucher's disease
Renal impairment

Cancer of the breast and bone
Cirrhosis
Hyperparathyroidism
Thrombocytosis
Cancer metastasis to the bone

Notes

adrenal angiography (Adrenal arteriography)

Type of test X-ray with contrast dye

Normal findings Normal adrenal artery vasculature

Test explanation and related physiology

The adrenal gland and its arterial system are visualized by the injection of radiopaque dye into the adrenal arteries. Both benign and malignant tumors of the adrenal glands can be detected easily by this technique. Bilateral adrenal hyperplasia can also be diagnosed.

Contraindications

- Patients with allergies to shellfish or iodinated dye
- Patients with atherosclerosis
- Patients who are pregnant
- Patients with bleeding disorders

Potential complications

- Allergic reactions to iodinated dye
  These may vary from mild flushing, itching, and urticaria to severe, life-threatening anaphylaxis (evidenced by respiratory distress, drop in blood pressure, shock). In the unusual event of anaphylaxis the patient is treated with diphenhydramine (Benadryl), steroids, and epinephrine. Oxygen and endotracheal equipment should be on hand for immediate use.
- Hemorrhage from the puncture site used for arterial access
- Embolism from dislodgement of an atherosclerotic plaque
- Infarction from dislodgement of an atherosclerotic plaque
- Fatal episode of severe hypertension
  In patients with pheochromocytoma (a catecholamine-producing tumor of the adrenal medulla) a fatal episode of severe hypertension can be precipitated by the dye injection. Propranolol (Inderal), a beta-adrenergic blocker, and phenoxybenzamine (Dibenzyline), an alpha-adrenergic blocker, are given for several days before the study to avoid the precipitation of a malignant hypertensive episode.

- Hemorrhage within the adrenal gland
  This may cause necrosis of the gland, leading to Addison's disease (adrenal insufficiency).

Procedure and patient care

Before

- Explain the procedure to the patient. Allay any fears and allow the patient to verbalize concerns.
- Ensure that written and informed consent for this procedure is in the patient's chart.
- Inform the patient that a warm flush may be felt when the dye is injected.
- Assess the patient for allergies to iodinated dye. Inform the radiologist if an allergy to iodinated contrast is suspected. The radiologist may prescribe a Benadryl and steroid preparation to be administered before testing. Usually, hypoallergenic non-ionic contrast will be used during the test.
- Determine if the patient has been taking anticoagulants.
- Keep the patient NPO after midnight on the day of the test.
- Mark the site of the patient's peripheral pulses with a pen before catheterization. This will permit quicker assessment of the pulses after the procedure.
- Administer preprocedural medications as ordered.
- If the patient is suspected of having a pheochromocytoma, administer propranolol and phenoxybenzamine as ordered to prevent a potentially fatal hypertensive episode.

During

- In the angiography room, place the patient on an x-ray table in the supine position.
- Note the following procedural steps:

  1. The patient is usually sedated with meperidine and atropine.
  2. The groin is prepared and draped in a sterile manner.
  3. The catheter is passed into the femoral artery and advanced into the aorta.
  4. With fluoroscopic visualization, the catheter is manipulated into the inferior adrenal artery, a branch of the renal artery, for dye injection.
  5. The x-ray films are taken.

6. The catheter is removed, and a pressure dressing is applied to the puncture site.

- Note that this procedure is usually performed by an angiographer (radiologist) in approximately 1 hour.
- During the dye injection, remind the patient that an intense burning flush may be felt throughout the body but lasts only a few seconds.
- Tell the patient that the only other discomfort is the groin puncture necessary for arterial access.

After

- Observe the arterial puncture site frequently for hematoma, hemorrhage, or absence of pulse.
- Assess the patient's extremities for signs of ischemia (numbness, tingling, pain, absence of peripheral pulses, loss of function).
- Compare the pulses with the preprocedural baseline values.
- Compare the color and temperature of the extremity with those of the uninvolved extremity.
- Assess the pulse and vital signs frequently because embolism or bleeding require immediate intervention.
- Keep the patient on bed rest for 12 to 24 hours to allow for complete healing of the arterial puncture.
- Apply cold compresses to the puncture site if needed to reduce swelling or discomfort.
- Have patient drink fluids after the study to prevent diuretic-induced dehydration caused by the dye.

Abnormal findings

Pheochromocytomas   Adrenal carcinomas
Adrenal adenomas   Bilateral adrenal hyperplasia

Notes

adrenal venography

Type of test   X-ray with contrast dye

Normal findings   Normal adrenal veins and normal adrenal vein hormone assay

Test explanation and related physiology

Adrenal venography is a radiologic test performed to obtain blood samples from the adrenal vein and allow localization of adrenal pathology. Once the vein is identified, a catheter can be placed in the vein and blood can be selectively obtained from each adrenal gland.

In patients with Cushing's syndrome the blood is analyzed for plasma cortisol. If the plasma cortisol level in the blood obtained from one side is much higher than that of the other, a unilateral adrenal tumor is causing the Cushing's syndrome. If, on the other hand, plasma cortisol levels are bilaterally elevated, one can safely conclude that the Cushing's syndrome is caused by bilateral adrenal hyperplasia.

In patients with a pheochromocytoma the adrenal venous blood is analyzed for catecholamines. If the catecholamine level on one side is much higher than that of the other, a unilateral pheochromocytoma exists on the side with the elevated levels. If blood obtained from both sides is equally elevated, the patient probably has bilateral adrenal pheochromocytoma. If the adrenal venous blood samples are not elevated on either side in a patient who has elevated peripheral blood catacholamine levels, the pheochromocytoma exists outside the adrenal gland (extraadrenal pheochromocytoma).

The venous blood can also be evaluated for aldosterone, androgens, and other substances.

Contraindications

- Patients with allergies to shellfish or iodinated dye
- Patients with bleeding disorders

Potential complications

- Allergic reaction to iodinated dye
  Allergic reactions may vary from mild flushing, itching, and urticaria to severe, life-threatening anaphylaxis (evi-

denced by respiratory distress, drop in blood pressure, shock). In the unusual event of anaphylaxis the patient is treated with diphenhydramine (Benadryl), steroids, and epinephrine. Oxygen and endotracheal equipment should be on hand for immediate use.
- Adrenal hemorrhage or necrosis caused by the pressure of the dye injection
  This may cause Addison's disease (adrenal insufficiency).
- Cellulitis
- Thrombophlebitis
- Bacteremia

Procedure and patient care

Before

- Explain the procedure to the patient.
- Ensure that a written and informed consent for this procedure has been obtained.
- Assess the patient for allergies to iodine dye. Inform the radiologist if an allergy to iodinated contrast is suspected. The radiologist may prescribe a Benadryl and steroid preparation to be administered before testing. Usually, hypoallergenic non-ionic contrast will be used during the test.
- Administer propranolol (Inderal), a beta-adrenergic blocker, and phenoxybenzamine (Dibenzyline), an alpha-adrenergic blocker, for the patient with a suspected pheochromocytoma. This prevents a potentially fatal catecholamine-induced hypertensive episode.

During

- Bring the fasting patient to the angiography laboratory (usually in the radiology department).
- Place the patient in the supine position on the x-ray table.
- Note the following procedural steps:
  1. The patient's groin is prepared and draped in a sterile manner.
  2. After the venous puncture site is locally anesthetized, the femoral vein is catheterized.
  3. The catheter is passed into the adrenal vein.
  4. Dye is injected to visualize the adrenal veins and to ensure that the catheter is in the adrenal vein.

5. Blood is obtained and sent to the chemistry laboratory for assays.

- Note that this procedure is usually performed by an angiographer (radiologist) in approximately 1 hour.
- Tell the patient that the only discomfort is the groin puncture necessary for arterial access.

After

- Evaluate the patient's vital signs frequently for signs of bleeding or hemorrhage.
- Assess the patient with a suspected pheochromocytoma for signs and symptoms of a hypertensive episode. If such an episode occurs, notify the physician immediately to obtain an order for appropriate alpha- and beta-adrenergic blocking agents.
- Assess the groin site for redness, pain, swelling, and bleeding with each vital sign check.
- Apply cold compresses to the puncture site if needed to reduce discomfort or swelling.

Abnormal findings

Unilateral adrenal tumor
Bilateral adrenal tumor
Unilateral pheochromocytoma

Bilateral pheochromocytoma
Extraadrenal pheochromocytoma

Notes

adrenocorticotropic hormone (ACTH, Corticotropin)

Type of test Blood

Normal findings

AM: 15-100 pg/ml or 10-80 ng/L (SI units)
PM: <50 pg/ml or <50 ng/L (SI units)

Test explanation and related physiology

The serum ACTH study is a test of anterior pituitary gland function that affords the greatest insight into the causes of either Cushing's syndrome or Addison's disease. In the patient with Cushing's syndrome an elevated ACTH level can be caused by a pituitary ACTH-producing tumor or a nonpituitary (ectopic) ACTH-producing tumor, usually in the lung, pancreas, thymus, or ovary. ACTH levels greater than 200 pg/ml usually indicate ectopic ACTH production. If the ACTH level is below normal in a patient with cushingoid symptoms, an adrenal adenoma or carcinoma is probably the cause of the hyperfunction.

In patients with Addison's disease an elevated ACTH level indicates primary adrenal gland failure, as in adrenal gland destruction caused by infarction, hemorrhage, or autoimmunity; surgical removal of the adrenal gland; congenital enzyme deficiency; or adrenal suppression after prolonged ingestion of exogenous steroids. If the ACTH level is below normal in a patient with Addison's disease, hypopituitarism is most probably the cause of the hypofunction.

One must be aware that there is a diurnal variation of ACTH levels. Evening samples are usually one half to two thirds of the morning specimen.

Interfering factors

- Stress (psychological or physical) can artifically increase levels.
- Recently administered radioisotope scans can affect levels.

Procedure and patient care

Before

- Explain the procedure to the patient. Allow plenty of time to answer questions so that stress is diminished as much as possible.

- Keep the patient NPO after midnight the day of the test.
- Evaluate the patient for high stress levels that would invalidate the test results.

During

- Collect approximately 20 ml of heparinized venous blood in a green-top tube.
- Chill the blood tube to prevent enzymatic degradation of ACTH.

After

- Place the blood on ice and send immediately to the chemistry laboratory.
- Apply pressure or a pressure dressing to the venipuncture site.
- Assess the venipuncture site for bleeding.

Abnormal findings

Increased levels

Addison's disease (primary adrenal insufficiency)
Cushing's disease (pituitary-dependent adrenal hyperplasia)
Ectopic ACTH syndrome
Stress
Adrenogenital syndrome (congenital adrenal hyperplasia

Decreased levels

Secondary adrenal insufficiency (pituitary insufficiency)
Cushing's syndrome
Hypopituitarism
Adrenal adenoma or carcinoma
Steroid administration

Notes

adrenocorticotropic hormone stimulation test (ACTH stimulation test, Cosyntropin test)

Type of test Blood

Normal findings

Rapid test: increase of more than 7 μg/dl above baseline
24-hour test: greater than 40 μg/dl
3-day test: greater than 40 μg/dl

Test explanation and related physiology

Exogenous ACTH is given to the patient, and the ability of the adrenal glands to respond to ACTH stimulation is measured by plasma cortisol levels. Patients with cushingoid symptoms caused by bilateral adrenal hyperplasia will have an exaggerated response to the ACTH stimulation. However, hyperfunctioning adrenal tumors, which are usually autonomous and relatively insensitive to changes in ACTH levels, are associated with little or no cortisol increase above baseline values in these patients.

This test is even more valuable in the patient suspected of having Addison's disease (adrenal insufficiency). An appropriate increase in plasma cortisol levels after the infusion of ACTH shows that the adrenal gland is capable of functioning if stimulated. The cause of the adrenal insufficiency would lie within the pituitary gland (hypopituitarism, which is secondary adrenal insufficiency). If either little or no rise in cortisol levels occurs, the adrenal gland cannot secrete cortisol because of primary adrenal insufficiency, which may be caused by adrenal hemorrhage, infarction, autoimmunity, metastatic tumor, surgical removal of the adrenal glands, or congenital adrenal enzyme deficiency.

Interfering factor

- Response may be abnormal after prolonged steroid therapy.

Procedure and patient care

Before

- Keep patient NPO after midnight the day of the test.

During

Rapid test
- Obtain a baseline plasma cortisol level.
- Administer an IM injection of cosyntropin.
- Measure plasma cortisol levels 30 and 60 minutes after drug administration.

24-hour test
- Obtain a baseline plasma cortisol level.
- Start an IV infusion of synthetic cosyntropin in 1 L of normal saline.
- Administer the solution at the rate of 2 units per hour for 24 hours.
- After 24 hours, obtain another plasma cortisol level.

3-day test
- Obtain a baseline plasma cortisol level.
- Administer 25 units of cosyntropin IV over an 8-hour period on 2 to 3 consecutive days.
- At the end of the 3 days, obtain another plasma cortisol level.
- Collect plasma for cortisol levels in a red-top tube.

After

- Apply pressure or a pressure dressing to the venipuncture site.
- Check the venipuncture site for bleeding.

Abnormal findings

Hypopituitarism
Addison's disease

Adrenocortical tumors
Cushing's syndrome

Notes

AIDS serology (Acquired immunodeficiency serology, AIDS screen, HIV antibody test, Western blot test for HIV and antibody, Enzyme-linked immunosorbent assay [ELISA] for HIV and antibody)

Type of test Blood

Normal findings No evidence of HIV antigen or antibodies

Test explanation and related physiology

Tests used to detect the antibody to human immunodeficiency virus (HIV), which is the virus that causes acquired immunodeficiency syndrome (AIDS), were first licensed by the Food and Drug Administration (FDA) in 1985 for the screening of blood and plasma donors. The HIV virus is also known as human T-lymphotrophic virus, type III (HTLV-III), or the lymphadenopathy-associated virus (LAV). Since 1985, millions of HIV antibody tests have been performed in laboratories of blood and plasma collection centers, in counseling centers, and in clinical facilities for screening. Those at high risk for AIDS include sexually active homosexuals and bisexual men with multiple partners, intravenous drug abusers, persons receiving blood products containing HIV, and infants exposed to the virus during gestation and delivery. Accurate test results require attention to both the intrinsic quality of the tests and the technical ability of the technician performing the test.

Because of the medical and social significance of a positive test for HIV antibody, test results must be accurate and their interpretation correct. Therefore the U.S. Public Health Service has emphasized that an individual can be said to have serologic evidence of HIV infection only after an enzyme immunoassay (EIA) screening test is repeatedly reactive and another test, such as Western blot or immunofluorescence assay, validates the results.

The *enzyme-linked immunosorbent assay (ELISA),* which tests for antibodies to HIV in serum or plasma, is the most widely used serologic test for AIDS. It is important to note that ELISA detects *antibodies* to HIV. Since it does not detect viral antigens, it cannot detect infection in its earliest stage before antibodies are formed. ELISA is used for clinical diagnosis, screening blood and blood products, and testing individuals who believe they may be infected with AIDS.

The sensitivity (probability that the test results will be reactive if the specimen is a true positive) of the ELISA test is approximately 99% for blood from persons infected with HIV for 12 weeks or more. The probability of a false negative test is remote except during the first few weeks after infection, before detectable antibodies appear.

The specificity (probability that test results will be nonreactive if the specimen is a true negative) of the ELISA test is approximately 99% when repeatedly reactive tests are considered. To increase the specificity of serologic tests further, a supplemental test, most often the *Western blot,* is done to validate repeatedly reactive ELISA results. Sensitivity of the blot test is comparable to or greater than a repeatedly reactive ELISA. The testing sequence of a repeatedly reactive ELISA and a positive Western blot test is highly predictive of HIV infection.

Procedure and patient care

Before

- Explain the procedure to the patient.
- Obtain an informed consent if required by the institution.
- Tell the patient that no fasting or preparation is required.
- Maintain a nonjudgmental attitude toward the patient's sexual practices, and allow the patient ample time to express his or her concerns regarding test results.

During

- Observe universal blood and body precautions. Wear gloves when handling blood products from all patients.
- Collect 7 ml of peripheral venous blood in a red-top tube. The blood is usually sent to an outside laboratory for testing.
- If the patient wishes to remain anonymous, use a number with the patient's name and record it accurately.
- Note that if the ELISA test is repeatedly reactive (test is positive twice consecutively), the Western blot test is performed on the same blood sample.
- If the Western blot test is equivocal, collect a second serum specimen 2 to 4 months later for testing.

After

- Apply pressure or a pressure dressing to the venipuncture site.
- Assess the site for bleeding.
- Inform the patient to observe the venipuncture site for infection. AIDS patients are immunocompromised and susceptible to infection.
- Follow the institution's policy regarding test result reporting. Do not give results over the telephone. Remember that positive results may have devastating consequences.
- Explain to the patient that a positive Western blot test merely implies exposure to and presence of the AIDS virus within the body. It does not mean, however, that the patient has clinical AIDS disease. Not all patients with positive antibodies will acquire the disease.
- Encourage AIDS-positive patients to identify their sexual contacts so that they can be informed and tested.
- Inform the patient that subsequent sexual contact will put new partners at high risk for contracting AIDS.
- Provide patient education regarding safe sexual practices.

Abnormal findings
Increased levels

AIDS
AIDS-related complex (ARC)

Notes

alanine aminotransferase (ALT, Serum glutamic-pyruvic transaminase [SGPT])

Type of test Blood

Normal findings

Adult/child: 5-35 IU/L
Elderly: may be slightly higher than adult
Infant: may be twice as high as adult

Test explanation and related physiology

ALT is found predominantly in the liver. Lesser quantities are found in the kidneys, heart, and skeletal muscle. Injury or disease affecting the liver parenchyma will cause a release of this hepatocellular enzyme into the bloodstream, thus elevating serum ALT levels. Generally, most ALT elevations are caused by liver dysfunction. Therefore this enzyme is not only sensitive, but also quite specific in indicating hepatocellular disease.

Interfering factors

- Drugs that may cause increased ALT levels include acetaminophen, allopurinol, aminosalicylic acid (PAS), ampicillin, azathioprine, carbamazepine, cephalosporins, chlordiazepoxide, chlorpropamide, clofibrate, cloxacillin, codeine, dicumarol, indomethacin, isoniazid (INH), methotrexate, methyldopa, nafcillin, nalidixic acid, nitrofurantoin, oral contraceptives, oxacillin, phenothiazines, phenylbutazone, phenytoin, procainamide, propoxyphene, propranolol, quinidine, salicylates, and tetracyclines.

Procedure and patient care

Before

- Explain the procedure to the patient.
- Tell the patient that no fasting is required.

During

- Collect approximately 7 to 10 ml of blood in a red-top tube and send it to the laboratory for analysis.
- Indicate on the laboratory slip any medications that can affect test results.

After

- Apply pressure or a pressure dressing to the venipuncture site.
- Assess the venipuncture site for bleeding. Patients with liver dysfunction often have prolonged clotting times.

Abnormal findings
Increased levels

Hepatitis
Cirrhosis
Hepatic necrosis
Cholestasis
Hepatic ischemia
Hepatic tumor
Hepatotoxic drugs

Notes

aldolase

Type of test Blood

Normal findings

Adult: 3.0-8.2 Sibley-Lehninger U/dl or 22-59 mU at 37°
       C (SI units)
Child: approximately 2 times the adult values
Newborn: approximately 4 times the adult values

Test explanation and related physiology

Serum aldolase is very similar to the enzymes aspartate aminotransferase (AST, SGOT) (see p. 78) and creatinine phosphokinase (CPK) (see p. 248). Aldolase is an enzyme used in the glycolytic breakdown of glucose. As with AST and CPK, aldolase exists throughout the body in most tissues. This test is most useful in indicating muscular or hepatic cellular injury or destruction. The serum aldolase level is very high in patients with muscular dystrophies, dermatomyositis, and polymyositis. Levels are also increased in patients with gangrenous processes, muscular trauma, and muscular infectious diseases (e.g., trichinosis). Elevated levels are also noted in chronic hepatitis, obstructive jaundice, and cirrhosis.

Neurologic diseases causing weakness can be differentiated from muscular causes of weakness with this test. Normal values are seen in patients with such neurologic diseases as poliomyelitis, myasthenia gravis, and multiple sclerosis. Elevated aldolase levels are seen in the primary muscular disorders.

Interfering factors

- Drugs that may cause increased aldolase levels include hepatotoxic agents.
- Drugs that may cause decreased levels include phenothiazines.

Procedure and patient care

Before

- Explain the procedure to the patient.
- Note that a short period of fasting usually will provide more accurate test results.

During

- Collect 7 to 10 ml of blood in a red-top tube.
- Indicate on the laboratory slip any drugs that can affect test results.

After

- Apply pressure or pressure dressing to the venipuncture site.
- Observe the venipuncture site for bleeding.

Abnormal findings
Increased levels

Hepatocellular diseases (e.g., hepatitis)

Muscular diseases (e.g., muscular dystrophy, dermatomyositis, polymyositis)

Muscular trauma (e.g., severe crush injuries)

Muscular infections (e.g., trichinosis)

Gangrenous processes (e.g., gangrene of the bowel)

Decreased levels

Late muscular dystrophy

Notes

aldosterone assay

Type of test Blood, urine (24 hour)

Normal findings

Blood
Supine: 3-10 ng/dl or 0.08-0.3 nmol/L (SI units)
Upright: female—5-30 ng/dl or 0.14-0.8 nmol/L (SI units)
   male—6-22 ng/dl or 0.17-0.61 nmol/L (SI units)

Newborn: 5-60 ng/dl
1 week-1 year: 1-160 ng/dl
1-3 years: 5-60 ng/dl
3-5 years: <5-80 ng/dl

5-7 years: <5-50 ng/dl
7-11 years: 5-70 ng/dl
11-15 years: <5-50 ng/dl

Urine
2-16 µg/24 hr or 5.5-72 nmol/24 hr (SI units)

Test explanation and related physiology

Aldosterone, a hormone produced by the adrenal cortex, is a potent mineralocorticoid. Production of this enzyme is regulated by adrenocorticotropic hormone (ACTH), plasma sodium or potassium concentration, and the renin-angiotensin system. Aldosterone stimulates the renal tubules to absorb increased amounts of sodium (which causes water retention) and to secrete potassium. In this way, it regulates sodium, potassium, and water balance based on the body's needs.

Increased aldosterone levels are a major diagnostic finding in primary aldosteronism, in which a tumor of the adrenal cortex or bilateral adrenal hyperplasia causes increased production of aldosterone. The typical pattern for primary aldosteronism (Conn's syndrome) is an increased aldosterone level and a decreased renin level. The renin level is low because the increased aldosterone level "turns off" the renin-angiotensin mechanism. Patients with primary aldosteronism characteristically have hypertension and hypokalemia. Increased aldosterone levels are also present in secondary aldosteronism (caused by renal vascular occlusion or other renal disease), but renin levels are high.

The aldosterone assay can be done on a 24-urine specimen or on a plasma blood sample. The advantage of the 24-hour urine sample is that short-term fluctuations are eliminated. Plasma values are more convenient to sample, but they are affected by the short-term fluctuations. For example, lower aldosterone values occur in the afternoon, or having the patient in an upright position greatly increases the plasma aldosterone level. Therefore a 24-hour urine collection is much more reliable. Levels of both urine and plasma are increased by low-sodium diets and are decreased by high-sodium diets. Hypokalemia inhibits aldosterone secretion.

Interfering factors

- Strenuous exercise and stress can stimulate adrenocortical secretions and increase aldosterone levels.
- Excessive licorice ingestion can cause decreased levels because it produces an aldosterone-like effect.
- Values are influenced by posture, diet, and pregnancy.
- Drugs that may cause increased levels include diazoxide (Hyperstat), hydralazine (Apresoline), and nitroprusside (Nipride).
- Drugs that may cause decreased levels include fludrocortisone (Florinef) and propranolol (Inderal).

Procedure and patient care
Before

- Explain the procedure for the blood collection to the patient. Hospitalized patients will usually have the blood drawn before getting out of bed. Inform nonhospitalized patients when to arrive at the laboratory and how the amount of time in the upright position affects the test.
- Tell the patient that no fasting is necessary.
- Explain the procedure for collecting a 24-hour urine sample.
- Give the patient verbal and written instructions regarding dietary and medication restrictions.
- Instruct the patient to maintain a normal sodium diet (approximately 3 g per day) for at least 2 weeks before the blood or urine collection.
- Have the patient ask the physician whether or not drugs that alter sodium, potassium, and fluid balance (e.g., diuretics, antihypertensives, steroids, oral contraceptives) can be withheld. Test results will be more accurate if

these are suspended at least 2 weeks before either the blood or the urine test.
- Inform the patient that renin inhibitors (e.g., propranolol) should not be taken 1 week before the test.
- Tell the patient to avoid licorice for at least 2 weeks before the test because of its aldosterone-like effect.

During blood collection
- Collect approximately 5 to 10 ml of venous blood in a red-top or green-top tube.
- For hospitalized patients, draw the sample with the patient in the supine position *before* he or she arises.
- Note that sometimes a second specimen (upright sample) is collected 4 hours later after the patient has been up and moving about.
- Indicate on the laboratory slip if the patient was supine or standing during the venipuncture.
- Handle the blood specimen gently. Rough handling may cause hemolysis and alter the test results.
- Transport the specimen on ice to the laboratory.
- List on the laboratory slip any medications that can affect test results.

During urine collection
- Instruct the patient to begin the 24-hour urine collection after urinating.
- Discard this specimen and note this time as the start of the 24-hour collection.
- Collect urine passed over the next 24 hours.
- Instruct the patient to void before defecating so the urine is not contaminated by feces.
- Remind the patient not to put toilet paper in the collection container.
- Use a preservative with this 24-hour specimen.
- Keep the urine specimen on ice or refrigerate it during the 24 hours.
- Collect the last specimen as close as possible to the end of the 24 hours. Add this urine to the container.

After blood collection
- Apply pressure or a pressure dressing to the venipuncture site.
- Assess the venipuncture site for bleeding.

After urine collection
- Transport the urine specimen promptly to the laboratory.

Abnormal findings
Increased levels

Primary aldosteronism
Hyponatremia
Hyperkalemia
Stress
Cushing's syndrome
Malignant hypertension
Generalized edema (from
  congestive heart failure,
  nephrotic syndrome, cir-
  rhosis)
Renal ischemia
Bartter's syndrome
Pregnancy
Oral contraceptives
Diuretics
Steroid therapy

Decreased levels

Patients on a high-sodium
  diet
Hypernatremia
Hypokalemia
Addison's disease
Toxemia of pregnancy
Antihypertensive therapy
Diabetes mellitus

Notes

alkaline phosphatase (ALP)

Type of test Blood

Normal findings

Adult: 30-85 ImU/ml
Elderly: slightly higher than adults
Child/adolescent: < 2 years: 85-235 ImU/ml
                2-8 years: 65-210 ImU/ml
                9-15 years: 60-300 ImU/ml
                16-21 years: 30-200 ImU/ml

Test explanation and related physiology

Although ALP is found in many tissues, highest concentrations are found in the liver, biliary tract epithelium, and bone. The intestinal mucosa and placenta also contain ALP. This phosphatase enzyme is called *alkaline* because its function is increased in an alkaline environment. Detection of this enzyme is important for determining liver and bone disorders. Within the liver the ALP is present in the Kupffer cells. These cells line the biliary collecting system. Enzyme levels of ALP are greatly increased in both extrahepatic and intrahepatic obstructive biliary disease. Other liver abnormalities, such as metastatic carcinoma, primary liver tumors (hepatoma), and cirrhosis, can cause elevated ALP levels.

Bone is the most frequent extrahepatic source of ALP; new bone growth is associated with elevated ALP levels. Pathologic new bone growth occurs with osteoblastic metastatic (e.g., breast, prostate) tumor. Paget's disease, healing fractures, rheumatoid arthritis, and normal-growing bones are also sources of elevated ALP levels. Ingestion of heptotoxic drugs is associated with increased ALP levels.

Isoenzymes of ALP are also used to distinguish between liver and bone diseases. These isoenzymes are most easily differentiated by the heat stability test. The isoenzyme of liver origin (ALP_1) is heat stable. The isoenzyme of bone origin (ALP_2) is inactivated by heat.

Interfering factors

- Drugs that may cause elevated ALP levels include albumin made from placental tissue, allopurinol, antibiotics, azathioprine, colchicine, fluorides, indomethacin, isonia-

zid (INH), methotrexate, methyldopa, nicotinic acid, oral contraceptives, phenothiazine, probenecid, and tetracyclines.
- Drugs that may cause decreased levels include arsenicals, cyanides, fluorides, nitrofurantoin, oxalates, and zinc salts.

Procedure and patient care
Before

- Explain the procedure to the patient.
- Tell the patient that no fasting is usually required. Overnight fasting may be required for isoenzymes.

During

- Collect approximately 7 to 10 ml of blood in a red-top tube.
- List on the laboratory slip any medications that can affect test results.

After

- Apply pressure or a pressure dressing to the venipuncture site.
- Assess the venipuncture site for bleeding. Patients with liver dysfunction often have prolonged clotting times.

Abnormal findings
Increased levels

Cirrhosis
Paget's disease
Rheumatoid arthritis
Intrahepatic or extrahepatic biliary obstruction
Primary and metastatic liver tumors
Normal pregnancy (third trimester, early postpartum)
Normal bones of growing children
Intestinal ischemia or infarction
Metastatic tumor to the bone
Healing fractures
Hyperparathyroidism

Decreased levels

Hypothyroidism
Malnutrition
Milk-alkali syndrome
Pernicious anemia
Hypophosphatemia
Scurvy (vitamin C deficiency)
Celiac disease
Excess vitamin B ingestion

alpha₁-antitrypsin test (A1AT, ATT)

Type of test Blood

Normal findings >250 mg/dl

Test explanation and related physiology

Serum alpha₁-antitrypsin (α_1-antitrypsin) determinations are obtained when an individual has a family history of emphysema, since there is a familial tendency to have a deficiency of this antienzyme. Deficient or absent serum levels of this enzyme are found in some patients with the early onset of emphysema. These people usually develop severe, disabling emphysema. The exact mechanism by which an antitrypsin deficiency produces emphysema is unclear.

Genetic typing has shown that most persons have two M genes, designated as MM, and have alpha₁-antitrypsin levels greater than 250 mg/dl. Z and S genes are typically associated with alterations in serum levels of alpha₁-antitrypsin. Individuals are who are homozygous ZZ or SS always have serum levels less than 50 mg/dl and often have levels near zero. These people develop severe panacinar emphysema in the third or fourth decade of life. Their major clinical symptoms usually include progressive dyspnea with minimal coughing. Chronic bronchitis is prominent in those who smoke.

Individuals of the heterozygous state MZ or MS have serum levels of alpha₁-antitrypsin between 50 and 250 mg/dl. Approximately 5% to 14% of the adult population are in the heterozygous state, which is considered to be a risk factor for emphysema.

Interfering factors

- Serum levels of alpha₁-antitrypsin increase during pregnancy and with oral contraceptives.

Procedure and patient care

Before

- Explain the procedure to the patient.
- Note that no fasting is usually required. Verify this with the laboratory performing the study.

During

- Collect approximately 5 to 10 ml of blood.

After

- Apply pressure or a pressure dressing to the venipuncture site.
- Observe the venipuncture site for bleeding.
- If test results show the patient is at risk for developing emphysema, begin patient teaching. Include such factors as avoidance of smoking, avoidance of infection, avoidance of inhaled irritants, proper nutrition, adequate hydration, and education about the disease process of emphysema.

Abnormal findings

Increased levels

Inflammatory disorders
Cancer
Thyroid infections
Stress

Decreased levels

Early onset of emphysema
Cirrhosis
Hepatic injury
Nephrotic syndrome
Malnutrition
Hepatitis

Notes

alpha-fetoprotein (AFP, α_1-Fetoprotein)

Type of test Blood

Normal findings

Adult: <40 ng/ml or <40 µg/L (SI units)
Child (<1 year): <30 ng/ml
Ranges are stratified by weeks of gestation and vary according to different laboratories.

Test explanation and related physiology

Serum AFP levels are obtained to screen for neural tube defects (NTDs). AFP is a glycoprotein produced by the yolk sac and the fetal liver. Although serum AFP levels have detected myelomeningocele and anencephaly, widespread screening for serum AFP is not yet a routine aspect of prenatal care in the United States or Canada.

Serum AFP levels are very low in normal adults. AFP from fetal sources can be detected in the mother's blood after 10 weeks of gestation. Since peak levels occur between weeks 16 and 18, the AFP test is done at this time. When the serum AFP level is elevated, further evaluation (including a repeat serum AFP, ultrasound, and amniocentesis) must be done before an open NTD can be documented. Elevated serum AFP levels may also indicate abortion, multiple pregnancy, and intrauterine fetal death.

Increased AFP levels are also useful in the diagnosis of primary hepatocellular cancers, which secrete AFP. AFP levels greater than 500 ng/ml indicate primary liver cancer in most patients. Levels of AFP may also be elevated in patients with Hodgkin's disease, lymphoma, renal cell cancer, or testicular cancer. AFP levels are also useful in monitoring cancer treatment.

Interfering factors

- Fetal blood contamination can cause increased AFP levels.
- Multiple pregnancies can cause increased levels.
- Recent administration of radioisotopes can affect values.

Procedure and patient care
Before
- Explain the procedure to the patient.
- Tell the patient that no food or fluid restriction is required.

During
- Collect approximately 7 to 10 ml of blood in a red-top tube.

After
- Apply pressure or a pressure dressing to the venipuncture site.
- Assess the venipuncture site for bleeding.
- Include the gestational age on the laboratory slip.

Abnormal findings
Increased levels

Neural tube defect (NTD) (e.g., anencephaly, encephalocele, spina bifida, myelomeningocele)
Abortion
Multiple pregnancy
Intrauterine fetal death

Primary hepatocellular cancer
Cirrhosis
Hodgkin's disease
Lymphoma
Renal tumor
Testicular cancer
Hepatitis

Notes

ammonia level

Type of test Blood

Normal findings
Adult: 15-110 µg/dl or 47-65 µmol/L (SI units)
Child: 40-80 µg/dl
Newborn: 90-150 µg/dl

Test explanation and related physiology

Ammonia, a by-product of protein metabolism, is normally converted by the liver into urea and then secreted by the kidneys. With severe liver dysfunction or when the blood flow to the liver is altered (e.g., in portal hypertension), ammonia cannot be catabolized. The blood levels rise. These blood levels are used primarily as an aid in diagnosing hepatic encephalopathy or hepatic coma.

Interfering factors

- Drugs that may cause increased ammonia levels include acetazolamide, alcohol, ammonium chloride, barbiturates, and diuretics (loop, thiazide).
- Drugs that may cause decreased levels include broad-spectrum antibiotics (e.g., neomycin), lactulose, and potassium salts.

Procedure and patient care

Before

- Explain the procedure to the patient.
- Note that usually no fasting is required.

During

- Collect approximately 5 to 7 ml of blood in a green-top tube. Note that some institutions require that the specimen be sent to the laboratory in an iced container.
- List on the laboratory slip any drugs that can affect test results.
- Avoid hemolysis and send the specimen promptly to the laboratory.

After

- Apply pressure or a pressure dressing to the venipuncture site.
- Assess the venipuncture site for bleeding. Many patients with liver disease have prolonged clotting times.

Abnormal findings
Increased levels

Primary hepatic disease
Renal failure
Reye's syndrome
Severe heart failure with congestive hepatomegaly
Hemolytic disease of the newborn (erythroblastosis fetalis)
Hepatic encephalopathy
Hepatic coma
Pulmonary emphysema

Decreased levels

Essential and malignant hypertension

Notes

amniocentesis (Amniotic fluid analysis)

Type of test Fluid analysis

Normal findings Depend on the reason for the test

Test explanation and related physiology

Amniocentesis involves the placement of a needle through the patient's abdominal and uterine walls into the amniotic cavity to withdraw fluid for analysis. Studying amniotic fluid is vitally important in assessing the following:

1. *Fetal maturity status,* especially pulmonary maturity (when early delivery is preferred)
2. *Sex of the fetus.* For example, sons of mothers who are known to be carriers of X-linked recessive traits would have a 50:50 chance of inheritance.
3. *Genetic and chromosomal aberrations* (e.g., hemophilia, Down's syndrome, galactosemia)
4. *Fetal status affected by Rh isoimmunization.* Mothers with Rh isoimmunization will have a series of amniocentesis procedures during the second half of pregnancy to assess the level of bilirubin pigment in the amniotic fluid. The quantity of bilirubin in the amniotic fluid is used to assess the severity of hemolytic anemia in Rh-sensitized pregnancy. The higher the amount of bilirubin, the lower is the amount of fetal hemoglobin. Amniocentesis is usually initiated at 24 to 25 weeks. This allows assessment of the severity of the disease and the status of the fetus. Early delivery or blood transfusion may be indicated.
5. *Hereditary metabolic disorders* (e.g., cystic fibrosis)
6. *Anatomic abnormalities,* such as neural tube closure defects (myelomeningocele, anencephaly, spina bifida)
7. *Fetal distress,* detected by meconium staining of the amniotic fluid. This is caused by relaxation of the anal sphincter. In this case the normally colorless and pale, straw-colored amniotic fluid may be green tinged. Other color changes may also indicate fetal distress. For example, a yellow discoloration may indicate a blood incompatibility. A yellow-brown opaque ap-

pearance may indicate intrauterine death. A red color indicates blood contamination either from the mother or the fetus.

Fetal maturity is determined by analysis of the amniotic fluid for the following:

1. *Lecithin/sphingomyelin (L/S) ratio.* The L/S ratio is a measure of fetal lung maturity, which is determined by measuring the phospholipids in amniotic fluid. Lecithin is the major constituent of surfactant, an important substance required for alveolar ventilation. If surfactant is insufficient, the alveoli collapse during expiration. This results in atelectasis and respiratory distress syndrome (RDS), which is a major cause of death in immature babies. In the immature fetal lung the sphingomyelin concentration in amniotic fluid is higher than the lecithin concentration. At 35 weeks' gestation, the concentration of lecithin rapidly increases, whereas sphingomyelin concentration decreases. An L/S ratio of 2:1 (3:1 in diabetic mothers) or greater is a highly reliable indication that the fetal lung, and therefore the fetus, is mature. In such a case, after birth, the infant would be unlikely to develop RDS. Other tests in the phospholipid screen, including one for phosphatidyl glycerol, are becoming available and are more accurate than the L/S ratio, especially in diabetic pregnant women. Phosphatidyl glycerol appears at 36 weeks' gestation and increases until term.

   The amount of surfactant in amniotic fluid can be evaluated by a quick, inexpensive, simple technique called the *shake test,* also called *foam stability* or *rapid surfactant test.* This test, which is used to assess fetal lung maturity, is based on the principle that surfactant should prolong the stability of an emulsifier. For this test, a small amount of amniotic fluid is diluted with saline solution. Ninety-five percent ethyl alcohol is then added, and the mixture is shaken vigorously for about 30 seconds. The persistence of fine bubbles indicates the presence of surfactant. A dilutional table is used to determine the stage of lung maturity. The test result is positive when the fine bubbles (foam) are present.

A positive test has a high accuracy for indicating pulmonary maturity. If no foam is seen, the test is negative and the risk for RDS is high.

2. *Creatinine concentration.* Creatinine is excreted in the fetal urine and is used to assess fetal renal function and fetal muscle mass. The creatinine concentration rises sharply between the 34th and 36th week of gestation. Values of 2 mg/dl of amniotic fluid or greater usually correlate with a gestational age of at least 36 weeks and therefore indicate fetal maturity. The measurement of the creatinine concentration is much less reliable (60%) than the L/S ratio (90%); however, when the two measurements are combined, their accuracy is greater than that of either test performed separately.

3. *Bilirubin levels.* The amount of bilirubin in amniotic fluid is a measure of liver maturity and should decrease near term in a normal fetus. When the optical density (OD) of bilirubinoid pigments in amniotic fluid at 450 nm is 0.01 or less, the gestational age is greater than 38 weeks and the fetus is considered mature. Bilirubin level measurements are no longer routinely performed for determining fetal maturity because they are nonspecific (e.g., bilirubin levels indicating maturity may be present earlier in an Rh-sensitized pregnancy).

4. *Cytologic findings.* The sebaceous glands of the fetus begin to function and shed cells near term. As the fetus matures, the percentage of cells containing lipids increases. By staining amniotic fluid with Nile blue stain, lipid cells can be identified. When more than 20% of the fetal cells stain orange with 0.1% Nile blue sulfate, the gestational age is considered to be greater than 35 weeks. At this time the probable weight of the fetus is 2500 g. One advantage of this test is that it can be done without sophisticated laboratory equipment.

The L/S ratio is the single most accurate indicator of fetal maturity. Although the accuracy of the other studies is only 50% to 60%, they are used for comparative purposes.

Genetic and chromosomal studies performed on cells aspirated within the amniotic fluid can indicate the sex of the fetus (important in sex-linked diseases such as hemophilia) or any of the described genetic and chromosomal aberrations. Increased levels of alpha-fetoprotein (AFP) in the amniotic fluid may indicate a neural crest abnormality (see p. 30). Amniocentesis may be done on the premise that elective abortion should be performed if the fetus is severely defective.

Timing of the amniocentesis varies according to the clinical circumstances. With advanced maternal age and if chromosomal or genetic aberrations are suspected, the test should be done early enough (14 to 16 weeks' gestation) to allow safe abortion. This timing is essential because of the 2 weeks necessary for cell growth to determine the study's results. If information on fetal maturity is sought, performing the study during or after the 35th week of gestation is best. Placental localization by ultrasonography should be done before amniocentesis to avoid the needle passing into the placenta, possibly interrupting the placenta, and inducing bleeding or abortion.

Contraindications

- Patients with abruptio placentae
- Patients with placenta previa
- Patients with a history of premature labor (before 34 weeks' gestation, unless patient is receiving antilabor medication)
- Patients with an incompetent cervix

Potential complications

- Miscarriage
- Fetal injury
- Leak of amniotic fluid
- Infection (amnionitis)
- Abortion
- Premature labor
- Maternal hemorrhage with possible maternal Rh isoimmunization
- Amniotic fluid embolism
- Abruptio placentae
- Inadvertent damage to the bladder or intestines

Interfering factors

- Fetal blood contamination can cause falsely elevated AFP levels.
- Bilirubin levels may be falsely decreased if the specimen is exposed to light.
- Hemolysis of the specimen can alter results.
- Contamination of the specimen with meconium or blood may give inaccurate L/S ratios.

Procedure and patient care
Before

- Explain the procedure to the patient. Allay any fears and allow the patient to verbalize her concerns.
- Obtain an informed consent from the patient and spouse.
- Tell the patient that no food or fluid is restricted.
- Evaluate the mother's blood pressure and the fetal heart rate (FHR).
- Follow instructions regarding emptying the bladder, which depend on gestational age. Before 20 weeks' gestation, the bladder may be kept full to support the uterus. After 20 weeks, the bladder may be emptied to minimize the chance of puncture.
- Localize the placenta before the study by ultrasound to permit selection of a site that will avoid placental puncture.

During

- Place the patient in the supine position.
- Note the following procedural steps:

  1. The skin overlying the chosen site is prepared and usually anesthetized locally.
  2. A long needle with a stylet is inserted through the midabdominal wall and directed at an angle toward the middle of the uterine cavity (see Figure 1).
  3. The stylet is then removed, and a sterile plastic syringe is attached.
  4. After 5 to 10 ml of amniotic fluid is withdrawn, the needle is removed. (This fluid volume is replaced by newly formed amniotic fluid within 3 to 4 hours after the procedure.)
  5. The specimen is placed in a light-resistant container to prevent breakdown of bilirubin.

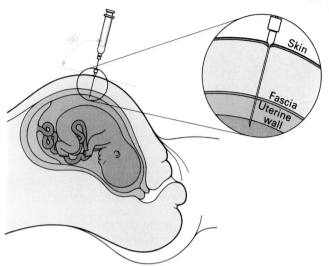

Figure 1 Amniocentesis. Ultrasound scanning is usually used to determine the placental site and to locate a pocket of amniotic fluid. The needle is then inserted. Three levels of resistance are felt as the needle penetrates the skin, fascia, and uterine wall. When the needle is placed within the uterine cavity, amniotic fluid is withdrawn.

6. The site is covered with an adhesive bandage.
7. If the amniotic fluid is bloody, the physician must determine whether the blood is maternal or fetal in origin. Kleinhauer-Boetke stain will stain fetal cells pink. Meconium in the fluid is usually associated with a compromised fetus.

- Note that this procedure takes approximately 20 to 30 minutes.
- Tell the patient that the discomfort associated with amniocentesis is usually described as a mild uterine cramping, which occurs when the needle contacts the uterus. Some women may complain of an "pulling" sensation as the amniotic fluid is withdrawn.
- Remember that many women are extremely anxious during this procedure.

After

- Place amniotic fluid in a sterile, siliconized glass container and transport it to a special chemistry laboratory for analysis. Sometimes the specimen may be sent by air mail to another commercial laboratory.
- Inform the patient that the results of this study are usually not available for at least 2 weeks.
- For women who have Rh-negative blood, administer RhoGAM because of the risk of immunization from the fetal blood.
- Assess FHR after the test to detect any ill effects related to the procedure. Compare to the preprocedural baseline value.
- If the woman felt dizzy or nauseated during the procedure, instruct her to lie on her left side for several minutes after the test before leaving the examining room.
- Observe the puncture site for bleeding or other drainage.
- Instruct the patient to call her physician if she has any fluid loss, bleeding, temperature elevation, abdominal pain or cramping, fetal hyperactivity, or unusual fetal lethargy.

Abnormal findings

Genetic or chromosomal aberrations (e.g., hemophilia, Down's syndrome, galactosemia)

Rh isoimmunization

Hereditary metabolic disorders (e.g., cystic fibrosis, Tay-Sachs disease)

Neural tube closure defects (e.g., myelomeningocele, anencephaly, spina bifida)

Meconium staining (fetal stress)

Immature fetal lungs

Sickle cell anemia

Thalassemia

Sex-linked disorders (e.g., hemophilia)

Notes

amnioscopy

Type of test Endoscopy

Normal findings Normal color of amniotic fluid; no meconium staining

Test explanation and related physiology

Amnioscopy is an endoscopic procedure that allows direct transcervical visualization of the amniotic fluid to detect meconium staining of the fluid. Fetal hypoxia results in passage of meconium through the rectum of the fetus. This meconium, which can be detected through the intact membranes with a vaginal speculum, may indicate fetal distress or death. Meconium is also present in some normal pregnancies. Therefore results must be evaluated within the overall clinical situation.

Amnioscopy is also used for fetal blood sampling for pH (see p. 345).

Contraindications

- Patients in labor
- Patients with premature membrane rupture
- Patients with active cervical infection (e.g., gonorrhea)

Potential complication

- Rupture of the placental membrane

Procedure and patient care
Before

- Explain the procedure to the patient.
- Ensure that an informed consent for this procedure is obtained, if required by the institution.
- Note that no fasting or sedation is required.

During

- Place the patient in the lithotomy position.
- Note the following procedural steps:
  1. The cervix is dilated to 2 cm, and an endoscope (amnioscope) is inserted into the cervical canal.

2. The color of the amniotic fluid is evaluated.
3. No fluid is obtained for laboratory analysis.

- Note that this procedure is performed by a physician in approximately 10 to 15 minutes.
- Inform the patient that the cervical dilation will cause some discomfort.

After

- Inform the patient that she may have vaginal discomfort and menstrual-type cramping.
- Assess the patient for rupture of the membrane and for uterine contractions.

Abnormal finding

Meconium staining of the amniotic fluid

Notes

amylase, blood

Type of test Blood

Normal findings 56-190 IU/L, 80-150 Somogyi units/dl, or 25-125 U/L (SI units) (Values may be slightly increased in normal pregnancy and in the elderly.)

Possible critical values More than three times the upper limit of normal (depending on the method)

Test explanation and related physiology

The serum amylase is an easily and rapidly performed test most specific for pancreatitis. Amylase is normally secreted from the pancreatic acinar cell into the pancreatic duct and then into the duodenum. Once in the intestine, it aids in the catabolism of carbohydrates to their component simple sugars. Damage to acinar cells (as in pancreatitis) or obstruction of the pancreatic duct flow (as in pancreatic carcinoma) will cause an outpouring of this enzyme into the intrapancreatic lymph system and the free peritoneum. Blood vessels draining the free peritoneum and absorbing the lymph pick up the excess amylase. An abnormal rise in the serum level of amylase occurs within 12 hours of the onset of disease. Because amylase is rapidly cleared by the kidney, serum levels return to normal 48 to 72 hours after the initial insult. Persistent pancreatitis, duct obstruction, or pancreatic duct leak (e.g., pseudocysts) will cause persistent elevated serum amylase levels.

Although serum amylase is a sensitive test for pancreatic disorders, it is not specific. Other nonpancreatic diseases can cause elevated amylase levels in the serum. For example, in a bowel perforation, intraluminal amylase leaks into the free peritoneum and is picked up by the peritoneal blood vessels. This results in an elevated serum amylase level. Also, a penetrating peptic ulcer into the pancreas will cause elevated amylase levels. Because salivary glands contain amylase, elevations can be expected in patients with parotiditis (mumps).

Patients with chronic pancreatic disorders (e.g., chronic pancreatitis) that have previously resulted in pancreatic cell destruction often do not have high amylase levels because less amylase is made within the pancreas.

Interfering factors
- IV dextrose solutions can cause a false negative result.
- Drugs that may cause increased serum amylase levels include aminosalicylic acid (PAS), aspirin, azathioprine, corticosteroids, dexamethasone, ethyl alcohol, glucocorticoids, iodine-containing contrast media, loop diuretics (e.g., furosemide), methyldopa, narcotic analgesics, oral contraceptives, and prednisone.
- Drugs that may cause decreased levels include citrates, glucose, and oxalates.

Procedure and patient care
Before
- Explain the procedure to the patient.
- Tell the patient that no fasting is required.

During
- Collect 5 to 7 ml of venous blood in a red-top tube.
- Indicate on the laboratory slip any medications that can affect test results.

After
- Apply pressure or a pressure dressing to the venipuncture site.
- Check the venipuncture site for bleeding.

Abnormal findings
Increased levels

Acute pancreatitis
Perforated peptic ulcer
Perforated bowel
Parotiditis (mumps)
Pulmonary infarction
Chronic relapsing pancreatitis

Penetrating peptic ulcer
Necrotic bowel
Acute cholecystitis
Ectopic pregnancy
Diabetic ketoacidosis

Notes

amylase, urine

Type of test Urine (24 hour)

Normal findings 3-35 IU/hr or 6-30 Wohlgemuth units/ml, up to 5000 Somogyi units/24 hr or 6.5-48.1 U/hr (SI units)

Test explanation and related physiology

Amylase is normally secreted from the pancreatic acinar cells into the pancreatic duct and then into the duodenum. Once in the intestine, it aids in the catabolism of carbohydrates to their component simple sugars. Destruction of acinar cells (as in pancreatitis) or obstruction to the pancreatic duct flow (as in pancreatitic carcinoma) will cause an outpouring of this enzyme into the bloodstream.

Because the kidney rapidly clears amylase, disorders affecting the pancreas will cause elevated amylase levels in the urine. The serum levels of amylase rise transiently. They usually return to normal 1 to 2 days after the onset of the disease. Levels of amylase in the urine, however, remain elevated 5 to 7 days after the onset of disease. This fact is important if one is to diagnose pancreatitis in patients who have had symptoms for 3 days or longer.

As with serum amylase, urine amylase is sensitive but not specific for pancreatitic disorders. Other diseases, such as parotiditis (mumps), cholecystitis, perforated bowel, penetrating peptic ulcer, ectopic pregnancy, and renal infarctions, can cause elevated urine levels. However, urine levels are usually highest with pancreatitis. A comparison of the renal clearance ratio of amylase to creatinine provides more diagnostic information than does either the urine amylase level or the serum amylase level alone. When the amylase/creatinine clearance ratio is 5% or more, the diagnosis of pancreatitis can be made with certainty. With ratios of less than 5% in a patient with elevated serum and urine amylase levels, nonpancreatic pathologic conditions should be suspected (e.g., perforated bowel, macroamylasemia).

Interfering factors

- Drugs that may increase urine amylase levels include aspirin, loop diuretics, and narcotic analgesics.

Procedure and patient care
Before

- Explain the procedure to the patient.
- Tell the patient that no fasting is required.
- Record the exact times of the urine collection.

During

- Instruct the patient to begin the 24-hour urine collection. Discard the initial specimen and start the 24-hour timing at that point.
- Collect all urine passed during the next 24 hours.
- A *2-hour spot urine* can be sent instead of the 24-hour urine collection.
- Show the patient where to store the urine specimen.
- Keep the specimen on ice or in a refrigerator during the collection period. No preservative is needed.
- Post the hours for urine collection in a prominent place to prevent accidental discarding of the specimen.
- Instruct the patient to void before defecating so that urine is not contaminated by stool.
- Remind the patient not to put toilet paper in the urine collection container.
- Collect the last specimen as close as possible to the end of the collection period. Add this urine to the container.
- List on the laboratory slip any medications that can affect test results.

After

- Send the urine specimen to the laboratory promptly.

Abnormal findings
Increased levels

Acute pancreatitis
Perforated bowel
Parotiditis (mumps)
Pulmonary infarction
Ectopic pregnancy

Chronic relapsing pancreatitis
Perforated peptic ulcer
Penetrating peptic ulcer
Necrotic bowel
Acute cholecystitis

Notes

angiotensin-converting enzyme (ACE, Serum angiotensin-converting enzyme [SACE])

Type of test Blood

Normal findings 23-57 U/ml (over age 20 years)

Test explanation and related physiology

ACE is found in pulmonary epithelial cells and converts angiotensin I to angiotensin II (a potent vasoconstrictor). For this reason the ACE levels may be used in the evaluation of hypertension. Elevated ACE levels are found in a high percentage of patients with sarcoidosis.

This test is primarily used in patients with sarcoidosis to evaluate the severity of the disease and the response to therapy. Elevated ACE levels also occur in conditions other than sarcoidosis, including Gaucher's disease (a rare familial disorder of fat metabolism), leprosy, alcoholic cirrhosis, active histoplasmosis, tuberculosis, Hodgkin's disease, myeloma, scleroderma, pulmonary embolism, and idiopathic pulmonary fibrosis.

Interfering factors

- Patients under 20 years of age normally have very high ACE levels.
- Steroid therapy can cause decreased ACE levels.

Procedure and patient care

Before

- Explain the procedure to the patient.
- Tell the patient that no fasting is required.

During

- Collect approximately 5 ml of blood in a red-top tube.
- Note on the laboratory slip if the patient is taking steroids.

After

- Apply pressure or a pressure dressing to the venipuncture site.
- Assess the venipuncture site for bleeding.

Abnormal findings
Increased levels

Sarcoidosis
Gaucher's disease
Leprosy
Alcoholic cirrhosis
Active histoplasmosis
Tuberculosis
Hodgkin's disease
Myeloma

Scleroderma
Pulmonary embolism
Idiopathic pulmonary fibrosis
Diabetes mellitus
Primary biliary cirrhosis
Amyloidosis
Hyperthyroidism

Notes

antegrade pyelography

Type of test X-ray with contrast dye

Normal findings Normal outline, size, and position of the ureters and bladder

Test explanation and related physiology

Occasionally a kidney with very poor dye excretion following intravenous pyelography (IVP) also cannot be adequately examined by retrograde pyelography because the ureter is impassable from below (e.g., from obstruction) or because a cystoscopic procedure is clinically contraindicated. For this patient the upper collecting system may be opacified by injection of contrast material via a percutaneous needle puncture of the renal pelvis or calyx. This test is usually done when attempts at retrograde catheterization (retrograde pyelography) have been unsuccessful. Antegrade pyelography is specifically indicated in the following conditions:

1. Localization of ureteral obstruction caused by a stricture, nonopaque stone, or tumor
2. Evaluation of ureteral obstruction after a urinary diversion procedure
3. Hydronephrosis in a child with poor IVP dye excretion to identify ureteropelvic and ureterovesical obstruction

Potential complications

- Hemorrhage from the needle
  The kidney is a highly vascular organ.
- Allergic reaction to iodinated dye
  This rarely occurs because the dye is not administered intravenously.

Procedure and patient care

Before

- Explain the procedure to the patient. Allay the patient's fears and allow time for the patient to verbalize concerns.
- Obtain an informed consent form.
- Check for allergy to iodine or shellfish. Inform the physician.

During

- Place the patient in a prone position.
- Note the following procedural steps:

1. The renal pelvis is localized by ultrasound or fluoroscopy.
2. Skin overlying the desired site is marked and prepared antiseptically.
3. With the patient under local anesthesia, the skin is incised and a needle with a stylet is inserted toward the renal pelvis.
4. With the patient suspending respiration, a smaller, thin-walled needle with a stylet is advanced through the needle into the lumen of the renal pelvis. Flexible tubing connects the syringe to the needle to aspirate urine.
5. Contrast material is injected to outline the upper collection system to the point of obstruction below.
6. Posteroanterior, oblique, and anteroposterior x-ray views are taken.

- Note that this test is performed by a radiologist or urologist in less than an hour.
- Inform the patient that the only uncomfortable aspect of this test is the local anesthesia used to numb the skin overlying the pelvis.

After

- Apply a small pressure dressing to the incision site.
- Assess the incision site for bleeding.
- Because the kidney is a highly vascular organ, check the vital signs as ordered to detect any evidence of bleeding.
- Note that antibiotic drugs are often recommended for several days to avoid infection, which may be caused by the instrumentation at a level above the ureteral obstruction.
- Evaluate for signs of an allergic reaction to dye (dyspnea, rash, tachycardia, hives).

Abnormal findings

Stone	Hydronephrosis
Tumor	Ureteropelvic obstruction
Ureteral obstruction	Ureterovesical obstruction

Notes

antidiuretic hormone (ADH, Vasopressin)

Type of test Blood

Normal values 1-5 pg/ml or <1.5 ng/L (SI units)

Test explanation and related physiology

ADH, also known as vasopressin, is formed by the hypo-thalamus and stored in the posterior pituitary gland. It con-trols the amount of water reabsorbed by the kidney. ADH release is stimulated by an increase in serum osmolality or a decrease in intravascular blood volume. Physical stress, sur-gery, and even high levels of anxiety may also stimulate ADH release. With a release of ADH, more water is reab-sorbed from the glomerular filtrate at the level of the distal convoluted renal tubule and collecting ducts. This increases the amount of free water within the bloodstream and causes a very concentrated urine. With low ADH levels, water is al-lowed to be excreted, producing hemoconcentration and a very dilute urine.

Diabetes insipidus occurs when ADH secretion is inade-quate or when the kidney is unresponsive to ADH stimula-tion. Inadequate ADH secretion is usually associated with central neurologic abnormalities such as trauma, tumor, or inflammation of the brain. Surgical ablation of the pituitary gland will also result in a neurologic form of diabetes insip-idus; such patients excrete large volumes of free water within a dilute urine. Therefore the blood is hemoconcentrated, causing the patient to have a strong thirst response.

Primary renal diseases may make the renal collecting sys-tem less sensitive to ADH stimulation. Again, in this in-stance a dilute urine created by excretion of high volumes of free water may occur.

High serum ADH levels are associated with the syndrome of inappropriate ADH secretion (SIADH). In response to this inappropriately high level of ADH secretion, water is re-absorbed by the kidneys greatly in excess of normal amounts. Thus the patient becomes very hemodiluted. Blood levels of important serum ions diminish, causing se-vere neurologic, cardiac, and metabolic alterations. The most frequent cause of SIADH is the paraneoplastic syndrome of ectopic ADH production. The most common tumors associated with SIADH include carcinoma of the lung, thymus lymphomas, leukemia, and carcinomas of the pancreas, urologic tract, and intestine. SIADH is also associated with pulmonary diseases (e.g., tuberculosis, bacterial pneumonia), severe stress (e.g., surgery, trauma), and brain tumors.

Interfering factors

- Patients with dehydration, hypovolemia, and stress may have increased ADH levels.
- Patients with overhydration, decreased serum osmolality, and hypervolemia may have decreased ADH levels.
- Use of a glass syringe or collection tube causes degradation of ADH.
- Drugs that elevate ADH levels include acetaminophen, barbiturates, cholinergic agents, estrogen, nicotine, oral hypoglycemic agents, some diuretics (e.g., thiazides), and tricyclic antidepressants.
- Drugs that decrease ADH levels include alcohol, beta-adrenergic agents, morphine antagonists, and phenytoin (Dilantin).

Procedure and patient care

Before

- Explain the procedure to the patient.
- Ensure that the patient is adequately hydrated. Tell the patient to fast from food for 12 hours.
- Evaluate the patient for high levels of physical or emotional stress.

During

- Collect approximately 7 ml of venous blood in a *plastic* red-top tube.
- Record on the laboratory slip any drugs that can alter test results.

After

- Apply pressure or a pressure dressing to the venipuncture site.
- Assess the venipuncture site for bleeding.
- Note that the laboratory personnel usually freeze the serum and send it to a reference laboratory for testing.

Abnormal findings
Increased levels

Syndrome of inappropriate ADH (SIADH)
Postoperative states
Severe physical stress (e.g., trauma, pain, prolonged mechanical ventilation)
Central nervous system tumors or infection
Pneumonia
Pulmonary tuberculosis
Brain tumors
Acute porphyria
Hypovolemia
Dehydration

Decreased levels

Neurogenic (or central) diabetes insipidus caused by central nervous system trauma, tumors, or infection
Surgical ablation of the pituitary gland
Nephrogenic diabetes insipidus caused by primary renal diseases
Overhydration
Decreased serum osmolality
Hypervolemia

Notes

antimitochondrial antibody and anti–smooth muscle antibody tests
(AMA and ASMA)

Type of test   Blood

Normal findings

No antimitochondrial antibodies (AMAs) at titers $> 1:5$
No anti–smooth muscle antibodies (ASMAs) at titers $> 1:20$

Test explanation and related physiology

The AMA and ASMA tests are used primarily to diagnose primary biliary cirrhosis and chronic hepatitis, respectively. They are also used to distinguish between surgical and non-surgical obstructive jaundice. Surgical or obstructive jaundice from extrahepatic biliary duct obstruction is not associated with the high elevations of these antibody levels. Normally the serum does not contain AMAs at a titer greater than $1:5$ and does not contain ASMAs at a titer greater than $1:20$.

AMAs are associated with liver and bile duct autoimmune diseases. AMA appears in most patients with primary biliary cirrhosis. These patients also have greatly elevated liver enzyme levels and a normal cholangiogram. Their liver biopsy is compatible with primary liver cirrhosis. For the AMA test these antibodies can be incubated with renal tubules, gastric mucosa, or other organs to which AMAs are known to react. Fluorescent-labeled antihuman antibodies are added and combine with the antibody-antigen immune complexes. This binding is examined under a ultraviolet microscope.

ASMAs are only present in approximately 30% of patients with primary biliary cirrhosis. However, most patients with chronic hepatitis have ASMAs. False positive ASMAs may be caused by infectious mononucleosis, acute hepatitis, or hepatomas. For the ASMA test the patient's serum is exposed to cut sections of smooth muscle. Fluorescent-labeled antihuman antibodies are then added and combine with the antibody-antigen immune complexes. This binding can be quantitated with an ultraviolet microscope.

Procedure and patient care

Before

- Explain the procedure to the patient.
- Tell the patient that no fasting or special preparation is required.

During

- Collect 7 to 10 ml of venous blood in a red-top tube.

After

- Apply pressure or a pressure dressing to the venipuncture site.
- Check the venipuncture site for bleeding. Jaundiced patients often have bleeding disorders associated with vitamin K deficiency.

Abnormal findings

Increased levels

Cirrhosis
Autoimmune-induced hepatitis
Chronic longstanding hepatic obstruction
Autoimmune disease (e.g., systemic lupus erythematosus, rheumatoid arthritis)

Pernicious anemia
Thyroiditis
Addison's disease

Notes

antinuclear antibody (ANA)

Type of test Blood

Normal findings No ANA detected in a titer with a dilution of greater than 1:32

Test explanation and related physiology

Many abnormal antibodies exist in patients with autoimmune (rheumatic) diseases. ANA is a protein antibody that reacts against cellular nuclear material. ANA is quite sensitive in detecting systemic lupus erythyematosus (SLE); positive results occur in approximately 95% of patients with this disease. However, many other rheumatic diseases and drugs can cause a false positive ANA test. ANA, therefore, is not a specific test for SLE. When a patient has a positive LE cell prep (see p. 491) and a positive ANA test, SLE is strongly suspected. Often the ANA test is used to screen patients with suspected SLE. If the ANA test is negative, the patient probably does not have SLE.

The test is usually performed by combining the patient's serum with nuclear material derived from a rat's liver or other such tissue. Flourescein-labeled antihuman serum is then mixed with the patient's serum and the rat's nuclear material. If positive, the radiolabeled antihuman antibody should attach to the patient's ANA. This fluorescein will then be seen under the ultraviolet microscope. The patient's serum is serially diluted, and the ANA test is carried out with each dilution. The most dilute serum in which ANA is detected is called the titer. The test is considered positive if ANA is found in a titer with a dilution of greater than 1:32.

Interfering factors

- Drugs that may cause a false positive ANA test include acetazolamide, aminosalicyclic acid, chlorprothixene, chlorothiazides, griseofulvin, hydralazine, penicillin, phenylbutazone, phenytoin sodium, procainamide, streptomycin, sulfonamides, and tetracyclines.
- Drugs that may cause a false negative test include steroids.

Procedure and patient care
Before

- Explain the procedure to the patient.
- Tell the patient that no fasting or preparation is required.

During

- Collect 7 to 10 ml of venous blood in a red-top tube.
- Indicate on the laboratory slip any drugs that can affect test results.

After

- Apply pressure or a pressure dressing to the venipuncture site.
- Assess the venipuncture site for bleeding.
- Because they are usually immunocompromised, instruct patients with an autoimmune disease to check for signs of infection at the venipuncture site. These patients often take steroids, which further compromise their immune system.

Abnormal findings
Increased levels

Systemic lupus erythemato-
  sus
Rheumatoid arthritis
Chronic hepatitis
Periarteritis (polyarteritis)
  nodosa
Dermatomyositis
Scleroderma

Infectious mononucleosis
Raynaud's disease
Sjögren's syndrome
Other immune diseases
Leukemia
Myasthenia gravis
Cirrhosis

Notes

antispermatozoal antibody (Sperm agglutination and inhibition, Sperm antibodies, Antisperm antibodies, Infertility screen)

Type of test Fluid analysis; blood

Normal findings Negative

Test explanation and related physiology

The antispermatozoal antibody test is an infertility screening test used to detect the presence of sperm antibodies. Antibodies directed toward sperm antigens can result in diminished fertility. In addition to a semen specimen, serum of both partners should be studied for sperm antibodies, since a relationship may exist between spermatozoal antibodies in women's serum and unexplained fertility.

Antisperm antibodies may be found in men with blocked efferent ducts in the testes or in those who have had a vasectomy. The reabsorption of sperm from the blocked ducts may result in the formation of autoantibodies to sperm.

Procedure and patient care

Before

- Explain the procedure to the patient.
- Inform the man that a semen specimen should be collected after avoiding ejaculation for at least 3 days.
- Give the male patient the proper container for the sperm collection.
- If the specimen is to be collected at home, be certain the patient is told that it must be taken to the laboratory for testing within 2 hours after collection.

During

- Collect a venous blood sample of approximately 7 to 10 ml from both the male and the female in red-top tubes.

After

- Apply pressure or a pressure dressing to the venipuncture sites.
- Check the venipuncture sites for bleeding.
- Instruct the couple when and how to obtain the test results.

A

Abnormal findings

Infertility
Blocked efferent ducts in the testes
Vasectomy

Notes

antistreptolysin O titer (ASO titer)

Type of test Blood

Normal findings
Adult/elderly: ≤160 Todd units/ml
Newborn: similar to mother's value
    6 months-2 years: ≤50 Todd units/ml
    2-4 years: ≤160 Todd units/ml
    5-12 years: 170-330 Todd units/ml

Test explanation and related physiology

The ASO titer is a serologic procedure that demonstrates the reaction of the body to infection caused by group A streptococci. It is used primarily in detecting poststreptococcal disease, such as glomerulonephritis, rheumatic fever, bacterial endocarditis, and scarlet fever.

The streptococcus organism produces an enzyme called streptolysin O, which has the ability to destroy (lyse) red blood corpuscles. Because streptolysin O is antigenic, the body reacts by producing ASO, a neutralizing antibody. ASO appears in the serum 1 week to 1 month after the onset of a streptococcal infection. A high titer is not specific for a certain type of poststreptococcal disease but merely indicates that a streptococcal infection is or has been present. When the ASO elevation is seen in a patient with glomerulonephritis or endocarditis, one can safely assume that the disease was caused by streptococcal infection. Subsequent testing may be done to detect the difference between the acute and convalescent blood sample.

Another immunologic test, *antideoxyribonuclease B (anti-DNase B)*, also detects antigens produced by group A streptococci. The anti-DNase B test is elevated in most patients with acute rheumatic fever and poststreptococcal glomerulonephritis.

Interfering factors
- Increased beta-lipoprotein levels inhibit streptolysin O and give a falsely high ASO titer.
- Drugs that may cause decreased ASO levels include antibiotics and adrenocorticosteroids.

Procedure and patient care
Before

- Explain the procedure to the patient.
- Tell the patient that no fasting is required.

During

- Collect approximately 5 to 10 ml of blood in a red-top tube.
- Avoid hemolysis of the blood specimen.
- Note on the laboratory slip any medications that can affect test results.

After

- Apply pressure or a pressure dressing to the venipuncture site.
- Observe the venipuncture site for bleeding.
- Note that repeat ASO testing may be done to determine the highest level of increase.

Abnormal findings
Increased levels

Streptococcal infection
Acute rheumatic fever
Acute glomerulonephritis

Bacterial endocarditis
Scarlet fever

Notes

antithyroglobulin antibody (Thyroid autoantibody, Thyroid antithyroglobulin antibody, Thyroglobulin antibody)

Type of test Blood

Normal findings Titer less than 1:100

Test explanation and related physiology

The serum antithyroglobulin titer evaluation detects the presence of thyroid antibodies formed in response to thyroglobulin released from the thyroid gland in certain destructive thyroid disorders. These autoantibodies combine with thyroglobulin and cause inflammation in the thyroid gland. These thyroid antibodies indicate the presence of an autoimmune disease and may be responsible for further destruction of the thyroid gland. This test is usually used in conjunction with the antithyroid microsomal antibody test (see p. 64).

This test is primarily used in a differential diagnosis of thyroid diseases such as Hashimoto's thyroiditis. The level must be extremely high to confirm the diagnosis of Hashimoto's thyroiditis.

Interfering factors

- Normal individuals, especially elderly women, may have antithyroglobulin antibody.

Procedure and patient care

Before

- Explain the procedure to the patient.
- Tell the patient that no fasting is required.

During

- Collect approximately 3 to 5 ml of blood in a red-top tube.

After

- Apply pressure or a pressure dressing to the venipuncture site.
- Assess the venipuncture site for bleeding.

Abnormal findings
Increased levels

Hashimoto's thyroiditis
Rheumatoid-collagen disease
Pernicious anemia
Thyrotoxicosis
Systemic lupus erythematosus

Rheumatoid arthritis
Hypothyroidism
Thyroid carcinoma
Sjögren's syndrome
Autoimmune hemolytic anemia
Myxedema

Notes

antithyroid microsomal antibody (Anti-
microsomal antibody, Microsomal antibody, Thyroid
autoantibody, Thyroid antimicrosomal antibody)

Type of test Blood

Normal findings Titer less than 1:100; present in 5%-
10% of healthy people

Test explanation and related physiology

This test is used to detect thyroid microsomal antibodies,
which are found in most patients with Hashimoto's thyroiditis. Microsomal antibodies are produced in response to microsomes escaping from the epithelial cells surrounding the
thyroid follicle. These escaped microsomes then act as antigens and give rise to antibodies, which have cytotoxic effects
on the thyroid follicle. This test is usually used in conjunction with the antithyroglobulin antibody test (see p. 62).

Procedure and patient care
Before

- Explain the procedure to the patient.
- Tell the patient that no fasting is required.

During

- Collect approximately 3 to 5 ml of venous blood in a
  red-top tube.

After

- Apply pressure or a pressure dressing to the venipuncture
  site.
- Assess the venipuncture site for bleeding.

Abnormal findings
Increased values

Hashimoto's thyroiditis
Myxedema
Thyroid carcinoma
Granulomatous thyroiditis
Systemic lupus erythemato-
sus

Rheumatoid arthritis
Autoimmune hemolytic
anemia
Nontoxic nodular goiter
Sjögren's syndrome

Notes

arteriography of the lower extremities
(Angiography)

Type of study X-ray with contrast dye

Normal findings

No evidence of occlusion from arteriosclerosis, embolus, or neoplasm

No evidence of aneurysmal dilation

No evidence of neovascularity associated with tumor

Normal vascular anatomy

Test explanation and related physiology

Lower extremity arteriography allows for accurate identification and location of occlusions within the femoral arterial system. After a catheter is placed in the femoral artery, radiopaque dye is injected. X-ray films are taken immediately in timed sequence to allow radiographic visualization of the arterial system of the lower extremities. Total or near-total occlusion of the flow of dye is seen in arteriosclerotic vascular occlusive disease. Embolic occlusions or acute atherosclerotic thrombi are seen as total occlusions of the artery. Arterial trauma, such as lacerations or intimal tears (laceration of the arterial inner lining), likewise appear as total or near-total obstructions to the flow of dye. Aneurysmal dilation of the artery or its branches can also be seen. Unusual arterial disorders such as Buerger's disease and fibromuscular dysplasia have classic arterial "beading," which is a pathognomonic arteriographic finding.

Lower extremity arteriography is usually done electively on patients who have symptoms and signs of peripheral vascular disease. However, emergency arteriography is needed when blood flow to an extremity has ceased suddenly. Immediate surgical therapy is needed and is most effective when the surgeon has knowledge of the etiology and location of the sudden occlusion. This knowledge can only be obtained by arteriography.

Contraindications

- Patients who are uncooperative or who find it difficult to stay still for several hours as arterial access is obtained
- Patients who are allergic to iodinated dye or shellfish

- Patients with renal failure because iodinated contrast is nephrotoxic
- Dehydrated patients because they are especially susceptible to dye-induced renal failure

Potential complications

- Hemorrhage at the site of arterial puncture
- Disruption of an arteriosclerotic plaque at the site of the arterial puncture, causing complete arterial occlusion
- Dissection of the intimal lining of the artery, causing complete arterial occlusion
- Allergic reactions to iodinated dye
  These vary from flushing, itching, and urticaria to severe, life-threatening anaphylaxis (evidenced by respiratory distress, drop in blood pressure, shock). In the event of anaphylaxis the patient is treated with diphenhydramine (Benadryl), steroids, and epinephrine. Oxygen and endotracheal equipment should be on hand for immediate use.
- Renal failure, especially in the elderly who are chronically dehydrated or have mild renal failure

Procedure and patient care
Before

- Explain the procedure to the patient.
- Obtain informed consent after explaining the risks to the patient.
- Allay the patient's fears and anxieties. Encourage the patient to verbalize concerns.
- Inform the patient of the discomfort in lying on a hard x-ray table, possibly for several hours. Consider obtaining permission to send an Egg-crate mattress with the patient to the x-ray department.
- Assess the patient's allergy to iodine dye. Inform the radiologist if an allergy to iodinated contrast is suspected. The radiologist may prescribe a Benadryl and steroid preparation to be administered before testing. Usually a hypoallergenic, non-ionic contrast is used during the test.
- Keep the patient NPO for at least 8 hours before the study except in an emergency.
- Administer appropriate pretest sedation if ordered.
- Ensure that appropriate coagulation studies have been obtained.

- Mark the patient's peripheral pulses before catheterization. This will permit quicker assessment after the procedure.

During

- Take the patient to the special studies arteriography laboratory of the x-ray department.
- Place the patient on a special movable x-ray table.
- Note the following procedural steps:

    1. Usually the skin overlying the arterial puncture is anesthetized before the needle puncture.
    2. A guide wire is placed through the needle, and the catheter is then inserted over the wire and into the artery.
    3. Under fluoroscopic guidance, the catheter wire is first threaded into the desired artery.
    4. Once this catheter is in position, radiographic dye is injected.
    5. Timed x-ray films are taken and then developed and reviewed by the radiologist. The interpretation is usually available the same day.
    6. The catheter is removed and pressure held on the puncture site for several minutes.

- Note that angiography is performed by a radiologist in approximately 1 to 3 hours.
- Tell the patient that an intense hot flush may be felt during injection of the dye and may last 15 to 30 seconds.
- Remind the patient of the discomfort in lying on the hard x-ray table for a long period.

After

- Monitor the patient's vital signs for signs of hemorrhage.
- Assess the peripheral arterial pulses in the extremity used for vascular access. Compare with the preprocedural baseline values.
- Make a neurologic assessment of the patient for any signs of catheter-induced embolic stroke (cerebrovascular accident).
- Observe the arterial puncture site frequently for signs of bleeding or hematoma.
- Maintain pressure at the puncture site with a sandbag or a 1 L IV bag.

- Keep the patient on bed rest for at least 8 hours following the procedure to allow for complete sealing of the arterial puncture site.
- Assess the extremities for signs of loss of blood supply (e.g., loss of pulses, numbness, pallor, tingling, pain, loss of motor function).
- Note and compare the color and temperature of the involved and uninvolved extremities.
- Administer mild analgesics for minor discomfort at the arterial puncture site. Notify the physician if the patient has severe, continuous pain.
- Have the patient drink fluids to prevent dehydration caused by the diuretic action of the dye.
- Evaluate for delayed reaction to the dye (dyspnea, rashes, tachycardia, hives). This usually occurs within 2 to 6 hours after the test. Treat the patient with antihistamines or steroids.

Abnormal findings

Arteriosclerotic occlusion
Embolic occlusion
Primary arterial diseases
(e.g., fibromuscular dysplasia, Buerger's disease)

Aneurysmal dilation of the involved artery or its branches
Aberrent arterial anatomy
Tumor neovascularity
Neoplastic arterial compression

Notes

arthrocentesis with synovial fluid analysis (Synovial fluid analysis, Joint aspiration)

Type of test Fluid analysis

Normal findings

Synovial fluid: clear and straw colored with few white
   blood cells (WBCs), no crystals, and a good mucin clot
Chemical test values (e.g., glucose determination): approximating those found in the bloodstream

Test explanation and related physiology

   Arthrocentesis is performed by inserting a sterile needle into a joint space, usually the knee, to obtain a specimen of synovial fluid for analysis. Synovial fluid is a liquid found in small amounts in the joints. Aspiration (withdrawal of the fluid) may be performed on any major joint, such as the knee, shoulder, hip, elbow, wrist, or ankle.

   Arthrocentesis is performed for many different reasons, such as to establish the diagnosis of infection, crystal-induced arthritis, synovitis, or neoplasms involving the joint. This procedure is also done to identify the cause of joint effusion, to follow the progression of joint disease, and to inject antiinflammatory medications, usually corticosteroids, into a joint area.

   A culture of the sample of synovial fluid is taken; the sample is also examined microscopically and chemically. Normal joint fluid is clear, straw colored, and quite viscous because of hyaluronic acid. Viscosity is reduced in patients with inflammatory arthritis. Viscosity can be grossly evaluated by forcing synovial fluid from a syringe. Fluid of high viscosity forms a "string" several inches long, in contrast to fluid of low viscosity, which drips similar to water.

   The *mucin clot test* correlates with the viscosity. The test is performed by adding acetic acid to joint fluid. The formation of a tight, ropy clot indicates qualitatively good mucin and the presence of adequate molecules of intact hyaluronic acid. The mucin clot is poor in quality and quantity in inflammatory joint diseases, such as rheumatoid arthritis. Synovial fluid should not form a fibrin clot because normal joint fluid does not contain fibrinogen. The fluid will clot only if blood entered the joint during the aspiration or an inflammatory effusion is present.

The synovial fluid glucose value is usually within 10 ml/dl of the serum glucose value. For proper interpretation the synovial fluid glucose and serum glucose samples should be drawn simultaneously after the patient has fasted for 6 hours. The synovial fluid glucose level falls with increasing inflammation. In septic arthritis the synovial fluid glucose value may be less than 50% of the serum glucose value. A low synovial glucose level may also be seen in patients with rheumatoid arthritis.

Cell counts should also be performed on the synovial fluid. Normally the joint fluid contains less than 200 WBCs/mm³. A very high percentage of neutrophils (more than 75%) is found in most patients with acute bacterial infectious arthritis.

Acid-fast stains for tubercle bacilli are also performed on the synovial fluid. Bacterial and fungal cultures are obtained when these diseases are suspected. Gonococci are a cause of joint infection. However, previous antibiotic therapy reduces the possibility of diagnosis by culture. Synovial fluid is also examined under polarized light for the presence of crystals. This permits a differential diagnosis between gout and pseudogout.

The synovial fluid can also be analyzed for complement levels. The complement level may be decreased in patients with systemic lupus erythematosus or rheumatoid arthritis. Decreased joint complement levels may be caused by consumption of the complement by the antigen-antibody complexes within the joint cavity.

Contraindications

- Patients with skin or wound infections in the area of the needle puncture because of the risk of sepsis

Potential complications

- Joint infection
- Hemorrhage in the joint area

Procedure and patient care

Before

- Explain the procedure to the patient.
- Obtain an informed consent if this is the institution's policy.

- Keep the patient NPO after midnight on the day of the test. This is done to prevent alterations of the chemical determinations (e.g., glucose) that may be performed with the study. However, this study may be done more conveniently in a physician's office without the patient fasting.

During

- Have the patient lie on his or her back with the joint fully extended.
- Note the following procedural steps:
  1. The skin is locally anesthetized to minimize pain.
  2. The area is aseptically cleansed, and a needle is inserted through the skin and into the joint space.
  3. Fluid is obtained for analysis. Sometimes the joint area may be wrapped with an elastic bandage to compress free fluid within a certain area, ensuring maximal collection of fluid.
  4. If a corticosteroid is to be administered, a syringe containing the steroid preparation is attached to the needle and the drug is injected.
  5. The needle is removed, and a pressure dressing may be applied to the site.
  6. Sometimes a peripheral venous blood sample is taken to compare chemical tests on the blood with chemical studies on the synovial fluid.

- Note that a physician performs this procedure in an office or at the patient's bedside in approximately 10 minutes.
- Tell the patient that the only discomfort associated with this test is the injection of the local anesthetic.
- Be aware that joint space pain may worsen after fluid aspiration, especially in patients with acute arthritis.

After

- Assess the joint for any pain, fever, or swelling, which may indicate infection.
- Apply ice to decrease pain and swelling.
- Keep a pressure dressing on the joint to avoid recollection of joint fluid or development of a hematoma.
- Tell the patient to avoid strenuous use of the joint for the next several days.

Abnormal findings

Infection
Arthritis
Synovitis
Neoplasms
Joint effusion

Septic arthritis
Systemic lupus erythemato-
    sus
Rheumatoid arthritis

Notes

arthrography (Arthrogram)

Type of test X-ray with contrast dye

Normal findings Normal bursae, menisci, ligaments, and articular cartilage of the joint

Test explanation and related physiology

Arthrography affords radiographic visualization of a joint after the injection of a radiopaque substance or air (or both) into the joint cavity to outline the soft tissue structures not normally seen on routine x-ray films. Bones with the meniscus, cartilage, and ligaments are clearly visualized with this procedure. Joint derangement and synovial cysts are also diagnosed with arthrography.

Arthrography is usually done on the knee and shoulder joints; however, it can also be done on other joints, such as the ankles, hips, wrists, or temporomandibular joint. This procedure is usually performed on patients with persistent, unexplained knee or shoulder pain.

Contraindications

- Patients who are pregnant
- Patients with active arthritis
- Patients with joint infection

Potential complications

- Infection at the puncture site
- Allergic reaction to the iodinated dye
  This rarely occurs because the dye is not administered intravenously.

Procedure and patient care

Before

- Explain the procedure to the patient.
- Obtain an informed consent if required by the institution.
- Tell the patient that no fasting or sedation is required.

During

- Place the patient in the supine position on the examining table.

- Note the following procedural steps:

1. The skin overlying the joint is aseptically cleansed and anesthetized.
2. A needle is inserted into the joint space.
3. Fluid is aspirated to minimize dilution of the contrast material, which could diminish the quality of the x-ray films.
4. With the needle still in place, the aspirating syringe is removed and a syringe containing dye is inserted.
5. The contrast agent is injected.
6. The needle is removed, and the joint is manipulated to help distribute the contrast material. The patient may be asked to walk a couple of steps or to pass the joint through range of motion exercises.
7. X-ray films are taken with the joint held in various positions.

- Note that the physician performs this procedure in approximately 30 minutes.
- Tell the patient that pressure or a tingling sensation may be felt as the contrast medium is injected and that some discomfort in the joint may occur.

After

- Assess the joint for swelling after the test. Apply ice if necessary.
- Administer a mild analgesic (e.g., aspirin, acetaminophen) if the patient has mild discomfort.
- Report any increase in pain or swelling to the physician.
- Inform the patient that crepitant noises (crackling tissue paper sounds) in the joint may be heard after the test. These symptoms are normal and usually disappear in 1 to 2 days. The sounds are caused by the air injected into the joint during the procedure.

Abnormal findings

Joint derangement
Cysts
Arthritis
Fractured knee meniscus
Cartilaginous diseases (e.g., chondromalacia)
Ligamentous injury
Synovial tumors
Synovitis

Notes

arthroscopy

Type of test Endoscopy

Normal findings Normal ligaments, menisci, and articular surfaces of the joint

Test explanation and related physiology

Arthroscopy is an endoscopic procedure that allows examination of the interior of a joint with a specially designed endoscope. Endoscopy is a highly accurate test because it allows direct visualization of the anatomic site. Although this technique can visualize many joints of the body, it is most often used to evaluate the knee for meniscus cartilage or ligament tears. It is also used in the differential diagnosis of acute and chronic disorders of the knee.

Physicians can now perform corrective surgery on the knee through the endoscope. Arthroscopy provides a safe, convenient alternative to open surgery (arthrotomy) because the surgical instruments can be passed directly through the arthroscope.

Arthroscopy is also used to monitor the progression of disease and the effectiveness of therapy. Visual findings may be recorded by attaching a video camera to the arthroscope.

Contraindications

- Patients with ankylosis because it is almost impossible to maneuver the instrument into a joint stiffened by adhesions
- Patients with local skin or wound infections because of the risk of sepsis

Potential complications

- Infection
- Hemarthrosis
- Swelling
- Thrombophlebitis
- Joint injury
- Synovial rupture

Procedure and patient care

Before

- Explain the procedure to the patient.
- Ensure that the physician has obtained a written consent for this procedure.
- Follow the routine, preoperative procedure of the institution.
- Keep the patient NPO after midnight on the day of the test.
- Instruct the patient who will use crutches after the procedure regarding the appropriate crutch gait. The patient should use crutches after arthroscopy until he or she can walk without limping.
- Shave the hair in the area 6 inches above and below the joint before the test (as ordered).

During

- Place the patient on his or her back on an operating room table.
- Note the following procedural steps:

  1. Local or general anesthesia is used.
  2. The leg is carefully scrubbed, elevated, and wrapped with an elastic bandage from the toes to the lower thigh to drain as much blood from the leg as possible.
  3. A tourniquet is placed on the patient's leg. If the tourniquet is not used, a fluid solution may be instilled into the patient's knee immediately before insertion of the arthroscope to distend the knee and help reduce bleeding.
  4. The foot of the table is lowered so that the patient's knee is at a 45-degree angle.
  5. A small incision is made in the skin around the knee.
  6. The arthroscope (a lighted instrument) is inserted into the joint space to visualize the inside of the knee joint.
  7. Although the entire joint can be viewed from one puncture site, making additional punctures for better visualization is often necessary.
  8. After the area is examined, biopsy or appropriate surgery can be performed.
  9. Before removing the arthroscope, the joint is irri-

gated. Pressure is then applied to the knee to remove the irrigating solution.

10. After a few stitches are placed into the skin, a pressure dressing is applied over the incision site.

- Note that this procedure is performed in the operating room by an orthopedic surgeon in approximately 15 to 30 minutes.
- Tell the patient who receives local anesthesia that he or she may have transient discomfort from the injection of the local anesthetic and from the pressure of the tourniquet on the leg.
- Inform the patient that a thumping sensation may be felt as the arthroscope is inserted into the joint and that the joint may be painful for a few days.

After

- Assess the patient's neurologic and circulatory status.
- Assess vital signs and observe the patient for signs of infection, including fever, swelling, increased pain, and redness or drainage at the incision site.
- Instruct the patient to elevate the knee when sitting and to avoid overbending the knee so that swelling is minimized.
- Inform the patient that he or she can usually walk with the assistance of crutches. However, this depends on the extent of the procedure and the physician's protocol.
- Tell the patient to minimize use of the joint for several days.
- Examine the incision site for bleeding.
- Apply ice to reduce pain and swelling.
- Inform the patient that the sutures will be removed in approximately 7 to 10 days.

Abnormal findings

Torn cartilage
Torn ligament
Patellar disease
Patellar fracture
Chondromalacia
Osteochondritis dissecans
Cysts (e.g., Baker's)

Synovitis
Osteoarthritis
Rheumatoid arthritis
Degenerative arthritis
Meniscal disease
Osteochondromatosis
Trapped synovium

Notes

aspartate aminotransferase (AST; formerly called Serum glutamic-oxaloacetic transaminase [SGOT])

Type of test Blood

Normal findings

Adult: 8-20 U/L, 5-40 IU/L, or 8-20 U/L (SI units);
   females tend to have slightly lower values than
   men.
Elderly: values slightly higher than adult
Child: values similar to adult
Newborn/infant: 15-60 U/L

Test explanation and related physiology

AST/SGOT is one of the enzymes tested in the cardiac enzyme series. This enzyme is found in very high concentrations within the heart muscle, liver cell, skeletal muscle cells and, to a lesser degree, in the kidneys and pancreas. Although not specific for myocardial injury, when observed with the enzymes creatinine phosphokinase (CPK, see p. 248) and lactic dehydrogenase (LDH, see p. 450), it is useful in diagnosis, quantitative analysis, and determination of timing of a recent myocardial infarction (MI). The AST level rises within 6 to 10 hours after MI, peaks at 12 to 48 hours, and returns to normal in 3 to 4 days, assuming further cardiac injury does not occur. Myocardial injuries such as angina, pericarditis, or rheumatic carditis do not increase the AST level.

As with CPK, serial determinations of AST are helpful in determining the timing, initiation, and resolution of MI. However, unlike the isoenzyme CPK-MB, it is much less specific for infarction of myocardial muscle cells.

Because AST also exists within the liver cells, diseases that affect the hepatocyte will cause elevated levels of this enzyme. Serum AST levels are often compared with alanine aminotransferase (ALT, see p. 18). The AST/ALT ratio is usually greater than 1.0 in patients with alcoholic cirrhosis, liver congestion, and metastatic tumor of the liver. Ratios less than 1.0 may be seen in patients with acute hepatitis, viral hepatitis, or infectious mononucleosis.

Patients with acute pancreatitis, acute renal diseases, or musculoskeletal diseases or trauma (e.g., IM injections) may have a transient rise in serum AST. Patients who have red blood cell abnormalities, such as acute hemolytic anemia and severe burns, can also have elevations of this enzyme. AST levels may be decreased in patients with beriberi or diabetic ketoacidosis and in pregnant patients.

Interfering factors

- Pregnancy may cause decreased AST levels.
- Exercise may cause increased levels.
- Drugs that may cause increased levels include antihypertensives, cholinergic agents, coumarin-type anticoagulants, digitalis preparations, erythromycin, isoniazid (INH), methyldopa, oral contraceptives, opiates, and salicylates.

Procedure and patient care

Before

- Explain the procedure to the patient.
- Discuss with the patient the need and reason for frequent venipunctures in diagnosing MI.
- Avoid giving the patient any IM injection.
- If possible, hold drugs that could interfere with test results for 12 hours before the test.

During

- Collect a venous sample of blood in a red-top tube. This is usually done daily for 3 days and then in 1 week. Rotate the venipuncture site.
- Avoid hemolysis.
- Indicate on the laboratory slip any drugs that can cause false positive results.
- Record the time and date of any IM injection given.
- Record the exact time and date when the blood test is performed. This aids in the interpretation of the temporal pattern of enzyme elevations.

After

- Apply pressure or a pressure dressing to the venipuncture site.
- Observe the venipuncture site for bleeding.

Abnormal findings

Increased levels

Myocardial infarction
Cardiac operations
Cardiac catherization and
 angioplasty
Hepatitis
Hepatic cirrhosis
Acute pancreatitis
Skeletal muscle trauma
Recent noncardiac surgery
Multiple trauma
Hepatic necrosis
Severe deep burn
Acute hemolytic anemia
Progressive muscular dys-
 trophy
Infectious mononucleosis
 with hepatitis
Recent convulsions
Hepatic infiltrative pro-
 cesses (e.g., tumor)
Primary muscle diseases
 (e.g., myopathy, myosi-
 tis)
Acute renal disease

Decreased levels

Beriberi
Diabetic ketoacidosis
Pregnancy

Notes

barium enema (BE, Lower GI series)

Type of test X-ray with contrast dye

Normal findings

Normal filling, contour, patency, and positioning of barium in the colon

Normal filling of the appendix and terminal ileum

Test explanation and related physiology

The BE study consists of a series of x-ray films of the colon. It is used to demonstrate the presence and location of polyps, tumors, and diverticula. Anatomic abnormalities (e.g., malrotation) can also be detected. Therapeutically the BE may be used to reduce nonstrangulated ileocolic intussusception in children.

The BE occasionally is used to assess filling of the appendix. When the clinical picture suggests possible appendicitis, failure of the appendix to fill with barium may support the diagnosis. Although the colon is the main organ evaluated by a BE, reflux of barium into the terminal ileum also will allow adequate visualization of the distal portion of the small intestine. Diseases that affect the terminal ileum, especially Crohn's disease (regional enteritis), can be identified.

In many instances, air is insufflated into the colon after the instillation of barium. This provides an air contrast to the barium. With the air contrast the colonic mucosa can be much more accurately visualized. This is called an *air-contrast barium enema*. It is used especially when small polyps are suspected. The accuracy of the regular BE in detecting small colonic tumors is approximately 60%. However, the accuracy of an air-contrast BE in detecting small colonic tumors exceeds 85%.

Contraindications

- Patients suspected of a perforation of the colon
  In these patients, diatrizoate (Gastrografin), a water-soluble contrast medium, is used.
- Patients who are unable to cooperate
  This test requires the patient to hold the barium in the rectum and colon. This is especially difficult for the elderly.

Potential complications

- Colonic perforation, especially when the colon is weakened by inflammation, tumor, or infection
- Barium fecal impaction

Interfering factors

- Barium within the abdomen from previous barium tests
- Significant residual stool within the colon
  This precludes adequate visualization of the entire bowel wall. Stool may be confused for polyps.
- Spasm of the colon
  Spasm can mimic the radiographic signs of a cancer. The use of IV glucagon minimizes spasm.

Procedure and patient care

Before

- Explain the procedure to the patient. Encourage the patient to verbalize questions and fears.
- Assist the patient with the bowel preparation, which varies among institutions. In the elderly, this preparation can be exhaustive and even cause severe dehydration. A typical preparation for most adults would include the following actions.

Day before examination

- Give the patient clear liquids for lunch and supper (no dairy products).
- Have the patient drink one glass of water or clear fluid every hour for 8 to 10 hours.
- Administer one full bottle (10 ounces) of magnesium citrate or X-Prep (extract of senna fruit) at 2 PM.
- Administer three 5 mg bisacodyl (Dulcolax) tablets at 7 PM.
- Keep the patient NPO after midnight the day of the test.

Day of examination

- Keep the patient NPO.
- Administer a bisacodyl suppository at 6 AM and/or a cleansing enema.
- Note that pediatric patients will have individualized bowel preparations.
- Note that special preparations will be ordered for the patient with an ileostomy or colostomy.
- Determine whether the bowel is adequately cleansed. When the stool is similar to clear water, preparation is

adequate. If large, solid fecal waste is still being evacu-
ated, preparation is inadequate. Notify the radiologist,
who may want to extend the bowel preparation.
- Suggest that the patient take reading material to the x-ray
  department to occupy the time while expelling the barium.

During

- Note the following procedural steps:
    1. The test begins with placement of a balloon rectal
       catheter.
    2. The balloon on the catheter is inflated tightly against
       the anal sphincter to hold the barium within the co-
       lon.
    3. The patient is asked to roll in the lateral, supine, and
       prone positions.
    4. The barium is dripped into the rectum by gravity.
    5. The barium flow is followed by fluoroscopy.
    6. The colon is thoroughly examined as barium flow
       progresses through the large colon and into the ter-
       minal ileum.
    7. The barium is drained out.
    8. If an air-contrast BE has been ordered, air is insuf-
       flated into the large bowel.
    9. The patient is asked to expel the barium, and a
       postevacuation x-ray film is taken.
    10. The standard procedure for administering the barium
        through a colostomy is to instill the contrast medium
        through an irrigation cone placed in the stoma.
        When the x-ray series is completed, the barium is
        allowed to be expelled from the stoma. A gentle
        stream of clean water for irrigation is helpful in ex-
        pelling the residual barium.
- Note that this test usually is performed in the radiology
  department by a radiologist in approximately 45 minutes.
- Inform the patient that abdominal bloating and rectal
  pressure will occur during instillation of barium.

After

- Ensure that the patient defecates as much barium as possible.

- Inform the patient that bowel movements will be white. However, when all the barium has been expelled, the stool will return to normal color.
- Suggest the use of soothing ointments to the anal area to minimize any anorectal pain that may result from the aggressive test preparation.
- Encourage ingestion of fluids to avoid dehydration caused by the cathartics.
- Encourage rest after the procedure. The cleansing regimen and the BE procedure may be exhausting.
- Note that laxatives may be ordered to facilitate evacuation of barium.

Abnormal findings

Malignant tumors
Polyps
Diverticula
Inflammatory bowel diseases (e.g., ulcerative colitis, Crohn's disease)
Colonic stenosis secondary to ischemia, infection, or previous surgery
Perforated colon
Colonic fistula
Appendicitis
Extrinsic compression of the colon from extracolonic tumors (e.g., ovarian)
Extrinsic compression of the colon from an abscess

Notes

barium swallow

B

Type of test X-ray with contrast dye

Normal findings Normal size, contour, filling, patency, and positioning of the esophagus

Test explanation and related physiology

This barium contrast study is a more thorough study of the esophagus than that provided by most upper GI series (see p. 746). As in most barium contrast studies, defects in normal filling and narrowing of the barium column indicate tumor, strictures, or extrinsic compression from extraesophageal tumors or an abnormally enlarged heart and great vessels. Varices can also be seen as serpiginous, linear filling defects. Also, anatomic abnormalities such as hiatal hernia, Shatzski's rings, and diverticula (Zenker's or epiphrenic) can be seen.

In patients with esophageal reflux the radiologist may identify reflux of the barium from the stomach back into the esophagus.

Contraindications

- Patients with evidence of bowel obstruction
  Barium may create a stonelike impaction.
- Patients with a perforated viscus
  If barium were to leak, the degree and duration of infection is much worse. Usually, when perforation is suspected, diatrizoate (Gastrografin), a water-soluble contrast medium, is used.
- Patients whose vital signs are unstable
- Patients who are unable to cooperate for the test

Potential complication

- Barium-induced fecal impaction

Interfering factor

- Food within the esophagus, which prevents adequate visualization

Procedure and patient care

Before

- Explain the procedure to the patient.
- Instruct the patient not to take anything by mouth for at least 8 hours before the testing. Usually the patient is kept NPO after midnight on the day of the test.
- Assess the patient's ability to swallow. If the patient tends to aspirate, inform the radiologist.
- Accompany the hospitalized patient to the x-ray department if vital signs are not stable and the test still needs to be performed.

During

- Note the following procedural steps:
  1. The fasting patient is asked to swallow the contrast medium. Usually, this is barium sulfate in a milkshake-like substance. However, if a perforated viscus is possible, Gastrografin is used.
  2. As the patient drinks the contrast through a straw, the x-ray table is tilted in the near-erect position.
  3. The patient is asked to roll into various positions so that the entire esophagus can be adequately visualized.
  4. With fluoroscopy, the radiologist follows the barium column through the entire esophagus.

- Note that this procedure usually is performed in the radiology department by a radiologist in approximately 15 to 20 minutes.
- Tell the patient that no discomfort is associated with this test.

After

- Inform the patient of the need to evacuate all the barium. Cathartics are recommended. Initially, stools will be white and should return to normal color with complete evacuation.

Abnormal findings

Total or partial esophageal
   obstructions
Cancer
Scarred strictures
Lower esophageal rings

Esophageal motility disorders (e.g., presbyesophagus, diffuse esophageal spasm)
Diverticula

Peptic esophageal ulcers
Varices
Peptic or corrosive esoph-
 agitis
Achalasia

Chalasia
Extrinsic compression from
 extraesophageal tumors,
 cardiomegaly, or aortic
 aneurysm

Notes

Barr body analysis (Sex chromatin body, Chromatin-positive body)

Type of test Microscopic examination

Normal findings Depends on the sex of the child

Test explanation and related physiology

Barr body (or Barr chromatin body) analysis studies may be performed when ambiguity of the newborn's genitalia makes it difficult to assign a sex to the infant. This test is also done to detect sex chromosomal abnormalities, such as Turner's syndrome and Klinefelter's syndrome.

The Barr body is a chromatin mass derived from one of the X chromosomes. The number of Barr bodies is one less than the total number of X chromosomes in the cell nucleus. Therefore females (XX) normally have one Barr body and are considered chromatin positive. Normal males (XY) have no Barr bodies and are chromatin negative. A female with Turner's syndrome (XO) would have no Barr body. These females are characterized by ovarian dysgenesis, amenorrhea, and the lack of secondary sexual maturation. A male with Klinefelter's syndrome (XXY) would have one Barr body. Klinefelter's syndrome is the most common form of male hypogonadism, which is caused by a chromosomal abnormality that results in primary testicular failure. An XXX female would have two Barr bodies.

Interfering factors

- Buccal smear specimens may show false lowering of sex chromatin bodies if specimens are taken during the first week of life or during adrenocorticosteroid or estrogen therapy.
- Poor slide preparation can obscure test results.

Procedure and patient care
Before

- Explain the procedure to the patient or parents.

During

- Note the following procedural steps:

    1. Sex chromatin analysis can be performed using any cell in the body. The most easily obtained cells are from the buccal mucosa. The oral mucosa is scraped, and the cells are smeared onto a glass slide.
    2. After chemical fixation and staining, the cells are studied.
    3. Assessment of the results, together with the secondary sexual characteristics and the genitalia of the patient, permit presumptive diagnosis of certain sex chromosomal abnormalities.
    4. If necessary, the results can be confirmed by chromosomal *karyotyping* (systematic arrangement of photographed chromosomes to demonstrate structure and number).

- Note that a buccal smear is performed by a technician in less than 5 minutes. A pathologist studies the slide smear.
- Tell the patient that no or minimal discomfort is associated with this test.

After

- Inform the patient how and when to obtain the test results.

Abnormal findings

Chromsomal abnormalities (e.g., Turner's syndrome, Klinefelter's syndrome)

Notes

Bence Jones protein

Type of test Urine

Normal findings No Bence Jones protein present

Test explanation and related physiology

Bence Jones proteins are lightweight immunoglobulins typically found in patients with multiple myeloma. These proteins are most notably made by the plasma cell in these patients. They may also be associated with tumor metastases to the bone, chronic lymphocytic leukemias, and amyloidosis. These immunoglobulins are rapidly cleared by the kidney and are excreted into the urine. Because the Bence Jones protein is rapidly cleared from the blood by the kidney, it is very difficult to detect in the blood; therefore only urine is used for this study. Normally the urine should contain no Bence Jones proteins.

Interfering factor

- Dilute urine may yield a false negative result.

Procedure and patient care

Before

- Explain the procedure to the patient.
- Instruct the patient not to contaminate the urine specimen with toilet paper or stool.

During

- Instruct the patient to collect an early morning specimen of at least 50 ml of uncontaminated urine in a container.

After

- Immediately transport the specimen to the laboratory.
- If it cannot be taken to the laboratory immediately, refrigerate the specimen because heat-coagulable proteins can decompose, causing a false positive test.

Abnormal findings
Increased levels

Multiple myeloma (plasma-cytoma)

Various metastatic tumors

Chronic lymphocytic leukemia

Amyloidosis

Notes

bilirubin, blood

Type of test Blood

Normal findings

Adult/elderly/child

Total bilirubin: 0.1 to 1.0 mg/dl or 5.1-17.0 μmol/L (SI units)

unconjug Indirect bilirubin: 0.2-0.8 mg/dl or 3.4-12.0 μmol/L (SI units)

conjug Direct bilirubin: 0.1-0.3 mg/dl or 1.7-5.1 μmol/L (SI units)

Newborn total bilirubin: 1-12 mg/dl or 17.1-20.5 μmol/L (SI units)

Test explanation and related physiology

Bile, which is formed in the liver, is made up of many constituents, including bile salts, phospholipids, cholesterol, bicarbonate, water, and bilirubin. Bilirubin metabolism begins with the breakdown of red blood cells (RBCs) in the reticuloendothelial system. Hemoglobin is released from RBCs and broken down to heme and globin molecules. Heme is then catobolized to form biliverdin, which is transformed to bilirubin. This form of bilirubin is called *unconjugated* (indirect) bilirubin. In the liver the indirect bilirubin is conjugated with a glucuronide, resulting in a *conjugated* (direct) bilirubin. The conjugated bilirubin is then excreted from the liver cells and into the intrahepatic canaliculi, which eventually lead to the hepatic ducts, to the common bile duct, and into the bowel.

Jaundice is the discoloration of body tissues caused by abnormally high blood levels of bilirubin. This yellow discoloration is recognized when the total serum bilirubin exceeds 2.5 mg/dl. Jaundice results from a defect in the normal metabolism or excretion of bilirubin. This defect can occur in any stage of heme catabolism.

Physiologic jaundice of the newborn occurs if the newborn's liver is immature and does not have enough conjugating enzymes. This results in a high circulating blood level of unconjugated bilirubin, which can pass through the blood-brain barrier and deposit in the brain cells of the newborn. This can cause encephalopathy *(kernicterus)*.

If the defect in bilirubin metabolism occurs after glucuronide addition, *conjugated (direct) hyperbilirubinemia* will result. Obstruction of the bile duct by a gallstone is the classic example of obstructed bilirubin excretion causing a direct hyperbilirubinemia.

Once the jaundice is recognized, either clinically or chemically, it is important, for therapy, to differentiate whether it is predominantly caused by unconjugated or conjugated bilirubin. This in turn will help differentiate the etiology of the defect. In general, jaundice caused by hepatocellular dysfunction (such as hepatitis) is caused by unconjugated bilirubin. This usually cannot be repaired surgically. On the other hand, jaundice resulting from extrahepatic dysfunction (e.g., gallstones or tumor blocking the bowel duct) is caused by elevated conjugated bilirubin levels. This type of jaundice can usually be resolved surgically.

The total serum bilirubin level is the sum of the conjugated (direct) and unconjugated (indirect) bilirubin. Normally the unconjugated bilirubin makes up 70% to 85% of the total bilirubin. In jaundiced patients, when more than 50% of the bilirubin is conjugated, it is considered a conjugated hyperbilirubinemia from gallstones, tumor, inflammation, or scarring. Unconjugated hyperbilirubinemia exists when less than 15% to 20% of the total bilirubin is conjugated. Diseases that typically cause this form of jaundice include accelerated erythrocyte (RBC) hemolysis, hepatitis, or drugs.

Interfering factors

- Blood hemolysis and lipemia can produce erroneous results.
- Drugs that may cause increased levels of total bilirubin include allopurinol, anabolic steroids, antibiotics, antimalarials, ascorbic acid, azathioprine, chlorpropamide (Diabinese), cholinergics, codeine, dextran, diuretics, epinephrine, meperidine, methotrexate, methyldopa, monoamine oxidase (MAO) inhibitors, morphine, nicotinic acid (large doses), oral contraceptives, phenothiazines, quinidine, rifampin, salicylates, steroids, sulfonamides, theophylline, and vitamin A.
- Drugs that may cause decreased levels of total bilirubin

include barbiturates, caffeine, penicillin, and salicylates (high dose).

Procedure and patient care
Before
- Explain the procedure to the patient.
- Note that fasting requirements vary among different laboratories. Some require keeping the patient NPO after midnight the day of the test except for water.

During
- Collect 5 to 7 ml of venous blood in a red-top tube.
- Use a heel puncture for blood collection in infants.
- Prevent hemolysis of blood during phlebotomy.
- Do *not* shake the tube because inaccurate test results may occur.
- Protect the blood sample from bright light. Prolonged exposure (more than 1 hour) to sunlight or artificial light can reduce bilirubin content.
- List on the laboratory slip any drugs that can affect test results.

After
- Apply pressure or a pressure dressing to the venipuncture site.
- Assess the venipuncture site for bleeding. Patients who are jaundiced can have prolonged clotting times.

Abnormal findings
Increased levels

Dubin-Johnson syndrome
Erythroblastosis fetalis
Cirrhosis
Hepatitis
Drug reactions
Hemolytic jaundice
Large-volume blood transfusion
Resolution of a large hematoma
Extensive replacement of the liver by tumor

Bile duct obstruction from tumor, inflammation, gall stone, scarring, or surgical trauma
Pernicious anemia
Sickle cell anemia
Transfusion reaction
Crigler-Najjar syndrome
Hemolytic anemia

Notes

bilirubin, urine

Type of test Urine

Normal findings No bilirubin in urine

Test explanation and related physiology

Bile, which is formed in the liver, is made up of many constituents, including bile salts, phospholipids, cholesterol, bicarbonate, water, and bilirubin. Bilirubin metabolism begins with the breakdown of red blood cells (RBCs) in the reticuloendothelial system. Hemoglobin is released from RBCs and broken down to heme and globin molecules. Heme is then catabolized to form biliverdin, which is transformed to bilirubin. This form of bilirubin is called *unconjugated* (indirect) bilirubin. In the liver the indirect bilirubin is conjugated with a glucuronide, resulting in a *conjugated* (direct) bilirubin. The conjugated bilirubin is then excreted from the liver cells and into the intrahepatic canaliculi, which eventually lead to the hepatic ducts, to the common bile duct, and into the bowel.

Jaundice is the discoloration of body tissues caused by abnormally high blood levels of bilirubin. This yellow discoloration is recognized when the total serum bilirubin exceeds 2.5 mg/dl. Jaundice results from a defect in the normal metabolism or excretion of bilirubin. This defect can occur in any stage of heme catabolism.

Physiologic jaundice of the newborn occurs if the newborn's liver is immature and does not have enough conjugating enzymes. This results in a high circulating blood level of unconjugated bilirubin, which can pass through the blood-brain barrier and deposit in the brain cells of the newborn. This can cause encephalopathy *(kernicterus)*.

If the defect in bilirubin metabolism occurs after glucuronide addition, *conjugated (direct) hyperbilirubinemia* will result. Obstruction of the bile duct by a gallstone is the classic example of obstructed bilirubin excretion causing a direct hyperbilirubinemia.

Once the jaundice is recognized, either clinically or chemically, it is important, for therapy, to differentiate whether it is predominantly caused by unconjugated or conjugated bilirubin. This in turn will help differentiate the etiology of the defect. In general, jaundice caused by hepatocellular dysfunction (e.g., hepatitis) is caused by unconjugated bilirubin. This usually cannot be repaired surgically. On the other hand, jaundice resulting from extrahepatic dysfunction (e.g., gallstones or tumor blocking the bowel duct) is caused by elevated conjugated bilirubin levels. This type of jaundice can usually be resolved surgically.

When the defect in bilirubin metabolism occurs after conjugation, elevated levels of conjugated bilirubin occur. Unlike the unconjugated form, conjugated bilirubin is water soluble and can be excreted into the urine. Therefore the finding of bilirubin in the urine suggests disease affecting bilirubin metabolism after conjugation or defects in excretion (e.g., gallstones).

Interfering factors

- Bilirubin is not stable in urine, especially when exposed to light.
- Drugs that may cause increased bilirubin levels include allopurinol, antibiotics, barbiturates, chlorpromazine, diuretics, ethoxazene (Serenium), oral contraceptives, phenazopyridine (Pyridium), steroids, and sulfonamides.
- Drugs that can cause false negative results include indomethacin (Indocin) and ascorbic acid (vitamin C).

Procedure and patient care

Before

- Explain the procedure to the patient.
- Tell the patient that no food or drink restrictions are necessary.

During

- Note that this is a spot urine test.
- Collect at least 10 ml of urine for quick, simple testing.
- Use reagent strips (e.g., Multistix) or tablets (e.g., Icotest) for quick, simple testing.

Multistix

- Note that this is a firm plastic strip with seven separate areas for testing pH, protein, glucose, ketones, bilirubin, blood, and urobilinogen.
- For testing bilirubin, obtain a fresh urine specimen and examine it as soon as possible.

- Immerse the dipstick in the well-mixed urine and remove immediately to avoid dissolving other reagents.
- Tap the dipstick against the rim of the urine container to remove excess urine.
- Hold the strip horizontally and compare it with the color chart on the label of the bottle after 20 to 30 seconds, according to directions. Results are given in the range of 0 to +3.

Icotest tablets
- Place 5 drops of urine on the special test mat.
- Add 2 drops of water. The bilirubin test is positive if the mat turns blue or purple within 30 seconds.
- Note that this test is considered more sensitive than reagent strips for the detection of bilirubin.
- Whether using strips or tablets or if sending the urine to the laboratory, list any medications that can affect test results.

After

- Do not reuse reagent strips or Icotest tablets.

Abnormal findings
Increased levels

Extrahepatic obstruction caused by:

Gallstones   Surgical trauma
Tumor   Cirrhosis
Inflammation   Hepatitis
Stricture

Notes

bleeding time (Ivy bleeding time)

Type of test Blood

Normal findings 1-9 minutes (Ivy method)

Possible critical values >12 minutes

Test explanation and related physiology

The bleeding time test is used to evaluate the vascular and platelet factors associated with hemostasis. When vascular injury occurs, the first hemostatic response is a spastic contraction of the lacerated microvessels. Next, platelets adhere to the wall of the vessel at the area of laceration in an attempt to plug the hole. Failure of either of these processes results in a prolonged bleeding time.

For this study a small, standard superficial incision is made in the forearm, and the time required for the bleeding to stop is recorded. This is called the bleeding time. Normal values vary according to the method used. The method most often used today is the Ivy bleeding time test.

Prolonged values occur in the following:

1. Decreased platelet counts caused by marrow failure (e.g., after radiotherapy or chemotherapy)
2. Infiltration of marrow by primary or metastatic tumor or fibrosis
3. Consumption of platelets during disseminated intravascular coagulation (DIC)
4. Increased platelet destruction, as in primary and secondary thrombocytopenia and hypersplenism
5. Inadequate platelet function caused by medications such as nonsteroidal antiinflammatory agents
6. Inadequate platelet function caused by von Willebrand's disease, uremia, or leukemia
7. Increased capillary fragility secondary to collagen vascular disease, Cushing's disease, or Henoch-Schönlein syndrome (purpura)
8. Ingestion of antiinflammatory drugs (e.g., aspirin, indomethacin)

Contraindications

- Patients with known low platelet counts
- Patients who are unable to cooperate
- Patients who cannot have a blood pressure cuff placed on the arm (e.g., those with cellulitis)
- Patients with a history of keloid formation
- Patients with senile skin changes
- Patients who have had a mastectomy
  Avoid the arm on that side.

Potential complications

- Skin infection
- Excessive bleeding from test site

Interfering factors

- Drugs that may cause increased bleeding times include anticoagulants, dextran, indomethacin, salicylates, streptokinase, and warfarin.

Procedure and patient care

Before

- Explain the procedure to the patient.
- Obtain a consent form if required by the institution.
- Tell the patient that no fasting is required.
- Obtain a drug history to detect if the patient has recently had aspirin, anticoagulants, or any other medications that can affect test results.

During

- Note the following procedural steps:

  1. The skin of the inner part of the forearm is cleansed with alcohol or povidone-iodine (Betadine).
  2. A blood pressure cuff is applied on the arm above the elbow, inflated to 40 mm Hg, and maintained at this pressure during the study.
  3. A small laceration is then made 1 mm deep into the skin, and the time is recorded.
  4. Bleeding ensues, and the blood is wiped clean at 30-second intervals.
  5. When no new bleeding occurs, the time is again noted.
  6. The interval from the beginning to the end of bleeding is calculated; this is the bleeding time.

7. The blood pressure cuff is then removed, and an adhesive is applied to the patient's arm.
8. If bleeding persists more than 10 minutes, the test is stopped and a pressure dressing is applied.

- Indicate on the laboratory slip any medications that can affect test results.
- Note that this test is usually performed by a laboratory technician in less than 10 minutes.
- Inform the patient that minor discomfort may occur with this test because of the skin laceration.

After

- Apply pressure or pressure dressing to the puncture site.
- Assess the puncture site for bleeding.

Abnormal findings
Prolonged times or increased values

Bone marrow failure
Primary or metastatic tumor infiltration of bone marrow
Disseminated intravascular coagulation (DIC)
Thrombocytopenia
Hypersplenism
von Willebrand's disease

Collagen vascular disease
Cushing's disease
Henoch-Schönlein syndrome
Severe liver disease
Clotting factor deficiencies
Hemophilia
Capillary fragility
Leukemia

Notes

blood culture and sensitivity

Type of test Blood

Normal findings Negative

Test explanation and related physiology

Blood cultures are obtained to detect the presence of bacteria in the blood. Bacteremia is usually intermittent and transient, except in endocarditis or suppurative thrombophlebitis. Bacteremia is usually accompanied by chills and fever; thus the blood culture should be drawn when the patient manifests these signs. It is important that at least two culture specimens be obtained from two different sites. If one produces bacteria and the other does not, it is safe to assume that the bacteria in the first culture are a contaminant and not the infecting agent. When both cultures are producing the infecting agent, bacteremia exists. If the patient is receiving antibiotics, the laboratory should be notified. The blood culture specimen should be taken shortly before the next dose of the antibiotic is administered. A resin that binds antibiotics can be added to the specimen, thereby allowing growth and identification of any bacteria.

Culture specimens drawn through an IV catheter are frequently contaminated, and tests using them should not be performed unless catheter sepsis is suspected. In these situations, blood culture specimens drawn through the catheter help identify the causative agent more accurately than a culture specimen from the catheter tip.

All cultures should be performed before antibiotic therapy is initiated. Otherwise the antibiotic may interrupt the organism's growth in the laboratory. Often, however, the physician will want to institute antibiotic therapy before the culture results are reported. In these instances a *Gram stain* of the specimen smeared on a slide is most helpful and can be reported in less than 10 minutes. Overwhelming bacteremia must be present to identify bacteria on a blood specimen Gram stain. All forms of bacteria are grossly classified as Gram positive (blue staining) or Gram negative (red staining). Knowledge of the organism's shape (e.g., spheric or rod shaped) can also be very helpful in its identification.

With knowledge of the Gram stain results the physician can institute a reasonable antibiotic regimen based on past experience as to which organism might be present. Most organisms require approximately 24 hours to grow in the laboratory, and a preliminary report can be given at that time. Often, 48 to 72 hours are required for growth and identification of the organism. Cultures may be repeated after antibiotic therapy to assess for complete resolution of the infection.

Interfering factors

- Contamination of the blood specimen, especially by skin bacteria, may occur.
- Drugs that may alter test results include antibiotics.

Procedure and patient care

Before

- Explain the procedure to the patient.
- Tell the patient that no fasting is required.

During

- Carefully prepare the proposed venipuncture site with povidone-iodine (Betadine). Allow the skin to dry.
- Clean the tops of the vacutainer tubes or culture bottles with povidone-iodine and allow them to dry. (Some laboratories suggest cleaning with 70% alcohol after cleaning with Betadine and air drying.)
- Collect approximately 10 to 15 ml of venous blood by venipuncture from each site in a 20 ml syringe.
- Discard the needle on the syringe and replace with a second sterile needle before injecting the blood sample into the culture bottle.
- Inoculate the anaerobic bottle first if both anaerobic and aerobic cultures are needed.
- Mix gently after inoculation.
- Label specimen with patient's name, date, time, and tentative diagnosis.
- Indicate on the laboratory slip any medications that can affect test results.

After

- Transport the culture bottles immediately to the laboratory (at least within 30 minutes).

- Notify the physician of any positive results so that appropriate antibiotic therapy can be initiated.

Abnormal finding

Bacteremia

Notes

blood gases (Arterial blood gases [ABGs])

Type of test Blood

Normal findings

pH

   Adult/child: 7.35-7.45
   Newborn: 7.32-7.49
   2 months-2 years: 7.34-7.46

P_{CO_2}

   Adult/child: 35-45 mm Hg
   Child <2 years: 26-41 mm Hg

HCO_3^-

   Adult/child: 21-28 mEq/L
   Newborn/infant: 16-24 mEq/L

P_{O_2}

   Adult/child: 80-100 mm Hg
   Newborn: 60-70 mm Hg

O_2 saturation

   Adult/child: 95%-100%
   Elderly: 95%
   Newborn: 40%-90%

Possible critical values

   pH: <7.25, >7.55
   P_{CO_2}: <20, >60
   HCO_3^-: <15, >40
   P_{O_2}: <40
   O_2 saturation: 75% or lower

Test explanation and related physiology

   Measurement of ABGs provides valuable information in assessing and managing a patient's respiratory and metabolic (renal) disturbances.

   pH. The pH is inversely proportional to the actual hydrogen ion concentration. Therefore, as the hydrogen ion concentration decreases, the pH increases, and vice versa. The pH is a measure of alkalinity (pH >7.4) and acidity (pH <7.35). In respiratory or metabolic alkalosis the pH is elevated. In respiratory or metabolic acidosis the pH is decreased.

P_{CO_2}. The P_{CO_2} is a measure of the partial pressure of carbon dioxide in the blood. P_{CO_2} is referred to as the *respiratory* component in acid-base determination because this value is primarily controlled by the lungs. As the CO_2 level increases, the pH decreases. Therefore the CO_2 level and the pH are inversely proportional.

The P_{CO_2} level is elevated in primary respiratory acidosis and decreased in primary respiratory alkalosis (Table 1). Because the lungs are used to compensate for primary metabolic acid-base derangements, P_{CO_2} levels are affected by metabolic disturbances as well. In metabolic acidosis the lungs attempt to compensate by "blowing off" CO_2 to raise pH. In metabolic alkalosis the lungs attempt to compensate by retaining CO_2 to lower pH (Table 2).

HCO_3^-. The bicarbonate ion (HCO_3^-) is a measure of the *metabolic* (renal) component of the acid-base equilibrium. This ion can be measured directly by the bicarbonate value or indirectly by the CO_2 content (see p. 147). As the HCO_3^- level increases, the pH also increases. Therefore the relationship of bicarbonate to pH is directly proportional. HCO_3^- is elevated in metabolic alkalosis and decreased in metabolic acidosis (Table 1). The kidneys are also used to compensate for primary respiratory acid-base derangements. For example, in respiratory acidosis the kidneys attempt to compensate by reabsorbing increased amounts of HCO_3^-. In respiratory alkalosis the kidneys excrete HCO_3^- in increased amounts in an attempt to lower pH through compensation (Table 2).

P_{O_2}. An indirect measure of the oxygen content of the arterial blood, P_{O_2} is the tension (pressure) of oxygen dissolved in the plasma. The P_{O_2} level is decreased in:

1. Patients who are unable to oxygenate the arterial blood because of O_2 diffusion difficulties (e.g., pneumonia, shock lung)
2. Patients who have premature mixing of venous blood with arterial blood (e.g., in congenital heart disease)
3. Patients who have underventilated and overperfused pulmonary alveoli (pickwickian syndrome), that is,

TABLE 1 Normal values for arterial blood gases and abnormal values in uncompensated acid-base disturbances

Acid-base disturbances	pH	Pco$_2$ (mm Hg)	HCO$_3^-$ (mEq/L)	Common cause
None (normal values)	7.35-7.45	35-45	22-26	
Respiratory acidosis	↓	↑	Normal	Respiratory depression (drugs, central nervous system trauma) Pulmonary disease (pneumonia, chronic obstructive pulmonary disease, respiratory underventilation)
Respiratory alkalosis	↑	↓	Normal	Hyperventilation (emotions, pain, respirator overventilation)
Metabolic acidosis	↓	Normal	↓	Diabetes, shock, renal failure, intestinal fistula
Metabolic alkalosis	↑	Normal	↑	Sodium bicarbonate overdose, prolonged vomiting, nasogastric drainage

TABLE 2 Acid-base disturbances and compensatory mechanisms

Acid-base disturbance	Mode of compensation
Respiratory acidosis	Kidneys will retain increased amounts of HCO_3^- to increase pH.
Respiratory alkalosis	Kidneys will excrete increased amounts of HCO_3^- to lower pH.
Metabolic acidosis	Lungs "blow off" CO_2 to raise pH.
Metabolic alkalosis	Lungs retain CO_2 to lower pH.

obese patients who cannot ventilate properly when in the supine position

O_2 saturation. Oxygen saturation is an indication of the percentage of hemoglobin saturated with O_2. When 95% to 100% of the hemoglobin carries O_2, the tissues are adequately provided with O_2. As the Po_2 level decreases, the percentage of hemoglobin saturation also decreases. This decrease (see an oxyhemoglobin dissociation curve) is linear to a certain value. However, when the Po_2 level drops below 60 mm Hg, small decreases in the Po_2 level will cause large decreases in the percentage of hemoglobin saturated with O_2. At O_2 saturation levels of 70% or lower, the tissues are unable to extract enough O_2 to carry out their vital functions.

Procedure and patient care
Before
- Explain the procedure to the patient.
- Notify the laboratory before drawing ABGs so that the necessary equipment can be calibrated before the blood sample arrives.
- Perform the *Allen test* to assess collateral circulation before performing the arterial puncture on the radial artery.
- To perform the Allen test, make the patient's hand blanch by obliterating both the radial and the ulnar pulses.
- Then release the pressure over the ulnar artery only. If flow through the ulnar artery is good, flushing will be seen immediately. The Allen test is then positive, and the radial artery can be used for puncture.

- If the Allen test is negative (no flushing), repeat it on the other arm.
- If both arms give a negative result, choose another artery for puncture.
- Note that the Allen test ensures collateral circulation to the hand if thrombosis of the radial artery should follow the puncture.

During

- Note that the arterial blood can be obtained from any area of the body where strong pulses are palpable, usually from the radial, brachial, or femoral artery.
- Cleanse the arterial site.
- Attach a 20-gauge needle to a syringe containing about 0.2 ml of heparin.
- After drawing 3 to 5 ml of blood, remove the needle and apply pressure to the arterial site for 3 to 5 minutes.
- Expel any air bubbles in the syringe.
- Cap the syringe and gently rotate to mix the blood and heparin.
- Indicate on the laboratory slip if the patient is receiving oxygen therapy or is attached to a ventilator.
- Note that an arterial puncture is performed by laboratory technicians, respiratory inhalation therapists, nurses, or physicians in approximately 10 minutes.
- Tell the patient that the arterial puncture is associated with more discomfort than a venous puncture.

After

- Place the arterial blood on ice and immediately take it to the chemistry laboratory for analysis.
- Apply pressure or a pressure dressing to the arterial puncture site.
- Assess the puncture site for bleeding. Remember: an artery rather than a vein has been stuck.
- If the patient has an abnormal clotting time or is taking anticoagulants, apply pressure for a longer period (approximately 15 minutes).

Abnormal findings

See Table 1.

Notes

blood smear (Peripheral blood smear, Red blood cell morphology, RBC smear)

B

Type of test Blood

Normal findings

Normal quantity of red and white blood cells (RBCs, WBCs) and platelets

Normal size, shape, and color of RBCs

Normal WBC differential count

Test explanation and related physiology

When adequately prepared and examined microscopically by an experienced technologist, a smear of the peripheral blood is the most informative of all hematologic tests. All three hematologic cell lines (RBCs, WBCs, platelets) can be examined.

Microscopic examination of the RBCs can reveal variation in RBC size (anisocytosis), shape (poikilocytosis), color, or intracellular content. Classification of RBCs according to these variables is most helpful in identifying the causes of anemia.

RBC size
  Microcytes (small RBC)
    Iron deficiency
    Hereditary spherocytosis
    Thalassemia
  Macrocytes (larger size)
    Vitamin B_{12} or folic acid deficiency
    Reticulocytosis secondary to increased erythropoiesis (RBC production)
    Occasional liver disorder
    Postsplenectomy anemia
RBC shape
  Spherocytes (small and round)
    Hereditary spherocytosis
    Acquired immunohemolytic anemia
  Elliptocytes (crescent or sickle shaped)
    Hereditary elliptocytosis
    Sickle cell anemia

Leptocytes, or "target cells" (thin and with less hemoglobin)
  Hemoglobinopathies
  Thalassemia
Spicule cell
  Uremia
  Liver disease
  Bleeding ulcer

RBC color
  Hypochromic (pale)
    Iron deficiency
    Thalassemia
    Cardiac disease
  Hyperchromasia (more colored)
    Concentrated hemoglobin, usually caused by dehydration

RBC intracellular structure
  Nucleus (Because the RBC maturation process results in loss of the nucleus, nucleated RBCs [normoblasts] seen in the peripheral smear indicate increased RBC production.)
    "Normal" for infant's blood
    Physiologic response to RBC deficiency (as in hemolytic anemias, sickle cell crisis, transfusion reaction, and erythroblastosis fetalis)
    Physiologic response to hypoxemia (as in congenital heart disease and congestive heart failure)
    Marrow-occupying neoplasm or fibrotic tissue (as in myeloma and leukemia)
  Basophilic stippling (refers to bodies enclosed or included in the cells)
    Lead poisoning
    Reticulocytosis
  Howell-Jolly bodies (small, round remnants of nuclear material)
    Postsplenectomy
    Hemolytic anemia
    Megaloblastic anemia
  Heinz bodies (small, irregular particles of hemoglobin)
    Drug-induced RBC injury
    Hemoglobinopathies
    Hemolytic anemia

The WBCs are examined for total quantity, differential count, and degree of maturity. An increased number of immature WBCs may indicate leukemia. A decreased WBC count indicates failure of marrow to produce WBCs, caused by drugs, chronic disease, neoplasia, or fibrosis.

Finally, an experienced cell examiner can estimate platelet number (see p. 563) on a peripheral blood smear.

Procedure and patient care

Before

- Explain the procedure to the patient.
- Tell the patient that no fasting is required.

During

- Collect a drop of blood from a finger stick or heel stick and place it on a slide.
- If necessary, perform a venipuncture and collect the blood in a lavender-top tube.
- Note that a blood smear is first studied with an automated calculator programmed to recognize abnormal blood cell shapes and so on. A more accurate smear is performed by a technologist. Low counts may be "hand counted" to ensure accuracy. The most accurate smear requires review by a pathologist.

After

- Apply pressure or a pressure dressing to the venipuncture site.
- Assess the venipuncture site for bleeding.

Abnormal findings

See listing under "Test explanation and related physiology."

Notes

blood typing

Type of test Blood

Normal findings Compatibility

Test explanation and related physiology

With blood typing, ABO and Rh antigens can be detected in the blood of prospective blood donors and potential blood recipients. This test is also used to determine the blood type of expectant mothers and newborns. Human blood is grouped according to the presence or absence of these antigens. The two major antigens, A and B, form the basis of the ABO system (group A red blood cells [RBCs] contain A antigens; group B RBCs contain B antigens; group AB RBCs have both A and B antigens; group O RBCs have neither A nor B antigens) (Table 3). The presence or absence of Rh antigens on the RBCs determines the classification of Rh positive or Rh negative.

All pregnant patients should have a blood typing and Rh factor determination. If the pregnant patient's blood is Rh negative or type O (the most common type), the husband's blood should also be typed. If his blood is Rh positive or type AB, the woman's blood should be examined for the presence of Rh antibodies (by the indirect Coombs' test, see p. 235). If the initial screening is negative (no antibodies to Rh found), the test is repeated at weeks 30 and 36 of pregnancy. If these tests are also negative, no risk is involved to the fetus. If the test is positive, the fetus has been affected by

TABLE 3 Blood typing

Blood type	Antigen	Antibody
Group A	A	B
Group B	B	A
Group AB (universal receiver)	A, B	None
Group O (universal donor)	None	A, B

maternal hemolysis of the fetal RBCs. The severity of the hemolytic anemia is then evaluated by the quantity of bilirubin in the amniotic fluid (see amniocentesis, p. 34).

ABO and Rh typing is also performed during pregnancy to advise the mother whether or not she is a candidate for RhoGAM (Rh immunoglobulin) after the delivery. RhoGAM will prevent any further fetal hemolytic problems during subsequent pregnancies.

Blood transfusions are actually transplantations of tissue (blood) from one person to another. It is important that the recipient does not have antibodies to the donor's RBCs and that the donor does not have antibodies to the recipient's RBCs. If either of these conditions exists, there will be a hypersensitivity reaction, which can vary in severity from mild fever to anaphylaxis with severe intravascular hemolysis. Although typing for the major ABO and Rh antigens does not guarantee that no reaction will occur, it does greatly reduce the possibility of such a reaction.

Many potential minor antigens are not routinely detected during blood typing. If allowed to go unrecognized, these minor antigens can also initiate a blood transfusion reaction. Therefore blood is not only typed but also cross-matched to identify a mismatch of blood caused by minor antigens. Cross-matching consists of the mixing of the recipient's serum with the donor's RBCs in saline solution followed by the addition of Coombs' serum (indirect Coombs' test, see p. 235).

Procedure and patient care

Before

- Explain the procedure to the patient.
- Tell the patient that no fasting is required.

During

- Collect approximately 7 to 14 ml of venous blood in a red-top tube. (This may vary among laboratories.)
- Avoid hemolysis.
- Appropriately label the blood tube before sending it to the laboratory.

After

- Apply pressure or a pressure dressing to the venipuncture site.
- Assess the venipuncture site for bleeding.

Abnormal findings

None

Notes

bone marrow biopsy (Bone marrow examination, Bone marrow aspiration)

B

Type of test Microscopic examination of tissue

Normal findings Active erythroid cell line, myeloid and lymphoid cell lines, and megakaryocyte (platelet) production

Test explanation and related physiology

By examination of a bone marrow specimen, the hematologist can fully evaluate hematopoiesis. Examination of the bone marrow reveals the number, size, and shape of the red and white blood cells (RBCs, WBCs) and megakaryocytes (platelet precursors) as these cells evolve through various stages of development in the bone marrow. Samples of the bone marrow can be obtained by either aspiration or surgical removal. Microscopic examination includes estimation of cellularity, determination of the presence of fibrotic tissue or neoplasms (both primary and metastatic), and estimation of iron storage.

For the estimation of cellularity, the specimen is examined and the relative quantity of each cell type is determined. This is more accurately performed on a biopsy specimen than on an aspirate because the aspirate may not be truly representative of the entire marrow. Leukemias or leukemoid drug reactions are suspected when increased numbers of leukocyte precursors are present. Physiologic marrow leukemoid compensation for infection will also be recognized by finding an increased number of leukocyte precursors. Decreased numbers of marrow leukocyte precursors occur in patients with myelofibrosis, metastatic neoplasia, or agranulocytosis; in the elderly; and following radiation therapy or chemotherapy.

Increased numbers of marrow RBC precursors occur with polycythemia vera or as physiologic compensation to hemorrhagic or hemolytic anemias. Decreased numbers of marrow RBC precursors occur with erythroid hypoplasia following chemotherapy, radiation therapy, administration of other toxic drugs, iron deficiency, or marrow replacement by fibrotic tissue or neoplasms.

Increased numbers of platelet precursors (megakaryocytes)

are seen in the marrow of patients following acute hemorrhage or some forms of chronic myeloid leukemia. This increase may also be compensatory in patients with secondary hypersplenism associated with portal hypertension or other conditions. Decreased megakaryocytes occur in patients who have had radiation therapy, chemotherapy, or other drug therapy and in patients with neoplastic or fibrotic marrow infiltrative diseases. Patients with aplastic anemia also have decreased megakaryocytes.

Lymphocyte precursors are increased in chronic or viral infections (e.g., mononucleosis), lymphocytic leukemia, and lymphoma. Plasma cells (plasmocytes) are increased in patients with multiple myelomas, Hodgkin's disease, hypersensitivity states, rheumatic fever, and other chronic inflammatory diseases.

Estimation of cellularity can also be expressed as a ratio of myeloid (WBC) to erythroid (RBC) cells (M/E ratio). The normal M/E ratio is approximately 3:1. The M/E ratio is greater than normal in those diseases mentioned previously in which increased leukocyte precursors are present or in which erythroid precursors are decreased. The M/E ratio is below normal when either leukocyte precursors are decreased or erythroid precursors are increased. A more detailed listing of diseases affecting the M/E ratio can be found in most hematology textbooks.

Drug-induced or idiopathic myelofibrosis can be detected by examination of the bone marrow. Using special stains, one can estimate iron stores with a marrow biopsy. Although fibrosis or neoplasia can occasionally be detected in aspiration studies, biopsy is the best method. Leukemias, multiple myelomas, and polycythemia vera can easily be detected in biopsy specimens. Similarly, lymphomas and other metastatic tumors (e.g., cancers of the breast, kidney, and lung) can be seen.

Contraindications

- Patients with acute coagulation disorders because of the risk of excessive bleeding
- Patients who cannot cooperate and remain still during the procedure

Potential complications

- Hemorrhage, especially if the patient has a coagulopathy
- Infection, especially if the patient is leukopenic
- Inadvertent puncture of the heart or great vessels when the test is done on the sternum

Procedure and patient care

Before

- Explain the procedure to the patient.
- Obtain a written and informed consent for this procedure.
- Encourage the patient to verbalize fears because many patients are anxious concerning this study.
- Assess the coagulation studies. Report any evidence of coagulopathy to the physician.
- Obtain an order for sedatives if the patient appears extremely apprehensive.
- Remind the patient to remain very still throughout the procedure.

During

- Note the following procedural steps for *bone marrow aspiration,* which is performed on the sternum, iliac crest, anterior or posterior iliac spines, and proximal tibia (in children):

  1. The procedure is usually performed at the patient's bedside using local anesthesia.
  2. A preferred site is the posterior iliac crest with the patient placed prone or on the side.
  3. The area overlying the bone is prepared and draped in a sterile manner.
  4. The overlying skin and soft tissue, along with the periosteum, is infiltrated with lidocaine.
  5. A large-bore needle containing a stylus is slowly advanced through the soft tissue and into the outer table of the bone.
  6. Once inside the marrow, the stylus is removed and a syringe is attached.
  7. One-half to 2 ml of bone marrow is aspirated, smeared on slides, and allowed to dry.
  8. The slides are sprayed with a preservative and taken to the pathology laboratory.

- Note the following procedural steps for *bone marrow biopsy:*
  1. The skin and soft tissues overlying the bone are incised.
  2. A core biopsy instrument is "screwed" into the bone.
  3. The biopsy specimen is obtained and sent to the pathology laboratory for analysis.

- Note that aspiration is performed by a trained nurse or physician. Bone marrow biopsy specimen removal is usually performed by a physician. The duration of these studies is approximately 20 minutes.

- Inform the patient that he or she may have some apprehension when pressure is applied to puncture the outer table of the bone during biopsy specimen removal or aspiration.

- Tell the patient that he or she probably will feel pain during lidocaine infiltration and pressure when the syringe plunger is withdrawn for aspiration.

After

- Apply pressure to the puncture site to arrest minimal bleeding. Apply an adhesive bandage.
- Observe the puncture site for bleeding. Ice packs may be used to help control bleeding.
- Assess for tenderness and erythema, which may indicate infection. Report this to the physician.
- Evaluate the patient for signs of shock (increased pulse rate, decreased blood pressure) and pain.
- Normally, place the patient on bed rest for 30 to 60 minutes after the test.
- Note that some patients complain of tenderness at the puncture site for several days after this study. Mild analgesics may be ordered.

Abnormal findings

Neoplasms	Acute hemorrhagic marrow
Infection	hyperplasia
Myelofibrosis	Anemias
Agranulocytosis	Mononucleosis
Polycythemia vera	Lymphoma

Multiple myelomas
Hodgkin's disease
Hypersensitivity states
Rheumatic fever

Chronic inflammatory diseases
Leukemias

B

Notes

bone scan

Type of test Nuclear scan

Normal findings No evidence of abnormality

Test explanation and related physiology

The bone scan permits examination of the skeleton by a scanning camera after IV injection of a radionuclide material. The degree of radionuclide uptake is related to the metabolism of the bone. Normally a uniform concentration should be seen throughout the bones of the body. An increased uptake of isotope is abnormal and may represent tumor, arthritis, fracture, degenerative bone and joint changes, osteomyelitis, bone necrosis, osteodystrophy, and Paget's disease. These areas of concentrated radionuclide uptake are often called "hot spots" and are detectable months before an ordinary x-ray film can reveal the pathology.

The major reason a bone scan is performed is to detect metastatic cancer to the bone. All malignancies capable of metastasis may reach the bone, especially those of the prostate, breast, lung, kidney, urinary bladder, and thyroid gland. Bone scans may be serially repeated to document the tumor's response to antineoplastic therapy.

Bone scans also provide valuable information in the evaluation of patients with trauma or unexplained pain. Bone scanning is much more sensitive than routine x-ray films in detecting small and difficult-to-find fractures, especially in the spine, ribs, face, and small bones of the extremities. Bone scans are also used to determine the age of a fracture. If a fracture is seen on a plain x-ray film, and if the uptake around that fracture is not increased on a bone scan, the injury is said to be an "old" fracture exceeding several months in age.

Although the bone scan is extremely sensitive, unfortunately it is not very specific. Fractures, infections, tumors, and arthritic changes all appear similar.

Contraindications

- Patients who are pregnant because of the risk of fetal damage
- Patients who are lactating because of the risk of contaminating the infant

Procedure and patient care
Before

- Explain the procedure to the patient.
- Assure patients that they will not be exposed to large amounts of radioactivity because only tracer doses of the isotope are used.
- Tell the patient that no fasting or sedation is required.

During

- Note the following procedural steps:

  1. The patient receives an IV injection of an isotope, usually sodium pertechnetate (technetium-99m) in a peripheral vein.
  2. The patient is encouraged to drink several glasses of water between the time of radioisotope injection and the scanning. This facilitates renal clearance of the circulating tracer not picked up by the bone. The waiting period before scanning is approximately 1 to 3 hours.
  3. The patient is instructed to urinate.
  4. The patient is positioned in the supine position on the scanning table in the nuclear medicine department.
  5. A radionuclide detector is placed over the patient's body and records the radiation emitted by the skeleton.
  6. This information is translated into a two-dimensional view of the skeleton, which is then visualized on a Polaroid or x-ray film.
  7. The patient is repositioned in the prone and lateral positions during the test.

- Note that this scan is performed by a nuclear medicine technician in 30 to 60 minutes. It is interpreted by a physician trained in nuclear medicine imaging.
- Tell the patient that the injection of the radioisotope causes slight discomfort.
- Inform patients in significant pain that lying on the hard scanning table can be uncomfortable.

After

- Because only tracer doses of radioisotope are used, remember that no precautions need to be taken to prevent radioactive exposure to other personnel or family.

- Assure the patient that the radioactive substance is usually excreted from the body within 6 to 24 hours.
- Encourage the patient to drink fluids to aid in the excretion of the radioactive substance.
- Observe the injection site for redness or swelling.

Abnormal findings

Primary and metastatic tumors of the bone
Fracture
Degenerative arthritis
Rheumatoid arthritis

Osteomyelitis
Bone necrosis
Renal osteodystrophy
Paget's disease

Notes

brain scan (Cisternal scan, Cerebral blood flow)

Type of test Nuclear scan

Normal findings No areas of increased radionuclide uptake within the brain

Test explanation and related physiology

Brain scanning allows for the detection of pathologic cerebral conditions by nuclear counter scanning of the patient's cranial contents after the IV administration of a radioisotope. This study is performed in patients who have frequent and severe headaches, stroke (cerebrovascular accident, CVA) syndrome, seizure complaints, or other neurologic complaints. Normally the blood-brain barrier does not allow the blood to come in direct contact with brain tissue. Frequently used isotopes (e.g., technetium-99m pertechnetate, mercury-201, radioiodinated albumin) are unable to cross this blood-brain barrier. However, in localized pathologic conditions, this normal barrier is disrupted. The isotopes are then preferentially localized or concentrated in abnormal regions of the brain.

The precise cause of the disruption of the blood-brain barrier can be any of various pathologic processes. Unfortunately the brain scan is not a specific indicator of the exact pathologic process. Study of the location, size, and shape of the abnormality, along with the timing of the scan, may help specify the pathologic process.

Timing of brain scanning in relation to the onset of CVA-like symptoms is usually significant. For example, in cerebral infarction, scanning performed soon after the onset of symptoms may be normal and then become abnormal 2 weeks later. This combination is virtually pathognomonic of infarction. Scanning patients with cerebral thrombosis without infarction may never reveal abnormalities. Tumors and abscesses will show abnormalities on the initial scan.

The injection of isotopes followed by immediate scanning can be used to detect changes in the dynamics of cerebral blood flow by comparing one side of the brain to the other. For example, cerebrovascular occlusive disease is characterized by a decreased flow rate, in contrast to an arteriovenous

(AV) malformation, which is associated with an increased flow rate.

Cisternal scans may be performed by injecting radioactive material into the subarachnoid space and then taking serial scans of the head. These scans are useful in evaluating ventricular size and patency of the cerebrospinal fluid (CSF) pathways and reabsorbtion. Normally, because only a small amount of CSF enters the ventricles, their uptake of radioactive material should be minimal. However, blocks in the CSF pathways may prevent this reabsorption, and thus large amounts of isotopes may appear in the ventricles. Cisternal scans may also be used to evaluate CSF leakage in patients with recurrent meningitis and to evaluate hydrocephalus.

In general, computed tomography (CT) scans, magnetic resonance imaging (MRI) scans, and carotid duplex scans have replaced the brain scan in diagnostic neurology.

Contraindications

- Patients who are pregnant
- Patients who cannot cooperate during the testing

Procedure and patient care

Before

- Explain the procedure to the patient.
- Administer blocking agents as ordered before scanning. For example, potassium chloride prevents an inordinate amount of technetium uptake by the choroid plexus, which would simulate a pathologic cerebral condition. Similar solutions (e.g., potassium iodine, Lugol's solution) may be given orally to block thyroid uptake. Blocking agents are not necessary with the use of technetium-99m diethylenetriamine penta-acetic acid (DTPA).
- Check for allergy to iodine if an iodinated solution will be used.
- Consider having a sedative ordered for agitated patients.

During

- Note the following procedural steps:

  1. After administration of the radioisotope, the patient is placed in the supine, lateral, and prone positions while a counter is placed over the head.
  2. The radioisotope counts are anatomically displayed and photographed while the patient remains very still.

3. When cerebral flow studies are performed, the counter is immediately placed over the head.
4. The counts are anatomically recorded in timed sequence to follow the isotope during its first flow through the brain.
5. Another scan is obtained later (½ to 2 hours) for identification of pathologic tissues.

- Note that this study is performed by a technician in the nuclear medicine department in approximately 35 to 45 minutes.
- Tell the patient that no discomfort is associated with this study other than the peripheral IV puncture required for injection of the radioisotope.

After

- Assure the patient that the radioactive material is usually excreted from the body within 6 to 24 hours.
- Because only tracer doses of radioisotopes are used, remember that no precautions need to be taken to prevent radioactive exposure to other personnel or family.
- Encourage the patient to drink fluids to aid the excretion of the isotope from the body.
- Observe the injection site for redness and swelling.

Abnormal findings

Cerebral neoplasm
Brain abscess
Acute cerebral infarction
Subdural hematoma
Cerebral thrombosis
Cerebrovascular occlusive disease
Cerebral hemorrhage

Hematoma
AV malformation
Aneurysm
CSF leakage
Hydrocephalus
Cancer metastasis to the brain

Notes

bronchography (Bronchogram, Laryngography)

Type of test X-ray with contrast dye

Normal findings Normal tracheobronchial tree

Test explanation and related physiology

A bronchogram is an x-ray examination of the tracheo-bronchial tree produced after the instillation of an iodinated dye into the bronchi via a catheter or bronchoscope. Positioning of the patient and the catheter allows the radiopaque material to coat all portions of the tracheobronchial tree so that their outline can be recorded on a chest x-ray film. X-ray films are taken to demonstrate the outline and structure of the trachea, bronchi, and the entire tracheobronchial tree.

Bronchography is indicated to diagnose bronchiectasis, to identify obstruction in the distal bronchi, and to detect congenital or acquired forms of tracheobronchial malformation. Bronchography may be used in the evaluation of patients for possible surgery and in those patients with recurring, localized pneumonia or severe hemoptysis. Bronchography should not be performed when patients have an exacerbation of cough or sputum production. The test should be performed after the symptoms are treated and when mucous secretions are minimal. Because of the alterations in pulmonary function and occasional inflammatory reactions induced by this procedure, studying one lung at a time is safer than studying both. The indications for bronchography have diminished since the development of flexible fiberoptic bronchoscopy has provided direct visualization of the tracheobronchial tree.

Contraindications

- Patients who are pregnant
- Patients with acute infections
- Patients with respiratory insufficiency

Potential complications

- Bronchospasm or laryngospasm
- Allergic reaction to iodinated dye
  This rarely occurs because the dye is not administered intravenously.

Interfering factors

- Excessive coughing or sputum production can inhibit bronchiolar filling and can cause premature explusion of the contrast material.

Procedure and patient care

Before

- Explain the procedure to the patient. Allay any concerns and allow the patient to express any fears.
- Obtain informed consent if required by the institution.
- Check for allergies to iodine dye and shellfish.
- Keep the patient NPO after midnight the day of the test.
- Instruct the patient to perform thorough mouth care the night before and the morning of the test to minimize the risk of introducing bacteria into the lungs during the procedure.
- Consider postural drainage to promote expulsion of mucus or exudate from the lungs.
- Remove and safely store the patient's dentures, glasses, or contact lenses.
- Administer the preprocedural medications as ordered. Medications may include atropine to decrease secretions and to minimize vagally induced bradycardia and diazepam (Valium) for its sedative effect.
- Instruct the patient not to swallow the local anesthetic sprayed into the throat. Provide an emesis basin for expectoration.
- Inform the patient to make every effort to suppress coughing during the procedure. Coughing will prevent adequate bronchiolar filling and will also expel the contrast substance before the test is completed. Rapid, shallow breathing will help to suppress the cough reflex. If the patient has a productive cough, an expectorant is administered and postural drainage is performed for 1 to 3 days before the procedure.

During

- Place the patient in a sitting position.
- Note the following procedural steps:

  1. After spraying a local anesthetic into the patient's nose or mouth to suppress the gag reflex, a catheter or bronchoscope is passed into the trachea.

2. The pharynx, larynx, and major bronchi are anesthetized before introduction of the radiopaque dye.
3. The position of the patient and the placing of the catheter allow the radiologist to fill regions of interest selectively with radiopaque material.
4. The positions assumed by the patient are usually the reverse of those used in postural drainage.
5. Multiple x-ray views are obtained.

- Note that bronchography is performed by a radiologist in approximately 45 minutes.
- Inform the patient of the discomfort usually associated with this test.

After

- Perform postural drainage, if indicated, to help remove the radiopaque dye from the tracheobronchial tree.
- Instruct the patient not to eat or drink anything until the tracheobronchial anesthesia has worn off and the gag reflex returns, usually in approximately 2 hours.
- Observe the patient closely for evidence of impaired respiration or laryngospasm. Vocal chords may go into spasm after intubation. Emergency resuscitation equipment should be readily available.
- Encourage the patient to cough, which will help clear the tracheobronchial tree.
- Inform the patient that a slight temperature elevation often occurs for 2 to 3 days after the test.
- Inform the patient a sore throat also often develops. This can be relieved by gargling or by taking throat lozenges.
- Note that follow-up x-ray films may be taken later to ascertain if any dye remains in the tracheobronchial tree.
- Tell the patient that normal activities may usually be resumed 24 hours after the test.

Abnormal findings

Bronchiectasis
Bronchial obstruction
Tracheobronchial malformation

Notes

bronchoscopy

Type of test Endoscopy

Normal findings Normal larynx, trachea, bronchi, and alveoli

Test explanation and related physiology

Bronchoscopy permits endoscopic visualization of the larynx, trachea, and bronchi by either a flexible fiberoptic bronchoscope or a rigid bronchoscope. *Diagnostic* uses of bronchoscopy include:

1. Direct visualization of the tracheobronchial tree for abnormalities (e.g., tumors, inflammation, strictures)
2. Biopsy of specimens from observed lesions
3. Aspiration of "deep" sputum for culture and sensitivity and cytology determinations

Therapeutic uses of bronchoscopy include:

1. Aspiration of retained secretions in patients with airway obstruction or postoperative atelectasis
2. Control of bleeding within the bronchus
3. Removal of foreign bodies that have been aspirated
4. Brachytherapy, which is endobronchial radiation therapy using an iridium wire placed via the bronchoscope
5. Palliative laser obliteration of bronchial neoplastic obstruction

The *rigid bronchoscope* is a wide-bore metal tube that permits visualization of only the larger airways. It is mainly used for the removal of large foreign bodies. Its use has radically diminished since the advent of the newer flexible fiberoptic bronchoscope. However, recently a slight resurgence has occurred in the use of rigid bronchoscopy with the emergence of laser therapy. Laser therapy can now be done through the bronchoscope to burn out endotracheal lesions.

Because of its smaller size and its flexibility, the *flexible fiberoptic bronchoscope* has increased the diagnostic reach of bronchoscopy to the smaller bronchi. This newer scope has an accessory lumen through which cable-activated instruments can be used for removing biopsy specimens of pathologic lesions. Also, the collection of bronchial washings (obtained by flushing the airways with saline solution), pulmonary toilet, and the instillation of anesthetic agents can be carried out through this extra lumen. Double-sheathed, plugged-protected brushes can also be passed through this accessory lumen. Specimens for cytology and bacteriology can be obtained with these brushes. This allows more accurate determination of pulmonary infectious agents.

Contraindications

- Patients with hypercapnia and severe shortness of breath who cannot tolerate interruption of high-flow oxygen

Potential complications

- Fever
- Hypoxemia
- Laryngospasm
- Bronchospasm
- Pneumothorax
- Aspiration
- Hemorrhage (after biopsy)

Procedure and patient care

Before

- Explain the procedure to the patient. Allay any fears and allow the patient to verbalize any concerns.
- Obtain informed consent for this procedure.
- Keep the patient NPO for 4 to 8 hours before the test to reduce the risk of aspiration.
- Instruct the patient to perform good mouth care to minimize the risk of introducing bacteria into the lungs during the procedure.
- Remove and safely store the patient's dentures, glasses, or contact lenses before administering the preprocedural medications.
- Administer the preprocedural medications as ordered. Atropine is used to prevent vagally induced bradycardia and to minimize secretions. Meperidine is used to sedate the patient and relieve anxiety.
- Reassure the patient that he or she will be able to breath during this procedure.
- Instruct the patient not to swallow the local anesthetic

sprayed into the throat. Provide a basin for expectoration of the lidocaine.

During

- Note the following procedural steps for *fiberoptic bronchoscopy:*

  1. This test is performed by a pulmonary specialist or a surgeon at the bedside or in an appropriately equipped room.
  2. The patient's nasopharynx and oropharynx are anesthetized topically with lidocaine spray before the insertion of the bronchoscope.
  3. The patient is placed in the sitting or supine position, and the tube is inserted through the nose or mouth and into the pharynx.
  4. After the tube passes into the larynx and through the glottis, more lidocaine is sprayed into the trachea to prevent the cough reflex.
  5. The tube is passed farther, well into the trachea, bronchi, and the first- and second-generation bronchioles for systematic examination of the bronchial tree (Figure 2).
  6. Biopsy specimens and washings are taken if pathology is suspected.
  7. If bronchoscopy is performed for pulmonary toilet (removal of mucus), each bronchus is aspirated until clear.

- Note the following procedural steps for *rigid bronchoscopy:*

  1. This test is usually performed in the operating room with the patient under heavy sedation or general anesthesia.
  2. The patient is placed in the supine position with the neck hyperextended.
  3. The tube is inserted through the mouth and larynx and then into the trachea.

- Note that this procedure is performed by a physician in approximately 30 to 45 minutes.
- Tell the patient that because of sedation, no discomfort is usually felt.

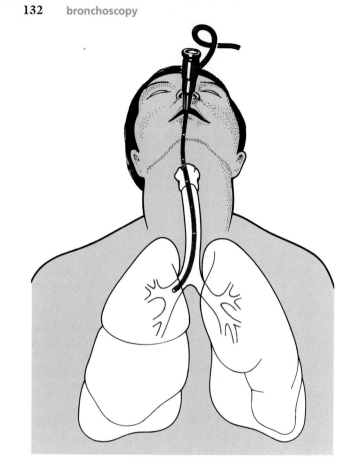

Figure 2 Bronchoscopy. A bronchoscope is inserted through the trachea and into the bronchus.

After

- Instruct the patient not to eat or drink anything until the tracheobronchial anesthesia has worn off and the gag reflex has returned, usually in approximately 2 hours.
- Observe the patient's sputum for hemorrhage if biopsy specimens were removed. A small amount of blood streaking may be expected and is normal for several

hours. Large amounts of bleeding can cause a chemical pneumonitis.

- Observe closely for evidence of impaired respiration or laryngospasm. The vocal cords may go into spasms after intubation. Emergency resuscitation equipment should be readily available.
- Inform the patient that postbronchoscopy fever often develops within the first 24 hours.
- If tumor is suspected, collect a postbronchoscopy sputum sample for a cytology determination.
- Inform the patient that warm saline gargles and lozenges may be helpful if a sore throat develops.

Abnormal findings

Tumor
Inflammation
Strictures
Tuberculosis

Hemorrhage
Foreign body
Abscesses
Infection

Notes

CA-125 tumor marker

Type of test Blood

Normal findings 0-35 U/ml

Test explanation and related physiology

The detection, extent of disease, and response to treatment of ovarian cancer can be determined by the use of CA-125. This tumor marker has a high degree of sensitivity and specificity for ovarian cancer and has proved to be of great benefit for clinicians. Just as alpha-fetoprotein (AFP) and human chorionic gonadotropin (HCG) are accurate tumor markers for germ cell tumors of the ovary, CA-125 is an extremely accurate tumor marker for epithelial tumors of the ovary.

CA-125 can be used in many ways. It is especially helpful in making the diagnosis of ovarian cancer. For example, CA-125 can be used in women who have abdominal distention, ascites, and a palpable pelvic mass. In these patients a greatly elevated CA-125 level is strong confirmation that the underlying etiology is an epithelial ovarian malignancy.

CA-125 serum tumor marker is also used to determine response to therapy. Serial comparative testing will show a progressive decline in CA-125 levels for patients responding to treatment. Also, CA-125 tumor markers can predict whether or not a second-look (repeat) diagnostic laparotomy will be positive. A second-look laparotomy will detect a residual tumor in 97% of patients whose CA-125 level is greater than 35 U/ml, whereas only 56% of ovarian cancer patients whose CA-125 level is less than 35 U/ml will have a positive second-look laparotomy.

Finally, CA-125 determinations can be used in posttreatment surveillance of ovarian cancer patients. If a patient has had complete response as a result of radiation therapy, chemotherapy, or surgery, a delayed rise in CA-125 level may be an early predictor of a recurrent tumor. CA-125 serum tumor marker has not yet been used as a screening test for the asymptomatic population; however, this is presently being studied.

Other tumors and benign processes can cause elevated

CA-125 levels. In 20% of patients with colon cancer and in 60% of patients with upper gastrointestinal cancers, CA-125 levels exceed 35 U/ml.

Interfering factors

- Pregnancy and normal menstruation may cause mild elevations of CA-125 levels.
- Patients with benign peritoneal diseases (e.g., cirrhosis, endometriosis) will have mildly increased levels.

Procedure and patient care

Before

- Explain the procedure to the patient.
- Tell the patient that no fasting or sedation is required.

During

- Collect 7 to 10 ml of blood in a red-top tube.
- Have the blood sent to a central diagnostic laboratory for determination of CA-125 level. The results are available to the local hospital in 3 to 7 days.

After

- Apply pressure or a pressure dressing to the venipuncture site.
- Observe the venipuncture site for bleeding.

Abnormal findings

Increased levels

Ovarian cancer
Metastatic peritoneal carcinomatosis
Endometriosis
Cirrhosis
Peritonitis

Pregnancy
Other gynecologic tumors
Colon cancer
Upper gastrointestinal cancers

Notes

CA 15-3 tumor marker

Type of test Blood

Normal findings <22 U/ml

Test explanation and related physiology

CA 15-3 is a tumor-associated serum marker available for diagnosing and monitoring the treatment of breast cancer. Until now, no other good tumor marker has been available for breast cancer patients. Carcinoembryonic antigen (CEA, see p. 151), the most widely used tumor marker, is limited by poor sensitivity and specificity for patients with disease. Most recently the monoclonal antibody technology has permitted the development of CA 15-3 antigen.

CA 15-3 is not as sensitive in the diagnosis of primary breast cancer as other tumor markers are for their respective tumors. That is, CA 15-3 levels are not high in patients whose presenting symptoms are limited, localized breast cancers or who have a small tumor burden. On the other hand, patients with metastatic breast cancer do have greatly elevated levels. Therefore the usefulness of CA 15-3 as a screening technique in early breast cancers, the most common cancer of women, is quite limited. Benign breast or ovarian disease and other nonbreast malignancies also can cause elevated CA 15-3 levels.

CA 15-3 is useful in monitoring the patient's response to therapy for metastatic breast cancer. A partial or complete response to treatment will be confirmed by declining levels. Likewise, a persistent rise of CA 15-3 levels despite therapy strongly suggests progressive disease.

CA 15-3 levels cannot be used in the surveillance of patients who have had a complete response to breast cancer as a result of surgery, radiation therapy, or chemotherapy. The high sensitivity but lack of specificity noted with this marker often inappropriately suggests recurrent disease when other benign processes exist.

Procedure and patient care
Before

- Explain the procedure to the patient.
- Tell the patient that no fasting is required.

During

- Collect 7 to 10 ml of venous blood in a red-top tube.
- Have the blood sample sent to a central diagnostic laboratory for CA 15-3 determinations. The results are available to the local hospital in 7 to 10 days.

After

- Apply pressure or a pressure dressing to the venipuncture site.
- Observe the venipuncture site for bleeding.

Abnormal finding
Increased levels

Metastatic breast cancer

Notes

CA 19-9 tumor marker

Type of test   Blood

Normal findings   <37 U/ml

Test explanation and related physiology

CA 19-9 is a tumor marker used in diagnosis, evaluation of response to treatment, and surveillance of patients with pancreatic or hepatobiliary cancer. It is used primarily in the diagnosis of pancreatic carcinoma. For example, in a patient whose presenting symptom is a pancreatic mass or biliary obstruction, greatly elevated levels of CA 19-9 would confirm that pancreatic cancer exists. Likewise, patients whose presenting symptoms are ascites, jaundice, and an elevated CA 19-9 level may have a hepatobiliary cancer. CA 19-9 levels, however, may not be elevated in all patients with pancreatic carcinoma. Approximately 70% of patients with pancreatic carcinoma and 65% of patients with hepatobiliary cancer have elevated levels.

CA 19-9 levels are used in the posttreatment surveillance of those who have had pancreatic or hepatobiliary cancers. In the few patients with pancreatic or biliary cancer who have a good response to surgery, chemotherapy, or radiation therapy, a decline in serum levels of CA 19-9 will confirm this response. A rapid rise in CA 19-9 levels may be associated with a recurrent or progressive tumor growth. Mildly elevated levels may exist in patients with gastric cancer, colorectal cancer, and even in 6% to 7% of patients with nongastrointestinal malignancies. Patients who have pancreatitis, gallstones, cirrhosis, and cystic fibrosis can also have minimally elevated levels of CA 19-9.

Procedure and patient care

Before

- Explain the procedure to the patient.
- Tell the patient that no fasting is required.

During

- Collect 7 to 10 ml of blood in a red-top tube.
- Have the blood sent to a central diagnostic laboratory for

CA 19-9 determinations. The results are available to the local hospital in 7 to 10 days.

After

- Apply pressure or a pressure dressing to the venipuncture site.
- Observe the venipuncture site for bleeding.

Abnormal findings
Increased levels

Pancreatic carcinoma
Hepatobiliary carcinoma
Pancreatitis
Cholecystitis
Cirrhosis

Gastric cancer
Colorectal cancer
Gallstones
Cystic fibrosis

Notes

calcium, blood (Total/ionized calcium, Ca⁺⁺, Serum calcium)

Type of test Blood

Normal findings

Adult (total): 9.0-10.5 mg/dl or 2.25-2.75 mmol/L (SI units)

(ionized): 4.5-5.6 mg/dl or 1.05-1.30 mmol/L (SI units)

Elderly: values slightly decreased

Child (total): 8.8-10.8 mg/dl or 2.2-2.7 mmol/L (SI units)

Newborn (total): 9.0-10.6 mg/dl or 2.3-2.65 mmol/L (SI units)

Umbilical cord (total): 9.0-11.5 mg/dl or 2.25-2.88 mmol/L (SI units)

Possible critical values

<6 mg/dl (may lead to tetany)

>14 mg/dl (may lead to coma)

Test explanation and related physiology

The serum calcium test is used to evaluate parathyroid function and calcium metabolism by directly measuring the total amount of calcium in the blood. When the serum calcium level is elevated on at least three separate determinations, the patient is said to have hypercalcemia. Total calcium exists in the blood in its free (ionized) form and in its protein-bound form (with albumin). The serum calcium level is a measure of both. As a result, when the serum albumin level is low, the serum calcium level will also be low, and vice versa. As a rule of thumb, the total serum calcium level decreases by approximately 0.8 mg for every 1 g decrease in the serum albumin level.

The ionized form of calcium can also be measured. An advantage of measuring the ionized form is that it is unaffected by changes in serum albumin levels. Some physicians consider measurement of ionized calcium as more sensitive and reliable than that of total calcium in the detection of primary hyperparathyroidism. However, other physicians do not agree with this. Also, many laboratories do not have the equipment to perform the ionized calcium assay.

Interfering factors

- Vitamin D intoxication may cause increased serum calcium levels.
- Excessive ingestion of milk may cause increased levels.
- Drugs that may cause increased levels include calcium salts, hydralazine, lithium, thiazide diuretics, parathyroid hormone (PTH), thyroid hormone, and vitamin D.
- Drugs that may cause decreased levels include acetazolamide, anticonvulsants, asparaginase, aspirin, calcitonin, cisplatin, corticosteroids, heparin, laxatives, loop diuretics, magnesium salts, and oral contraceptives.

Procedure and patient care

Before

- Explain the procedure to the patient.
- Tell the patient that no fasting is required. (However, the serum calcium may be part of a multichemical analysis in which fasting is required for the other studies.)

During

- Collect approximately 7 ml of venous blood in a red-top tube.
- List on the laboratory slip any medications that can affect test results.

After

- Apply pressure or a pressure dressing to the venipuncture site.
- Assess the venipuncture site for bleeding.

Abnormal findings

Increased levels (hypercalcemia)

Metastatic tumor to the bone
Hyperparathyroidism
Vitamin D intoxication
Sarcoidosis
Milk-alkali syndrome
Addison's disease
Paget's disease of bone
Nonparathyroid PTH-producing tumors (e.g., lung and renal carcinomas)
Acromegaly

Decreased levels (hypocalcemia)

Hypoparathyroidism
Renal failure
Rickets
Osteomalacia

Hyperphosphatemia secondary to renal failure
Vitamin D deficiency
Malabsorption
Pancreatitis

Notes

calcium, urine (Urine calcium, Quantitative calcium)

Type of test Urine (24 hour)

Normal findings Vary with the diet

Normal diet: 100-300 mg/day or 2.50-7.50 mmol/day (SI units)

Low-calcium diet: 50-150 mg/day or 1.25-3.75 mmol/day (SI units)

Test explanation and related physiology

This quantitative test measures the amount of calcium excreted in the urine within 24 hours. (This test differs from the qualitative Sulkowitch's reagent test, which is rarely performed today.) Excretion of calcium in the urine is increased in most patients with primary hyperparathyroidism. Values are decreased in patients with hypoparathyroidism.

Disagreement exists as to whether the specimen should be collected with the patient who has a normal diet, a normal diet except for milk products, or a controlled diet limited to 100 to 200 mg of calcium. Therefore the reference values vary according to the type of diet.

Interfering factors

- Drugs that may increase urine calcium levels include antacids, anticonvulsants, carbonic anhydrase inhibitors, diuretics, and phosphates.
- Drugs that may cause decreased urine calcium levels include adrenocorticosteroids and oral contraceptives.

Procedure and patient care

Before

- Explain the procedure to the patient.
- Determine the diet regimen recommended by the specific laboratory.
- Give the patient written and oral instructions regarding dietary restrictions.

During

- Begin the 24-hour urine collection after the patient urinates. This is the start time of the collection.
- Discard the first sample.

- Collect all urine passed by the patient during the next 24 hours.
- Post the hours for urine collection in a prominent location.
- Remind the patient to void before defecating so that the urine is not contaminated by feces.
- Instruct the patient not to place toilet paper in the collection container.
- Encourage the patient to drink fluids during the 24 hours unless this is contraindicated for medical purposes.
- Collect the last specimen as close as possible to the end of the 24 hours.
- Indicate the time the last specimen was collected on the laboratory slip or urine container.
- Store the 24-hour collection in a plastic urine container or in an acid-washed glass bottle. Refrigerate or keep on ice.
- Note that some laboratories add a preservative to the container to prevent precipitation. Check with the laboratory.
- List on the laboratory slip any medications that can affect test results.

After

- Send the specimen to the laboratory as soon as it is completed.

Abnormal findings

Increased levels (hypercalciuria)

Primary hyperparathyroidism
Idiopathic hypercalciuria
Cushing's syndrome
Milk-alkali syndrome
Osteoporosis
Osteolytic bone disease
Renal tubular acidosis
Sarcoidosis
Vitamin D intoxication

Decreased values (hypocalciuria)

Hypoparathyroidism
Vitamin D deficiency
Malabsorption disorders
Renal osteodystrophy

Notes

caloric study (Oculovestibular reflex study)

Type of test Electrodiagnostic

Normal findings Nystagmus with irrigation

Test explanation and related physiology

Caloric studies are used to evaluate the vestibular portion of the eighth cranial nerve (CN VIII) by irrigating the external auditory canal with hot or cold water. Normally, stimulation with cold water causes rotary nystagmus (involuntary rapid eye movement) away from the ear being irrigated; hot water induces nystagmus toward the side of the ear being irrigated. If the labyrinth is diseased or CN VIII is not functioning (e.g., from tumor compression), no nystagmus is induced. This study aids in the differential diagnosis of abnormalities that may occur in the vestibular system, brainstem, or cerebellum. When results are inconclusive, electronystagmography (see p. 298) may be performed.

Contraindications

- Patients with a perforated eardrum
  However, cold air may be substituted for the fluid.
- Patients with an acute disease of the labyrinth (e.g., Ménière's syndrome)
  The test can be performed when the acute attack subsides.

Interfering factors

- Drugs such as sedatives and antivertigo agents can alter test results.

Procedure and patient care

Before

- Explain the procedure to the patient.
- Hold solid foods before the test to reduce the incidence of vomiting.

During

- Although the exact procedures for caloric studies vary, note the following steps in a typical test:

  1. Before the test the patient is examined for the presence of nystagmus, postural deviation (Romberg's sign), and past-pointing. This examination provides the baseline values for comparison during the test.
  2. The ear on the suspected side is irrigated first, since the patient's response may be minimal.
  3. After an emesis basin is placed under the ear, the irrigation solution is directed into the external auditory canal until the patient complains of nausea and dizziness or until nystagmus is seen. Usually this occurs in 20 to 30 seconds.
  4. If after 3 minutes no symptoms occur, the irrigation is stopped.
  5. The patient is tested again for nystagmus, past-pointing, and Romberg's sign.
  6. After approximately 5 minutes the procedure is repeated on the other side.

- Note that this procedure is usually performed by a physician in approximately 15 minutes.
- Tell the patient that he or she will probably experience nausea and dizziness during the test.

After

- Usually, place the patient on bed rest for approximately 30 to 60 minutes until nausea or vomiting subsides.
- Ensure patient safety related to dizziness.

Abnormal findings

Brainstem inflammation, infarction, or tumor
Cerebellar inflammation, infarction, or tumor
Vestibular or cochlear inflammation or tumor
Acoustic neuroma

Notes

carbon dioxide content (CO_2 content, CO_2
combining power)

Type of test Blood

Normal findings
Adult/elderly: 23-30 mEq/L or 23-30 mmol/L (SI units)
Child: 20-28 mEq/L
Infant: 20-28 mEq/L
Newborn: 13-22 mEq/L

Possible critical values ≤6 mEq/L

Test explanation and related physiology
   The serum CO_2 test is usually included with other assessments of electrolytes. This test is a measure of the bicarbonate ion (HCO_3^-) that exists in the serum. This anion is of secondary importance in electrical neutrality of extracellular and intracellular fluid; its major role is in acid-base balance. Levels of HCO_3^- are regulated by the kidneys. Increases occur with alkalosis; decreases occur with acidosis.

Interfering factors
- Drugs that may cause increased serum CO_2 and HCO_3^- levels include aldosterone, barbiturates, bicarbonates, ethacrynic acid, hydrocortisone, loop diuretics, mercurial diuretics, and steroids.
- Drugs that may cause decreased levels include methicillin, nitrofurantoin (Furadantin), paraldehyde, phenformin hydrochloride, tetracycline, thiazide diuretics, and triamterene.

Procedure and patient care
Before
- Explain the procedure to the patient.
- Tell the patient that no fasting is required.

During
- Collect approximately 7 to 10 ml of venous blood in a red-top or green-top tube.

After

- Apply pressure or a pressure dressing to the venipuncture site.
- Assess the venipuncture site for bleeding.

Abnormal findings

Increased levels

Severe vomiting
Aldosteronism
Emphysema
Metabolic alkalosis
Gastric suction
Renal failure
Salicylate toxicity
Diabetic ketoacidosis
Metabolic acidosis
Shock

Decreased levels

Severe diarrhea
Starvation

Notes

carboxyhemoglobin (COHb, Carbon monoxide)

Type of test Blood

Normal findings

Nonsmoker: less than 3%
Smoker: up to 12%
Newborn: up to 12%

Possible critical values >20%

20%-30%: dizziness, headache, disturbances in judgment
30%-40%: tachycardia, hyperpnea, hypotension, confusion
50%-60%: coma
Greater than 60%: death

Test explanation and related physiology

This test measures the amount of serum carboxyhemoglobin (COHb), which is formed by the combination of carbon monoxide (CO) and hemoglobin (Hb). CO combines with Hb 200 times more readily than oxygen (O_2) can combine with Hb (oxyhemoglobin). This greater affinity of CO for Hb results in less Hb bonds available to combine with O_2 and causes the patient to become hypoxic. CO poisoning is detecting by Hb analysis for COHb. A specimen should be drawn as soon as possible after exposure, since CO is rapidly cleared from the Hb by breathing normal air. This test may also be indicated to evaluate patients with complaints of headache, irritability, nausea, vomiting, vertigo, collapse, and coma. Patients exposed to smoke inhalation, exhaust fumes, and fires may also be evaluated by this study.

Principal sources of CO include tobacco smoke, petroleum and natural gas fuels, automobile exhaust, unvented natural gas heaters, and defective gas stoves. Continuous exposure to CO can lead to coma and death. The treatment of CO toxicity is administration of high concentrations of O_2.

Procedure and patient care

Before

- Explain the procedure to the patient or the family.
- Obtain the patient history related to any possible source of CO inhalation.

- Assess the patient for signs and symptoms of mild CO toxicity (e.g., headache, weakness, dizziness, malaise, dyspnea) and moderate to severe CO toxicity (e.g., severe headache, bright-red mucous membranes, cherry-red blood). Maintain patient safety precautions if confusion is present.

During

- Collect approximately 5 to 10 ml of venous blood in a lavender-top or green-top tube.

After

- Apply pressure or a pressure dressing to the venipuncture site.
- Assess the venipuncture site for bleeding.
- Treat the patient as indicated by the physician. Usually the patient receives high concentrations of O_2.
- Encourage respirations to allow the patient to clear CO from the Hb.

Abnormal finding

Carbon monoxide poisoning

Notes

C

carcinoembryonic antigen (CEA)

Type of test Blood

Normal findings <5 ng/ml or 0-2.5 μg/L (SI units)

Test explanation and related physiology

CEA is a protein that normally occurs in fetal gut tissue. By birth, detectable serum levels disappear. In the early 1960s CEA was found to exist in the bloodstream of adults who had colorectal tumors. Therefore the antigen was thought to be a specific indicator of the presence of colorectal cancer. Subsequently, however, this protein has been found in patients who have a variety of carcinomas (e.g., breast, pancreatic, gastric, hepatobiliary), sarcomas, and even many benign diseases (e.g., ulcerative colitis, diverticulitis, cirrhosis). Chronic smokers also have elevated levels of CEA.

Because the CEA level can be elevated in both benign and malignant diseases, it is not considered a specific test for colorectal cancer. As a result, CEA is not a reliable screening test for the detection of colorectal cancer. Its use is limited to determining the prognosis and monitoring the patient response to antineoplastic therapy. This is especially helpful in patients with breast and gastrointestinal cancers. The degree of increase in the CEA level on the initial test is an indicator of tumor burden and prognosis. A drastic reduction to normal CEA levels is expected with complete eradication of tumor. Therefore this test is used to determine the adequacy of treatment.

This test also is used in the surveillance of cancer patients. A steadily rising CEA level is occasionally the first sign of tumor recurrence. This fact makes CEA testing very valuable in the follow-up of patients who have had potentially curative therapy.

It is important to note that many patients who have advanced breast or gastrointestinal tumors may not have elevated CEA levels.

Interfering factors

- Smoking
- Benign diseases (e.g., cholecystitis, colitis, diverticulitis)
- Liver diseases (e.g., hepatitis, cirrhosis)

Procedure and patient care

Before

- Explain the procedure to the patient.
- Tell the patient that no fasting is required.

During

- Collect a peripheral blood specimen. The collecting tube varies according to the commercial laboratory. (The two most frequently used laboratories for this test are Abbott Laboratories and Roche Labs.)
- Indicate on the laboratory slip if the patient smokes or has diseases that can affect test results.

After

- Apply pressure or a pressure dressing to the venipuncture site.
- Observe the venipuncture site for bleeding.

Abnormal findings

Cancer (gastrointestinal, breast, lung)
Inflammation (colitis, cholecystitis, pancreatitis)

Cirrhosis
Peptic ulcer

Notes

cardiac catheterization (Coronary angiography, Angiocardiography, Ventriculography)

Type of test X-ray with contrast dye

Normal findings Normal heart muscle motion, normal coronary arteries, normal great vessels, and normal intracardiac pressures and volumes

Test explanation and related physiology

Cardiac catheterization is a procedure that allows the heart, great blood vessels, and coronary arteries to be studied. During the study a catheter is passed into the heart through a peripheral vein or artery, depending on whether catheterization of the right or left side of the heart is being performed. Through the catheter, pressures are recorded and radiographic dyes are injected. With the assistance of a computer, cardiac output and other measures of cardiac functions can be determined. Cardiac catheterization is indicated for the following reasons:

1. To identify, locate, and quantitate the severity of atherosclerotic occlusive coronary artery disease
2. To evaluate the severity of acquired and congenital cardiac valvular or septal defects
3. To determine the presence and the degree of congenital cardiac abnormalities, such as transposition of great vessels, patent ductus arteriosus, and anomalous venous return to the heart
4. To evaluate the success of previous cardiac surgery or balloon angioplasty
5. To evaluate cardiac muscle function
6. To identify and quantify ventricular aneurysms
7. To identify and locate acquired disease of the great vessels, such as atherosclerotic occlusion or aneurysms within the aortic arch
8. To evaluate patients with acute myocardial infarction and to facilitate infusion of streptokinase into the occluded coronary arteries
9. To insert a catheter to monitor right-sided heart pressures, such as pulmonary artery and pulmonary wedge pressures (See Table 4 for pressures and volumes used in cardiac monitoring.)

TABLE 4 Pressures and volumes used in cardiac monitoring

	Description	Normal values
Pressures		
Routine blood pressure	Routine brachial artery pressure	90-140/60-90 mm Hg
Systolic left ventricular pressure	Peak pressure in the left ventricle during systole	90-140 mm Hg
End diastolic left ventricular pressure	Pressure in the left ventricle at the end of diastole	4-12 mm Hg
Central venous pressure (CVP)	Pressure in the superior vena cava	2-14 cm H_2O
Pulmonary wedge pressure	Pressure in the pulmonary venules, an indirect measurement of left atrial pressure and left ventricular end diastolic pressure	Left atrial: 6-15 mm Hg
Pulmonary artery pressure	Pressure in the pulmonary artery	15-28/5-16 mm Hg
Aortic artery pressure	Same as routine blood pressure	

Volumes

End diastolic volume (EDV)	Amount of blood present in the left ventricle at the end of diastole	50-90 ml/m^2
End systolic volume (ESV)	Amount of blood present in the left ventricle at the end of systole	25 ml/m^2
Stroke volume (SV)	Amount of blood ejected from the heart in one contraction (SV = EDV − ESV)	45±12 ml/m^2
Ejection fraction (EF)	Proportion (fraction) of EDV ejected from the left ventricle during systole (EF = SV/EDV)	0.67 ± 0.07
Cardiac output (CO)	Amount of blood ejected by the heart in 1 minute	3-6 L/min
Cardiac index (CI)	Amount of blood ejected by the heart in 1 minute per square meter of body surface (CI = CO/Body surface area)	2.8-4.2 L/min/m^2 for a patient with 1.5 m^2 of body surface

Cardiac catheterizations are performed under sterile conditions. In right-sided heart catheterization, usually the subclavian vein or femoral vein is used for vascular access. In left-sided heart catheterization, usually the right femoral artery is cannulated. Alternatively, however, the brachial vein or brachial artery may be chosen. As the catheter is placed into the great vessels in the heart chamber, pressures are monitored and recorded. Blood samples for analysis of oxygen content are also obtained. The catheter is advanced with appropriate guidance into the desired position. After pressures are obtained, angiographic visualization of the heart chambers, valves, and coronary arteries is performed with the injection of radiographic dye.

Transluminal coronary angioplasty is a therapeutic procedure that can be performed during coronary angiography in medical centers where open heart surgery is available. During this procedure a specific, specially designed balloon catheter is introduced into the coronary arteries and placed across the stenotic area of the coronary artery. This area can then be dilated by controlled inflation of the balloon. The coronary arteriogram is then repeated to document the effects of the forceful dilation of the stenotic area.

Contraindications

- Patients who are unable to cooperate during the test
- Patients who would refuse surgery if a surgically amenable lesion were found
- Patients with an iodine dye allergy who have not received preventive medication for allergy
- Patients who are pregnant because of radiation exposure to the fetus

Potential complications

- Cardiac arrhythmias (dysrhythmias)
- Perforation of the heart myocardium
- Catheter-induced embolic stroke (cerebrovascular accident) or myocardial infarction
- Complications associated with the catheter insertion site, such as arterial thrombosis, embolism, or pseudoaneurysm
- Allergic reactions to iodinated dye
  These vary from flushing, itching, and urticaria to severe, life-threatening anaphylaxis (evidenced by respiratory dis-

tress, drop in blood pressure, shock). In the event of anaphylaxis the patient is treated with diphenhydramine
(Benadryl), steroids, and epinephrine. Oxygen and endotracheal equipment should be on hand for immediate use.
- Infection at the catheter insertion site
- Pneumothorax following subclavian vein catheterization
  of the right side of the heart

Procedure and patient care

Before

- Explain the procedure to the patient.
- Obtain a written permission from the fully informed pa-
  tient.
- Allay the patient's fears and anxieties regarding this test.
  Although this test creates tremendous fear in a patient, it
  is performed often and complications are rare.
- Instruct the patient to abstain from oral intake for at least
  4 to 8 hours before the test.
- Prepare the catheter insertion site by shaving and scrub-
  bing it.
- Determine whether the patient has an iodine dye allergy.
  If so, Benadryl and steroids should be provided several
  days before the test if possible. Also, non-ionic iodine
  contrast dye should be used during the test.
- Mark the patient's peripheral pulses with a pen before
  catheterization. This will facilitate postcatheterization assessment of the pulses of the affected and nonaffected
  extremities.
- Provide appropriate precatheterization sedation as ordered by the physician.
- Instruct the patient to void before going to the catheterization laboratory.
- Remove all valuables and dental prostheses before trans-
  porting the patient to the catheterization laboratory.
- Obtain IV access for delivery of IV fluids and cardiac
  drugs, if necessary.

During

- Take the patient to the radiology department.
- Note the following procedural steps:

    1. The chosen catheter insertion site is prepared and
       draped in a sterile manner.
    2. The desired vessel is punctured with a needle.

3. A wire is placed through the needle and into the catheter.
4. The angiographic catheter is threaded on top of the wire.
5. Once the catheter is in the desired location, the appropriate cardiac pressures and volumes are obtained.
6. Cardiac ventriculography is performed with controlled injection of contrast.
7. Each coronary artery is catheterized. Cardiac angiography is then carried out with a controlled injection of contrast material.
8. During the injection, x-ray films are rapidly performed.
9. The patient's vital signs must be monitored constantly during this procedure.
10. If *angioplasty* is performed, the cardiologist appropriately places the catheter and balloon at the stenotic area.
    a. As the EKG tracing is observed, the balloon is inflated and the stenotic areas forcefully dilated.
    b. If signs of myocardial ischemia develop, the balloon is immediately deflated.
    c. Usually, inflation of the balloon is continued only for a few seconds.
11. After obtaining all the required information, the catheter is removed.

- Note that this test is usually performed by a cardiologist in approximately 1 hour.
- Tell the patient that during the injection, he or she may experience a severe hot flush. This is extremely uncomfortable but lasts only a few seconds.
- Note that some patients have a tendency to cough as the catheter is placed into the pulmonary artery.
- Verbally support the patient as the x-ray films are taken, since the possibly loud noises may frighten the patient.

After

- Monitor the patient's vital signs.
- Apply pressure to the site of vascular access.
- Keep the patient on bed rest for 6 to 8 hours to allow for complete sealing of the arterial puncture.
- Keep the affected extremity extended and immobilized with sandbags to decrease bleeding.

- Assess the puncture site for signs of bleeding, hematoma, or absence of pulse.
- Assess the patient's pulses of both extremities. Compare to preprocedural baseline values.
- Encourage the patient to drink fluids to maintain adequate hydration. Dehydration may be caused by the diuretic action of the dye.
- Evaluate the patient for delayed reaction to the dye (dyspnea, rashes, tachycardia, hives). This usually occurs within the first 2 to 6 hours after the test. Treat with antihistamines or steroids.
- Instruct the patient that the test will be reviewed by the cardiologist and the results will be available in 1 or 2 days.

Abnormal findings

Anatomic variation of the cardiac chambers and great vessels

Coronary artery occlusive disease

Ventricular aneurysm

Ventricular mural thrombi

Intracardiac tumors

Aortic root arteriosclerotic or aneurysmal disease

Anomalies in pulmonary venous return

Acquired or congenital septal defects and valvular anomalies

Pulmonary emboli

Pulmonary hypertension

Notes

cardiac nuclear scanning (Myocardial scan, Cardiac scan, Nuclear cardiac scanning, Heart scan, Thallium scan, Dipyridamole-thallium scan)

Type of test Nuclear scan

Normal findings Normal myocardial ejection fraction and coronary perfusion

Test explanation and related physiology

Cardiac radionuclear scanning is a noninvasive and safe method of recognizing alterations of left ventricular muscle function and coronary artery blood distribution. Many different radiocompound materials can be used, most often technetium-99m pertechnetate, thallium-201, or technetium-99m pyrophosphate. When these compounds are injected intravenously and a radiation detector is placed over the heart, an image of the heart can be recorded and photographed.

In evaluation of the patency of the coronary arteries, the characteristic abnormality varies according to the type of radiocompound used. When thalliam is used, all normal myocardial cells take up the substance and show up on the photoscan. Ischemic or infarcted cells do not take up the substance and appear as "cold spots" devoid of nuclear material and surrounded by normal cells. Technetium pyrophosphate, on the other hand, is taken up only by the ischemic or infarcted cells. Therefore an acute myocardial infarction will show up as a "hot spot" on this type of cardiac photoscan.

For an evaluation of myocardial function, technetium pertechnetate or technetium-labeled albumin is used to measure the portion of blood ejected from the ventricle. Normally, greater than 65% of the blood is ejected from the ventricle during systole. Values less than that indicate decreased contractility of the heart, caused by ischemia or infarction or by cardiomyopathy. Computers can be synchronized with the electrocardiogram (ECG) during scanning. This computer-assisted *gated* (synchronized) cardiac scan can allow the myocardial wall to be photographed while in motion. This allows visualization of the myocardium during several cardiac cycles. Contractility of the myocardium can be determined. Further, the amount of blood ejected during systole can also be calculated. This form of determination of ventricular function is called *gated pool imaging* or the *gated pool ejection fraction* (GPEF). These imaging techniques can provide the same information as does radiographic ventriculography, which is performed during cardiac catheterization (see p. 153). However, the nuclear scans are noninvasive and much safer.

Thallium can also be used to assess myocardial ischemia during stress testing. In some cases no evidence of diminished blood supply to the myocardium is evident during the resting state. When stressed, however, evidence of myocardial ischemia can become quite obvious and is easily detected by *thallium stress testing*. In this form of nuclear cardiac scanning, thallium 201 is injected intravenously during exercise stress testing. The thallium accumulates in the myocardium in direct proportion to the regional myocardial blood flow. The normal myocardium will have much greater thallium activity than the ischemic myocardium. Comparing this stress testing to a resting thallium scan, one can see exercise-induced ischemia. This is called *exercise stress testing with thallium scanning*, or *thallium stress testing*. This test is not only beneficial in detecting coronary occlusive disease, but is also successful in assessing postoperative patency of a coronary bypass graft.

When exercise testing is not advisable, or the patient is unable to exercise to a level adequate to stress the heart, *dipyridamole-thallium scanning* can be substituted for thallium stress testing. Dipyridamole (Persantine) is a coronary vasodilator that simulates the exercise portion of nuclear stress testing. If one coronary artery is significantly occluded, a discrepancy in the coronary blood flow exists and can be visualized on the thallium gamma-detector scanning camera. This discrepancy is accentuated because the dipyridamole-induced vascular dilation steals the blood from the ischemic areas and diverts it to the open, dilated coronary vessels. However, caution must be taken because this can precipitate angina or myocardial infarction. This test should be performed only with a cardiologist in attendance. IV aminophylline can reverse the effect of dipyridamole. This scanning technique is usually performed on patients who have an orthopedic, arthritic, neurologic, or pulmonary limitation that precludes thallium stress testing.

Recently, *single-photon emission computed tomography* (SPECT) has been used to visualize the heart from several different angles. These images are then reconstructed using tomographic techniques, and three-dimensional images of the physiologic cardiac processes are obtained. Areas of myocardial ischemia can be seen with far greater resolution and accurately quantified.

Specific indications for cardiac nuclear scanning include:

1. Screening of adults for past and recent infarction
2. Evaluation of patients with chest pain and uninterpretable or equivocal ECG changes caused by drugs, bundle branch block, or left ventricular hypertrophy
3. Evaluation of myocardial perfusion before and after coronary artery bypass surgery
4. Quantification and surveillance of myocardial infarction
5. Evaluation of medical and surgical therapy for coronary artery perfusion
6. Evaluation of ventricular function in patients with myocardial disease
7. Evaluation of patients receiving cardiotoxic drugs (e.g., adriamycin chemotherapy)

Contraindications

- Patients who are uncooperative
- Patients who are pregnant because of fetal exposure to radionuclide material

Interfering factors

- Myocardial trauma
- Drugs, such as long-acting nitrates
- Recent nuclear scans (e.g., thyroid or bone scan)

Procedure and patient care
Before

- Explain the procedure to the patient.
- Instruct the patient that a short fasting period may be required.

During

- Take the patient to the nuclear medicine department.
- Note the following procedural steps:

1. An IV injection of radionuclide material is performed.
2. Depending on the radionuclide used, scanning is performed 15 minutes to 4 hours later.
3. A gamma ray detector is placed over the precordium.
4. The patient is placed in a supine position, the lateral position, and then both right and left oblique positions.
5. The gamma ray scanner records the image of the heart, and a photograph is immediately developed.
6. If exercise is required, the patient does this during the injection.

- Tell the patient that the only discomfort associated with this test is the venipuncture required for injection of the radioisotope.
- Note that myocardial scans are usually performed in less than 30 minutes by a nuclear medicine technician.

After

- Because only tracer doses of radioisotopes are used, note that no precautions need to be taken against radioactive exposure to personnel or family.
- Encourage the patient to drink fluids to aid in the excretion of the radioactive substance.
- Apply pressure or a pressure dressing to the venipuncture site.
- Assess the venipuncture site for bleeding.
- If stress testing was performed, evaluate the patient's vital signs at frequent intervals (as indicated).

Abnormal findings

Coronary artery occlusive disease
Decreased myocardial function associated with ischemia, myocarditis, cardiomyopathy, or congestive heart failure

Notes

carotid duplex scanning

Type of test Ultrasound

Normal findings Cartoid artery free of plaques and stenosis

Test explanation and related physiology

Carotid duplex scanning is a noninvasive ultrasonic test used on the extracranial carotid artery to detect occlusive disease directly. The duplex concept is based on the ability to define the carotid artery walls within a two-dimensional image and uses a pulse Doppler probe to evaluate flow velocities within the artery. With this technique, one can measure the amplitude and the wave form of the carotid arterial pulse. Further, a two-dimensional image of the carotid artery can be produced. As a result, one can directly visualize possibly stenotic or occluded arteries and the arterial flow disruption.

Procedure and patient care

Before

- Explain the procedure to the patient.
- Tell the patient that no special preparation is required.
- Assure the patient that the study is painless.

During

- Place the patient in the supine position with the head supported to prevent lateral motion.
- Note the following procedural steps:

  1. A water-soluble gel is used to couple the sound from the transducer to the skin surface.
  2. Images of the carotid artery and pulse wave form are obtained.

- Note that this test is performed by an ultrasound technologist in the ultrasound or radiology department in approximately 15 to 30 minutes.
- Tell the patient that no discomfort is associated with this test.

After

- Remove the water-soluble gel from the patient.

Abnormal finding

Carotid artery occlusive disease

Notes

cerebral angiography (Cerebral arteriography)

Type of test X-ray with contrast dye

Normal findings Normal cerebral vasculature

Test explanation and related physiology

Cerebral angiography provides radiographic visualization of the cerebral vascular system after the intraarterial injection of radiopaque dye into the carotid or vertebral arteries. This procedure is used for the detection of abnormalities of the cerebral circulation, such as aneurysms, occlusion, or arteriovenous (AV) malformations. A vascular tumor is seen as a mass containing multiple, small AV fistulas. A nonvascular tumor, abscess, or hematoma appears as an avascular mass, distorting the normal vascular location.

Contraindications

- Patients with allergies to shellfish or iodinated dye
- Patients with atherosclerosis
- Patients who are pregnant
- Patients with bleeding disorders

Potential complications

- Allergic reactions to iodinated dye
  These may vary from mild flushing, itching, and urticaria to severe, life-threatening anaphylaxis (evidenced by respiratory distress, drop in blood pressure, shock). In the unusual event of anaphylaxis the patient is treated with diphenhydramine (Benadryl), steroids, and epinephrine. Oxygen and endotracheal equipment should be on hand for immediate use.
- Hemorrhage from the puncture site used for arterial access
- Embolism because of dislodgement of an atherosclerotic plaque
- Infection at the catheter insertion site

Procedure and patient care

Before

- Explain the procedure to the patient.
- Ensure that written and informed consent for this procedure is in the patient's chart.

- Inform the patient that a warm flush may be felt when the dye is injected. Allay any fears and allow the patient to verbalize concerns.
- Assess the patient for allergies to iodine dye. Inform the radiologist if an allergy to iodinated contrast is suspected. The radiologist may prescribe a Benadryl and steroid preparation to be administered before the testing. Usually, hypoallergenic non-ionic contrast will be used during the test.
- Determine if the patient has been taking anticoagulants because of the potential complication of hemorrhage.
- Keep the patient from eating solid foods after midnight on the day of the test.
- Mark the patient's peripheral pulses with a pen before catheterization. This will facilitate assessment of pulses after the procedure.
- Perform a baseline neurologic assessment (eyes, speech, motor, strength).
- Administer the preprocedural medications as ordered.
- Remove all valuables and dental prostheses.

During

- Note the following procedural steps:
  1. The patient is usually sedated with atropine and meperidine (Demerol) before being taken to the angiography room in the radiology department.
  2. The patient is placed on an x-ray table in the supine position.
  3. Since access to the cerebral arteries is usually achieved through the femoral artery, the groin is prepared, shaved, and draped in a sterile manner.
  4. A catheter is followed under fluoroscopy as it passes into the desired artery.
  5. Radiopaque contrast material is injected, and the flow of blood through the cranial cavity is seen.
  6. Serial x-ray films are taken in timed sequence to show the arterial and venous phases of the cerebral circulation.
  7. After the x-ray films are completed, the catheter is removed and a pressure dressing is applied to the puncture site.
- Note that this procedure is usually performed by an angiographer (radiologist) in approximately 1 hour.

- During the dye injection, remind the patient that an intense burning flush may be felt throughout the body but lasts only a few seconds.
- Tell the patient that the only other discomfort is the groin puncture necessary for arterial access.

After

- Observe the arterial puncture site for hematoma, hemorrhage, or absence of pulse.
- Keep the affected extremity extended and immobilized with sandbags to decrease bleeding.
- Maintain a pressure dressing for the prescribed period.
- Assess the extremities for signs of ischemia (numbness, tingling, pain, absence of peripheral pulses, loss of function).
- Compare the pulses with the preprocedural baseline values.
- Compare the color and temperature of the involved and uninvolved extremities.
- Assess the pulse and vital signs frequently because embolism, bleeding, or adverse reactions may require immediate intervention.
- Keep the patient on bed rest for 12 to 24 hours to allow for complete sealing of the arterial puncture.
- Apply cold compresses to the puncture site if needed to reduce discomfort or swelling.
- Have the patient drink fluids to promote dye excretion by the kidneys and to prevent diuretic-induced dehydration.

Abnormal findings

Aneurysm   Abscess
Occlusion   Hematoma
AV malformation   Cerebral fistula
Tumor   Cerebral thrombosis

Notes

cervical mucus test (Fern test)

Type of test Fluid analysis

Normal findings Arborization, or ferning, of cervical mucus during midcycle

Test explanation and related physiology

The cervical mucus can be examined near midcycle and just before menstruation to detect ovulation. Because pregnancy is impossible without ovulation, this study is used in the evaluation of infertility to predict the day of ovulation and to determine whether or not ovulation occurs.

At ovulation the cervical mucus is clear, abundant, watery, and elastic. This elasticity, or *spinnbarkheit* (Figure 3), increases at ovulation. Excellent spinnbarkheit occurs when the mucus can be stretched at least 5 to 6 cm.

When the cervical mucus is spread on a clean glass slide and allowed to dry, a pattern of "arborization" or "ferning" occurs. This is caused by the increased levels of salt and water interacting with the glycoproteins in the mucus during ovulation. This pattern is correlated with estrogen activity and is therefore present in all ovulatory women at midcycle. When the cervical mucus is checked again immediately before menstruation, no ferning is found because of progesterone activity. Therefore, during a normal ovulatory cycle, the ferning of cervical mucus will occur at midcycle and no ferning will occur before menstruation.

Besides its absence in anovulatory premenopausal patients, ferning of the cervical mucus is also absent in postmenopausal, castrated, or normally pregnant women (because of the presence of fern-inhibiting progesterone).

Interfering factors

- Slides cleaned with tap water may produce false ferning. The slides used for the mucus must be washed in distilled water.
- Cervical trauma during this procedure may cause blood to mix with the mucus and inhibit ferning.

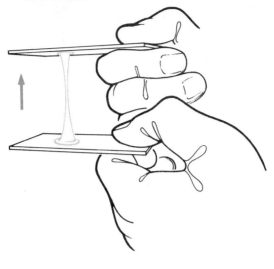

Figure 3 Spinnbarkheit (elasticity) of the cervical mucus increases at ovulation.

Procedure and patient care

Before

- Explain the procedure to the patient.
- Tell the patient that no fasting or sedation is required.

During

- Note that this procedure is performed at midcycle to detect estrogen-induced ferning and repeated approximately 7 days later to detect the progesterone inhibition of ferning.
- Note the following procedural steps:
  1. The patient is placed in the lithotomy position.
  2. A nonlubricated speculum is inserted into the vagina to expose the cervix.
  3. A cotton-tipped applicator is gently inserted into the cervical canal and rotated.

4. The mucus that adheres to the cotton swab is spread on the clean glass slide and allowed to dry at room temperature. No staining is used.
5. The dried spread of mucus is examined under the low-power lens of a microscope for the presence of ferning.

- Note that this procedure is performed by a physician in approximately 15 minutes.
- Tell the patient that the only discomfort associated with this study is the insertion of the speculum.

After

- Inform the patient that she is usually given the results immediately after the test.

Abnormal findings

Infertility
Pregnancy

Notes

chest tomography (Tomogram, Tomography of the lung)

Type of test X-ray

Normal findings Normal lungs and surrounding structures

Test explanation and related physiology

Tomography is a radiographic examination by which a sequence of x-ray films, each representing a "slice" of the lung at different depths, is taken. Usually the slices are made at 0.5 to 1.0 cm apart throughout the organ being studied. Tomography permits examination of a single layer or plane of tissue that would otherwise be obscured by the surrounding tissue on an ordinary film.

For tomography the x-ray tube and the film cassette are rapidly moved in opposite directions while the x-ray film is taken. This technique effectively blurs all the tissue planes except that plane, or slice, being studied.

Tomography is often a helpful adjunct to a routine chest x-ray examination for several reasons:

1. It may reveal properties of a lung lesion (e.g., cavitation, tumor margins) that are normally not seen on chest x-ray films.
2. It provides better visualization of many structures (e.g., the hilus, trachea, mediastinum) that are not clearly seen on a routine chest x-ray film.
3. It may demonstrate many small lesions (e.g., in metastasis) that are not normally seen on a routine chest x-ray film.

Indications for chest tomography have greatly decreased since the advent of computed tomography (CT) of the chest (see p. 223).

Contraindications

- Patients who are pregnant

Interfering factors

- Conditions (e.g., severe pain) that prevent the patient from taking and holding a deep breath

Procedure and patient care

Before

- Explain the procedure to the patient.
- Tell the patient that no fasting is required.
- Instruct the patient to put on an x-ray gown.
- Inform the patient to remove all metal objects (e.g., necklaces, pins) so they do not block visualization of part of the chest.
- Tell the patient that he or she will be asked to take a deep breath and hold it while x-ray films are being taken.
- Instruct men to ensure that their testicles are covered and women to have their ovaries covered with a lead shield to prevent radiation-induced abnormalities.

During

- Take the nonfasting patient to the radiology department as for a routine chest x-ray film.
- Note the following procedural steps:
  1. With the patient remaining completely still, an x-ray tube is rapidly moved back and forth while the film is rapidly moved in the opposite direction. Excursion of this movement regulates the plane of tissues photographed.
  2. Prone and supine positions may be required.
- Tell the patient that he or she will be unable to detect the fine, synchronized movements of x-ray tube and film.
- Note that a radiologist performs this test in approximately 15 minutes.
- Tell the patient that no discomfort is associated with chest tomography.

After

- Note that no special care is required following the test.

Abnormal findings

Lung tumors	Bronchiectasis
Tuberculosis	Bronchial occlusion
Lung abscess	Granulomas

Notes

chest x-ray (CXR, Chest radiography)

Type of test X-ray

Normal findings Normal lungs and surrounding structures

Test explanation and related physiology

The chest x-ray film is important in the complete evaluation of the pulmonary and cardiac systems. This procedure is often part of the general admission screening workup in adult patients. Much information can be provided by the chest x-ray film. One can identify or follow (by repeated chest x-ray films) the following:

1. Tumors of the lung (primary and metastatic), heart (myxoma), chest wall (soft tissue sarcomas), and bony thorax (osteogenic sarcoma)
2. Inflammation of the lung (pneumonia), pleura (pleuritis), and pericardium (pericarditis)
3. Fluid accumulation in the pleura (pleural effusion), pericardium (pericardial effusion), and lung (pulmonary edema)
4. Air accumulation in the lung (chronic obstructive pulmonary disease) and pleura (pneumothorax)
5. Fractures of the bones of the thorax
6. Diaphragmatic hernia

Most chest x-ray films are taken at a distance of 6 feet, with the patient standing. The sitting or supine position can also be used, but x-ray films taken with the patient in the supine position will not demonstrate fluid levels. A *posteroanterior* (PA) view, with the x-rays passing through the back of the body (posterior) to the front of the body (anterior), is taken first. Then a *lateral* view, with the x-rays passing through the patient's side, is taken.

Oblique views may be taken with the x-rays slanted at different angles as they pass through the body. *Lordotic* views provide visualization of the apices (rounded upper portions) of the lungs and are usually used for detection of tuberculosis. *Decubitus* films are taken with the patient in the recumbent lateral position to localize fluid in the pleural space (pleural effusion).

Chest x-ray studies are best performed in the radiology department. Studies using a portable x-ray machine may be done at the bedside and are often performed on critically ill patients who cannot leave the nursing unit.

Contraindications

- Patients who are pregnant

Interfering factors

- Conditions (e.g., severe pain) that prevent the patient from taking and holding a deep breath

Procedure and patient care

Before

- Explain the procedure to the patient.
- Tell the patient that no fasting is required.
- Instruct the patient to remove clothing to the waist and put on an x-ray gown.
- Inform the patient to remove all metal objects (e.g., necklaces, pins) so they do not block visualization of part of the chest.
- Tell the patient that he or she will be asked to take a deep breath and hold it while the x-ray films are taken.
- Instruct men to ensure that their testicles are covered and women to have their ovaries covered with a lead shield to prevent radiation-induced abnormalities.

During

- After the patient is correctly positioned, tell him or her to take a deep breath and hold it until the x-ray films are taken.
- Note that x-ray films are taken by a radiologic technologist in several minutes.
- Inform the patient that no discomfort is associated with chest radiography.

After

- Note that no special care is required following the procedure.

Abnormal findings

Lung tumors
Myxoma

Soft tissue sarcomas
Osteogenic sarcoma

Pneumonia
Pleuritis
Pericarditis
Pleural effusion
Pericardial effusion
Pulmonary edema
Chronic obstructive pulmonary disease (COPD)

Pneumothorax
Fractures
Diaphragmatic hernia
Atelectasis
Tuberculosis
Lung abscess
Scoliosis

Notes

chlamydial smear

Type of test Microscopic examination

Normal findings Negative

Test explanation and related physiology

Chlamydia trachomatis is now isolated more frequently in clinics for sexually transmitted diseases than either gonorrhea or syphilis. This organism causes the eye disease *trachoma*, which is the most common form of preventable blindness.

It is estimated that the incidence of chlamydial infections in infants is 28 per 1000 live births. This rate far exceeds that of herpes simplex and toxoplasmosis. Prenatal screening and treatment of pregnant women are beginning to be considered in many areas. This screening technique could prevent trachoma, ophthalmia neonatorum, inclusion conjunctivitis, chlamydial pneumonia, and genital tract infections (e.g., nonspecific urethritis).

Interfering factors

▪ Women presently having their routine menses

Procedure and patient care

Before

▪ Explain the procedure to the patient.

During

▪ Note the following procedural steps for *cervical culture:*

1. The female patient should refrain from douching and tub bathing before the cervical culture is performed.
2. The patient is placed in the lithotomy position.
3. A nonlubricated vaginal speculum is inserted to expose the cervix.
4. Cervical mucus is removed.
5. A sterile cotton-tipped swab is inserted into the endocervical canal and moved from side to side to obtain the culture.

▪ Note the following procedural steps for *urethral culture:*

1. The urethral specimen should be obtained from the man before voiding.

2. A culture is taken by inserting a sterile swab gently into the urethra.

- Note that these tests are performed by a physician or nurse in several minutes.
- Tell the patient that minimal discomfort is associated with these procedures.

After

- Treat patients with positive smears with antibiotics.
- Tell affected patients to have their sexual partners examined.

Abnormal finding

Chlamydial infection

Notes

chloride, blood (Cl⁻)

Type of test Blood

Normal findings

Adult/elderly: 90-110 mEq/L or 98-106 mmol/L (SI units)
Child: 90-110 mEq/L
Newborn: 96-106 mEq/L
Premature infant: 95-110 mEq/L

Possible critical values <80 or >115 mEq/L

Test explanation and related physiology

Chloride is the major extracellular anion. Its main purpose is to maintain electrical neutrality, mostly as a salt with sodium. It follows sodium losses and accompanies sodium excesses, thus affecting water balance. Chloride also serves as a buffer to assist in acid-base balance. As carbon dioxide increases, bicarbonate moves from the intracellular space to the extracellular space. To maintain electrical neutrality, chloride will shift back into the cell.

Hypochloremia and hyperchloremia rarely occur alone and usually parallel shifts in sodium levels (see p. 676). Signs and symptoms of hypochloremia include hyperexcitability of the nervous system and muscles, shallow breathing, hypotension, and tetany. Signs and symptoms of hyperchloremia include lethary, weakness, and deep breathing.

Interfering factors

- Drugs that may cause increased serum chloride levels include acetazolamide, ammonium chloride, androgens, chlorothiazide, cortisone preparations, estrogens, guanethidine, hydrochlorothiazide, methyldopa, and nonsteroidal antiinflammatory drugs.
- Drugs that may cause decreased levels include aldosterone, bicarbonates, corticosteroids, cortisone, hydrocortisone, loop diuretics, thiazide diuretics, and triamterene.

Procedure and patient care

Before

- Explain the procedure to the patient.
- Tell the patient that no fasting is required.

During

- Collect 5 to 10 ml of venous blood in a red-top or green-top tube.

After

- Apply pressure or a pressure dressing to the venipuncture site.
- Assess the venipuncture site for bleeding.

Abnormal findings

Increased levels (hyper-chloremia)

Dehydration
Renal tubular acidosis
Excessive infusion of normal saline
Cushing's syndrome
Eclampsia
Multiple myeloma
Kidney dysfunction
Metabolic acidosis
Hyperventilation
Anemia

Decreased levels (hypo-chloremia)

Overhydration
Congestive heart failure
Syndrome of inappropriate secretion of antidiuretic hormone (SIADH)
Vomiting
Gastric suction
Chronic respiratory acidosis
Salt-losing nephritis
Addison's disease
Burns
Metabolic alkalosis
Diuretic therapy
Hypokalemia

Notes

chloride, urine (Cl⁻)

Type of test Urine (24 hours)

Normal findings
Adult/elderly: 110-250 mEq/day or 110-250 mmol/day (SI units)
Child: 15-40 mmol/day
Infant: 2-10 mmol/day

Test explanation and related physiology
Chloride is the major extracellular anion. Its main purpose is to maintain electrical neutrality, mostly as a salt with sodium. It follows sodium losses and accompanies sodium excesses, thus affecting water balance. Chloride also serves as a buffer to assist in acid-base balance. As carbon dioxide increases, bicarbonate moves from the intracellular space to the extracellular space. To maintain electrical neutrality, chloride will shift back into the cell.

A 24-hour urine collection for chloride is useful for evaluating the electrolyte composition of urine and for evaluating acid-base imbalances.

Interfering factors
- Urine volume and perspiration can affect chloride levels.
- Dietary salt intake affects levels.
- Drugs that may cause increased levels include bromides, diuretics, and steroids.

Procedure and patient care
Before
- Explain the procedure to the patient.
- Tell the patient that no special diet is required.

During
- Instruct the patient to begin the 24-hour urine collection after voiding.
- Discard the initial specimen and start the 24-hour timing at that point.
- Collect all the urine passed during the next 24 hours.
- Show the patient where to store the urine container.

- Keep the specimen on ice or refrigerated during the entire 24 hours.
- Indicate the starting time on the urine container and laboratory slip.
- Post the hours for the urine collection in a prominent location to prevent accidental discarding of the specimen.
- Instruct the patient to void before defecating so that the urine is not contaminated by feces.
- Remind the patient not to put toilet paper in the collection container.
- Encourage the patient to drink fluids during the 24 hours.
- Instruct the patient to collect the last specimen as close as possible to the end of the 24 hours.

After

- Transport the urine specimen promptly to the laboratory.

Abnormal findings

Increased levels

Dehydration
Starvation
Salicylate toxicity
Diuretic therapy

Decreased levels

Addison's disease
Malabsorption syndrome
Prolonged gastric suction
Diarrhea
Congestive heart failure
Emphysema
Pyloric obstruction
Diaphoresis

Notes

cholangiography (Intravenous cholangiogram [IVC])

Type of test X-ray with contrast dye

Normal findings

Patent hepatic and common bile ducts with no obstruction
   and no filling defects
Common bile ducts <1 cm in diameter

Test explanation and related physiology

IV cholangiography provides visualization of the hepatic
and common bile ducts. If the cystic duct is patent, occasionally the gallbladder will be visualized. The IVC is used
to demonstrate stricture or tumor affecting the bile duct.
Gallstones can also be detected.

This test is performed by administering radiographic dye
intravenously. This dye is concentrated in the liver and secreted into the bile. With use of plain and tomographic x-ray
films, the common bile duct can usually be visualized. Since
the introduction of endoscopic retrograde cholangiopancreatography (ERCP, see p. 305) and percutaneous transhepatic cholangiography (PTC, PTHC, see p. 551), the indications for this test have greatly diminished.

Contraindications

- Patients with an allergy to iodine dyes
- Patients whose bilirubin level exceeds 3.5 mg/dl

Potential complication

- Adverse reaction or allergy to dye
   Allergic reactions vary from flushing, itching, and urticaria to severe, life-threatening anaphylaxis (evidenced by
   respiratory distress, drop in blood pressure, shock). In
   the event of anaphylaxis the patient will be treated with
   diphenhydramine (Benadryl), steroids, and epinephrine.
   Oxygen and endotracheal equipment should be on hand
   for immediate use.

Interfering factor

- Barium within the abdomen as a result of a previous upper gastrointestinal or barium enema precludes visualization of the biliary tree.

Procedure and patient care

Before

- Explain the procedure to the patient.
- Ensure that an informed consent for this procedure is obtained.
- Provide cartharties if ordered. Usually, two bisacodyl (Dulcolax) tablets are given the day before testing.
- Keep the patient NPO after midnight the day of the test.
- Be sure the bilirubin level is less than 3.5 mg/dl so that x-ray visualization will be possible.
- Inform the radiologist if an allergy to iodinated contrast is suspected. The radiologist may prescribe a Benadryl and steroid preparation to be administered before testing.

During

- Note the following procedural steps:
  1. In the radiology department, while in the supine position, the patient is given an IV infusion of iodine dye (cholangiograph).
  2. X-ray films of the right upper quandrant of the abdomen are taken intermittently for up to 8 hours, thus allowing the gallbladder, hepatic, and common bile ducts to fill.
  3. Frequently, tomography is used to allow better visualization of the duct system. Tomography is a technique of radiographic examination by which a sequence of x-ray films, each representing a "slice" of the bile duct at different depths, is taken. Usually, slices are made 0.5 cm apart throughout the right upper quandrant. Tomography permits examination of a single layer or plane of tissue that would otherwise be obscured by the surrounding structures on a plain x-ray film.

After

- Evaluate the patient for delayed reactions to the dye (dyspnea, rashes, tachycardia, hives). Delayed reactions usually occur 2 to 6 hours after the test. Treat the patient with antihistamines or steroids.
- Explain to the patient that dye is eventually excreted in the urine. Some patients may report slight dysuria after the IVC.

Abnormal findings

Obstruction of the bile ducts from tumor, gallstones, or
  stricture
Nonobstructing gallstones

Notes

cholecystography (Oral cholecystogram, Gallbladder series, GB series)

Type of test X-ray with contrast dye

Normal findings
Good visualization of gallbladder
No filling defects
No stones

Test explanation and related physiology
The oral cholecystogram provides x-ray visualization of the gallbladder after the oral ingestion of a radiopaque, iodinated dye that comes in the form of pills. Adequate visualization of the gallbladder requires concentration of this dye within the gallbladder. The following factors are necessary for adequate dye concentration within the gallbladder:

1. Ingestion of all the dye tablets.
2. Adequate absorption of the dye from the gastrointestinal tract. Vomiting or diarrhea may preclude this absorption.
3. Abstinence from a meal on the morning of the test. A fatty meal eaten before x-ray films would induce gallbladder emptying of the concentrated dye. No visualization of the gallbladder would occur.
4. Excretion of the dye into the bile. This excretion is inhibited by inadequate hepatocellular function or when the bilirubin level is greater than 2 mg/dl.
5. Patency of the cystic duct. The dye is secreted by the liver through the hepatic duct and enters the gallbladder through the cystic duct. Obstruction of the cystic duct (as found in acute cholecystitis) will prevent the dye from entering the gallbladder.
6. Concentration of the dye within the gallbladder. The mucosa of a chronically inflamed gallbladder is unable to absorb the bile waters and concentrate the dye adequately for visualization.

On x-ray film the biliary calculi (gallstones) are visualized as radiolucent shadows within a dye-filled gallbladder. Gallbladder polyps and tumors occasionally can also be seen as filling defects.

Occasionally the gallbladder will not visualize after a single dose of dye tablets is ingested. The test should then be repeated using a double dose. Nonvisualization after a double dose is reliable evidence of chronic cholecystitis as long as none of the previously listed factors necessary for adequate dye concentration have not been violated.

The oral cholecystogram is less accurate than the gallbladder ultrasound. It is also more cumbersome to perform. It may take several days to obtain an accurate result. Fasting is required. Gallbladder ultrasonography, on the other hand, can be done on an emergency basis. Although fasting is preferred, it is not necessary for ultrasonography. When positive, the accuracy of gallbladder ultrasound is unparalleled.

Contraindications

- Patients who are allergic to iodine dye
  This is a relative contraindication. Most patients who are allergic to iodine dye react only when the dye is administered intravenously.
- Patients who are pregnant
- Patients whose bilirubin is greater than 2 mg/dl
  The dye will not visualize the gallbladder.
- Patients who have another inflammatory process within the abdomen
  The absorption of the orally ingested dye is not adequate for visualization.
- Patients who have diarrhea or vomiting
  They cannot absorb the dye.

Potential complications

- Adverse reaction or allergy to dye
  This rarely occurs because the dye is not administered intravenously.

Interfering factors

- Barium within the abdomen (usually as a result of an upper GI series or barium enema) will preclude visualization of the gallbladder.
- Vomiting or diarrhea will affect absorption of the radiopaque dye.

Procedure and patient care
Before
- Explain the procedure to the patient.
- Instruct the patient as to the importance of ingesting the appropriate dose of the radiopaque dye.
- Be sure that the serum bilirubin level is less than 1.8 mg/dl.
- Instruct the patient to ingest a low-fat or fat-free meal the evening before testing.
- Assess for iodine dye allergy before administering radiopaque dye. The dye tablets are usually taken 2 hours after the dinner meal. Usually six 0.5 g iopanoic acid tablets are administered. These are best taken one tablet at a time at 5-minute intervals.
- Inform the radiologist if vomiting or diarrhea occurs after ingestion of the radiopaque dye tablets.
- Instruct the patient to remain NPO except for water after taking the contrast tablets.

During
- Note the following procedural steps:
  1. In the radiology department, several plain x-ray films of the patient's right upper quadrant are taken.
  2. If the patient is to receive a fatty meal, a palatable liquid is ingested.
  3. Repeat x-ray films of the right upper quadrant are performed.

- Note that the x-rays take only a few minutes to perform. They are interpreted by a radiologist, and the results are available later that day.
- Tell the patient that no discomfort is associated with the test.

After
- If the gallbladder does not visualize, note that the patient may be instructed to repeat the procedure with a double dose of radiopaque dye tablets.
- Inform the patient that the radiopaque dye is eventually excreted in the urine. Some patients may report slight dysuria following cholecystography.

Abnormal findings

Gallstones
Gallbladder polyps
Chronic cholecystitis

Cholesterolosis
Gallbladder cancer
Cystic duct obstruction

Notes

cholesterol

Type of test Blood

Normal findings Vary with age and testing center
Adult/elderly: 150-200 mg/dl or 3.90-6.50 mmol/L (SI units)
Child: 120-200 mg/dl
Infant: 70-175 mg/dl
Newborn: 53-135 mg/dl

Test explanation and related physiology

Cholesterol is the main lipid associated with arteriosclerotic vascular disease. Cholesterol, however, is required for the production of steroids, bile acids, and cellular membranes. Most of the cholesterol we eat comes from foods of animal origin. The liver metabolizes the cholesterol to its free form. Cholesterol is transported in the bloodstream by lipoproteins. Nearly 75% of the cholesterol is bound to low-density lipoproteins (LDLs), and 25% is bound to high-density lipoproteins (HDLs). Because cholesterol is the main lipid involved in arteriosclerotic disease, high levels of free and bound LDLs are associated with increased risk for arteriosclerotic vascular disease.

Since the liver is required to metabolize ingested cholesterol products, subnormal cholesterol levels are indicative of severe liver diseases. Malnutrition also is associated with low cholesterol levels.

The purpose of cholesterol testing is to identify the patients at risk for arteriosclerotic heart disease. Cholesterol testing is usually done as a part of lipid profile testing, which also evaluates lipoproteins (see p. 464) and triglycerides (see p. 736).

Interfering factors

- Pregnancy is usually associated with elevated cholesterol levels.
- Oophorectomy increases levels.
- Drugs that may cause increased levels include adrencorticotropic hormone (ACTH), anabolic steroids, beta-adrenergic blocking agents, corticosteroids, epinephrine,

oral contraceptives, phenytoin (Dilantin), sulfonamides, thiazide diuretics, and vitamin D.

- Drugs that may cause decreased levels include allopurinol, androgens, bile salt–binding agents, captopril, chlorpropamide, clofibrate, colchicine, colestipol, erythromycin, isoniazid, liothyrinone (Cytomel), lovastatin (Mevacor), MAO inhibitors, neomycin (oral), niacin, and nitrates.

Procedure and patient care

Before

- Instruct the patient to fast 12 to 14 hours after eating a low-fat diet before testing. Only water is permitted.
- Indicate to the patient that dietary intake at least 2 weeks before testing will affect results.

During

- Collect 5 to 10 ml of blood in a red-top tube.
- Indicate on the laboratory slip any drugs that may affect cholesterol levels.

After

- Apply pressure or a pressure dressing to the venipuncture site.
- Assess the venipuncture site for bleeding.
- Instruct patients with high levels regarding a low-cholesterol diet, exercise, and appropriate body weight.

Abnormal findings

Increased levels	Decreased levels
Hypercholesterolemia	Malabsorption
Hyperlipidemias	Malnutrition
Hypothyroidism	Hyperthyroidism
Uncontrolled diabetes mellitus	Cholesterol-lowering medication
Nephrotic syndrome	Pernicious anemia
Pregnancy	Liver disease
High-cholesterol diet	Anemia
Xanthomatosis	Sepsis
Hypertension	Stress
Myocardial infarction	
Atherosclerosis	
Biliary cirrhosis	
Stress	
Nephrosis	

chorionic villus sampling (CVS, chorionic villus biopsy [CVB])

Type of test Cell analysis

Normal findings No genetic or biochemical disorders

Test explanation and related physiology

CVS is a relatively new procedure that can be performed between 8 and 12 weeks of gestation for the early detection of genetic and biochemical disorders. With the exception of diagnosing neural tube disorders, it is hoped that CVS will eventually replace amniocentesis for early prenatal diagnosis. Because CVS detects congenital defects early, first-trimester therapeutic abortions can be done if indicated and desired.

For this study, a sample of chorionic villi is obtained for analysis. The villi in the chorion frondosum are present from 8 to 12 weeks and are believed to reflect fetal chromosome, enzyme, and DNA content. This permits a much earlier diagnosis of prenatal problems than amniocentesis, which cannot be done before 14 to 16 weeks.

Potential complications

- Accidental abortion
- Infection
- Bleeding

Procedure and patient care

Before

- Explain the procedure to the patient.
- Be certain that the physician has obtained a signed consent for the procedure.
- Tell the patient that no food or fluid restrictions are necessary.

During

- Note the following procedural steps:
  1. The patient is placed in the lithotomy position.
  2. A cannula is inserted into the cervix and uterine cavity.
  3. Under ultrasonic guidance, the cannula is rotated to the site of the developing placenta.

4. A syringe is attached, and suction is applied to obtain several samples of villi.

- Note that this procedure is performed by an obstetrician in approximately 5 minutes.
- Inform the patient that discomfort associated with this test is similar to that of a Pap smear.

After

- Note that some Rh-negative mothers may receive RhoGAM. RhoGAM is given because of the risk of immunization from the fetal blood, which could jeopardize the fetus.
- Monitor the vital signs and check the mother for signs of bleeding.
- Schedule the mother for an ultrasound in 2 to 4 days to affirm the continued viability of the fetus.
- Assess the vaginal area for discharge and drainage. Note color and amount.
- Assess the patient for signs of spontaneous abortion (e.g., cramps, bleeding).
- Inform the patient how she can obtain the results from her physician. Make sure that she understands that the results are usually not available for several weeks. (Results may be available much sooner at major medical centers that perform this test.)

Abnormal findings

Genetic and biochemical disorders

Notes

cisternal puncture

Type of test Fluid analysis

Normal findings

Pressure: less than 200 cm H_2O
Color: clear and colorless
Blood: none
Cells: no red blood cells; less than 5 lymphocytes/mm^3
Culture and sensitivity: no organisms present
Protein: 15-45 mg/dl cerebrospinal fluid (CSF) (up to 70 mg/dl in elderly adults and children)
Glucose: 50-75 mg/dl CSF or 60%-70% of blood glucose level
Chloride: 700-750 mg/dl
Lactic dehydrogenase (LDH): less than 2.0-7.2 U/ml
Cytology: no malignant cells
Serology for syphilis: negative
Glutamine: 6-15 mg/dl

Test explanation and related physiology

In certain conditions a spinal needle may be inserted into the cisterna magna for a cisternal puncture instead of into the subarachnoid space as in a lumbar puncture (see p. 478). This procedure is hazardous because of the proximity of the needle to the brainstem. A cisternal puncture may be indicated in the following conditions:

1. To obtain CSF for examination when it cannot be obtained at the lumbar level (e.g., because of infection, lumbar deformity)
2. To demonstrate a subarachnoid block by performing a cisternal puncture simultaneously with a lumbar puncture
3. For drainage of CSF when a lumbar puncture is contraindicated
4. To introduce contrast material or air for myelography
5. To perform encephalography

With the use of accurate central nervous system imaging (e.g., CT scan, MRI), the diagnostic role of this test has greatly diminished.

Contraindications

- Patients with increased intracranial pressure
- Patients with infection near the puncture site
  Meningitis can result from contamination with infected material.
- Patients who have a developmental anomaly at the level of the foramen magnum
- Patients with suspected lesions in the cisterna magna
- Patients who cannot cooperate and remain still during the procedure

Potential complications

- Meningitis
- Herniation of the brain

Procedure and patient care

Before

- Explain the procedure to the patient. Allay the patient's fears and allow time for verbalization of concerns.
- Obtain consent if required by the institution.
- Inform the patient that his or her head must be kept still during the procedure. Rotation of the neck could cause needle injury to the medulla.
- Tell the patient that no fasting or sedation is usually required.

During

- Note the following procedural steps:

  1. The occipital area at the back of the head is shaved and cleansed with an antiseptic.
  2. The patient is placed on his or her side with a pillow under the head to keep the head and spine aligned. The chin rests on the chest and is held in place by an assistant to prevent rotation.
  3. The needle is inserted approximately 4 to 5 cm between the first cervical vertebra and the rim of the foramen magnum.
  4. The insert (obturator) is removed, and CSF can be seen slowly dripping from the needle.
  5. The needle is then attached to a sterile manometer, and the pressure (opening pressure) is recorded. Before the pressure reading is taken, the patient is asked

to relax and straighten the legs to reduce the intraabdominal pressure, which causes an increase in CSF pressure.

6. Three sterile test tubes are filled with 5 to 10 ml of CSF.

7. The pressure (closing pressure) is measured.

- Note that the duration of the procedure is approximately 20 to 60 minutes.
- Tell the patient that this procedure is usually described as painful by most patients.

After

- Apply digital pressure and a bandaid to the puncture site.
- Assess the puncture site for drainage of blood or CSF at the puncture site.
- Observe the patient for respiratory complications (e.g., cyanosis, dyspnea, apnea) and irregularities in the heartbeat, which could indicate injury to the medulla.
- Encourage the patient to drink increased amounts of fluid to replace the CSF lost during the procedure.
- Tell the patient that headaches do not usually occur as a result of this procedure.
- Inform the patient that he or she can usually get out of bed in 2 to 3 hours if no problems occur.

Abnormal findings

Subarachnoid block
Brain neoplasm
Spinal cord neoplasm
Cerebral hemorrhage
Meningitis
Encephalitis
Degenerative cord or brain disease
Autoimmune disorders
Hepatic encephalopathy
Coma

Cerebral abscess
Viral or tubercular meningitis
Myelitis
Tumors
Neurosyphilis
Multiple sclerosis
Acute demyelinating polyneuropathy
Subarachnoid bleeding
Reye's syndrome

Notes

clostridial toxin assay (*Clostridium difficile*, antibiotic-associated colitis assay; Pseudomembranous colitis toxic assay)

Type of test Stool

Normal findings Negative (no *Clostridium* toxin identified)

Test explanation and related physiology

Clostridium difficile bacterial infection of the intestine may occur in patients who are immunocompromised or taking broad-spectrum antibiotics. The clostridial bacterium releases a toxin that causes necrosis of the colonic epithelium. The detection of this toxin in the stool is therefore diagnostic of clostridial enterocolitis (pseudomembranous colitis). Management of this antibiotic-associated colitis includes immediate cessation of the broad-spectrum antibiotics, IV replacement of fluid and electrolytes, and institution of metronidazole (Flagyl) and vancomycin (Vancocin) antibiotic therapy.

Procedure and patient care

Before

- Explain the method of stool collection to the patient. Be matter-of-fact to avoid embarrassment to the patient.
- Instruct the patient not to mix urine and toilet paper with the stool specimen.
- Handle the specimen carefully, as though it is capable of causing infection. If the nurse is assisting with the specimen collection, gloves should be worn.

During

- Ask the patient to defecate into a clean container. A rectal swab cannot be used because it collects inadequate amounts of stool.
- Note that a stool specimen also can be collected by protoscopy.
- Place the specimen in a closed container and then transport it to the laboratory to prevent deterioration of the toxin.

- If the specimen cannot be processed immediately, refrigerate it.

After

- Maintain enteric isolation precautions on all patients until appropriate therapy is completed.

Abnormal finding

Clostridial enterocolitis

Notes

clot retraction test (Whole blood clot retraction test)

Type of test Blood

Normal findings
50%-100% clot retraction in 1-2 hours
Complete retraction within 24 hours

Test explanation and related physiology
The clot retraction test is used to determine if bleeding disorders may be caused by thrombocytopenia (decreased platelet count). Platelets play a vital role in hemostasis and blood clotting. This test measures the role and degree of blood clot retraction. The clot should contract to one-half its original size within 1 to 2 hours. The retraction should be nearly complete in 4 hours and definitely completed within 24 hours.

If thrombocytopenia exists, the clot retraction will be slower and the clot formation will stay soft and watery. If fibrinolysins are present, no clot retraction will occur. This test is only reliable if the hematocrit and fibrinogen (factor I) concentration (Table 5) are within normal limits.

In addition to thrombocytopenia, poor whole blood clot retraction occurs in patients with thrombasthenia (abnormal platelets) and Waldenström's macroglobulinemia.

Contraindications
- Patients with low platelet counts
- Patients with hypofibrinogenemia
- Patients taking aspirin

Interfering factors
- Uremia
- Drugs that may alter test results include aspirin and non-steroidal antiinflammatory agents.

Procedure and patient care
Before
- Explain the procedure to the patient.
- Tell the patient that no fasting is required.

TABLE 5 Minimum concentration of coagulation factors required for adequate fibrin production

Factor	Minimal hemostatic level (mg/dl)	Blood components*
I	60-100	C, FFP, FWB
II	10-15	P, WB, FFP, FWB
V	5-10	FFP, FWB
VII	5-20	P, WB, FFP, FWB
VIII	30	C, FFP, VIII CONC
IX	30	FFP, FWB
X	8-10	P, WB, FFP, FWB
XI	25	P, WB, FFP, FWB

*Blood components capable of providing specific factor: *C,* cryoprecipitate; *FFP,* fresh frozen plasma; *FWB,* fresh whole blood (<24 hours old); *P,* unfrozen banked plasma; *WB,* banked whole blood; *VIII CONC,* factor VIII concentrate.

During

- Avoid excessive probing during the venipuncture if a coagulation disorder is suspected.
- Collect approximately 5 to 7 ml of venous blood in a red-top tube.
- Avoid hemolysis.
- Indicate on the laboratory slip if the patient is taking aspirin or a nonsteroidal antiinflammatory agent.

After

- Transport the specimen to the laboratory within 1 hour of collection.
- Apply pressure or a pressure dressing to the venipuncture site.
- Assess the venipuncture site for bleeding and bruising.

Abnormal findings
Increased clot retraction

Severe anemia
Hypofibrinogenemia

Decreased or poor clot retraction

Thrombocytopenia
von Willebrand's disease
Thrombasthenia (abnormal platelets)
Waldenström's macroglobulinemia

Notes

coagulating factors concentration (Factor assay, Coagulating factors, Blood clotting factors)

Type of test Blood

Normal findings 50%-200% of "normal"

Test explanation and related physiology

The coagulating factors concentration test measures the concentration of a specific coagulating factor in the blood. Testing is available to measure the quantity of the following factors:

I (fibrinogen)
II (prothrombin)
V (proaccelerin)
VII (proconvertin stable factor)
VIII (antihemophilic factor)
IX (Christmas factor)
X (Stuart factor)
XI (plasma thromboplastin antecedent)
XII (Hageman factor)

For example, fibrinogen (factor I) is essential to the blood-clotting mechanism because it is converted to fibrin by the action of thrombin during the coagulation process (Figure 4). Measurement of factor I is often referred to as a *quantitative fibrinogen*. When these factors exist in concentrations below their "minimal hemostatic level," clotting time will be prolonged. These minimal hemostatic levels vary according to the factor involved (see Table 5, p. 200). Common medical conditions associated with decreased factor concentrations are listed in Table 6. It is important to identify the exact factor or factors involved in the coagulating defect so that appropriate blood component replacement can be administered (Table 5).

Procedure and patient care

Before

- Explain the procedure to the patient.
- Tell the patient that no fasting is required.

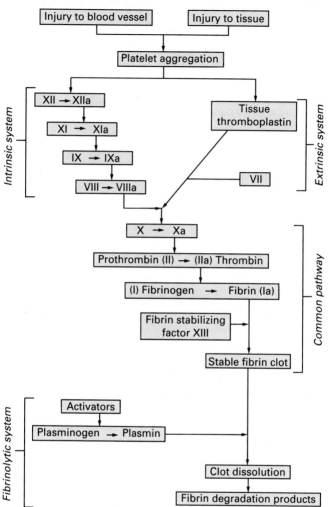

Figure 4 Process of hemostasis and fibrinolysis. Injury to blood vessel surface or tissue initiates platelet aggregation. Intrinsic or extrinsic system is activated and then activates common pathway of fibrin formation. Finally, fibrin is physiologically dissolved by fibrinolytic system.

TABLE 6 Conditions that may result in coagulation factor deficiency

Condition	Factor diminished
Liver disease	I, II, V, VII, IX, X, XI
Disseminated intravascular coagulation (DIC)	I, V, VIII
Fibrinolysis	I, V, VIII
Congenital deficiency	I, II, V, VII, VIII, IX, X, XI, XII
Heparin administration	II
Warfarin ingestion	II, VII, IX, X, XI
Autoimmune disease	VIII
Vitamin K deficiency or maldigestion	II, VII, IX, X, XI

During
- Collect approximately 7 to 10 ml of venous blood in a blue-top tube.

After
- Apply pressure or pressure dressing to the venipuncture site.
- Assess the venipuncture site for bleeding.
- Deliver the blood specimen to the laboratory as soon as possible.

Abnormal findings

See Table 6 for conditions that may result in a coagulation factor deficiency.

Notes

colonoscopy

Type of test Endoscopy

Normal findings Normal colon

Test explanation and related physiology

With the development of fiberoptic colonoscopy, the entire colon from anus to cecum can be examined in most patients. As with sigmoidoscopy, benign and malignant neoplasms, polyps, mucosal inflammation, ulceration, and sites of active hemorrhage can be visualized. Diseases such as cancer, polyps, ulcers, and arteriovenous (AV) malformations can be visualized. Cancers, polyps, and inflammatory bowel diseases can be biopsied through the colonoscope with cable-activated instruments. Sites of active bleeding can be coagulated with the use of laser, electrocoagulation, and injection of sclerosing agents.

This test is recommended for patients who have hemoccult positive stools, lower gastrointestinal bleeding, change in bowel habits, or those who are at high risk for colon cancer. The latter include patients with a strong personal or family history of prior colon cancer, polyps, or ulcerative colitis.

Contraindications

- Patients who are uncooperative
  As in all studies that require technical finesse, patient cooperation is essential to the successful completion of the test.
- Patients whose medical condition is not stable
  This test requires sedation, which may induce hypotension in the medically unstable patient.
- Patients who are bleeding profusely from the rectum
  The viewing lens will become covered with blood clots, preventing visualization of the lower intestinal tract.
- Patients who have a suspected perforation of the colon

Potential complications

- Bowel perforation
- Persistent bleeding from a biopsy site
- Oversedation resulting in respiratory depression

Interfering factors

- Poor bowel preparation
  The stool immediately obstructs the lens, thereby precluding adequate visualization of the colon.
- Active bleeding
  Blood obstructs the lens system and precludes adequate visualization of the colon.

Procedure and patient care

Before

- Explain the procedure to the patient.
- Fully inform the patient as to the risks of the procedure and obtain an informed consent.
- Instruct the patient as to the appropriate bowel preparation. One type is the 2-day bowel preparation, which uses clear liquids for 2 days along with a strong cathartic such as magnesium citrate and bisacodyl (Dulcolax). On the day of examination an enema is given. Recently a 1-day preparation using a Colyte bowel preparation has become more widely used. After the patient ingests a gallon of Colyte, enemas are not usually needed. Dulcolax tablets may be taken.
- Avoid an oral bowel preparation in patients who have upper gastrointestinal obstruction, suspected acute diverticulitis, or recent bowel resectional surgery.
- Ensure patients that they will be appropriately draped to avoid unnecessary embarrassment.
- Administer appropriate preendoscopy sedation, usually meperidine (Demerol) and diazepam (Valium). Often, atropine is ordered to minimize patient secretions.

During

- Note the following procedural steps:

  1. IV access is obtained.
  2. After a rectal examination indicates adequate bowel preparation, the patient is sedated.
  3. The patient is placed in the lateral decubitus position, and the colonoscope is placed into the rectum.
  4. Under direct visualization the colonoscope is directed to the cecum. Often a significant amount of manipulation is required to obtain this position.
  5. As in all endoscopy, air in insufflated to distend the bowel for better visualization.

6. Complete examination of the large bowel is carried out.
7. Polypectomy, biopsy, and other endoscopic surgery is performed after appropriate visualization.
8. When the laser or coagulator is used, the air is removed and carbon dioxide is used as an insufflating agent to avoid explosion.

- Note that this test is performed by a physician trained in gastrointestinal endoscopy in approximately 30 to 60 minutes.
- Tell the patient that minimal discomfort is associated with the test.

After

- Explain to patients that air has been insufflated into the bowel. They may experience flatulence or gas pains.
- Examine the abdomen for evidence of colon perforation (abdominal distention and tenderness).
- Assess the patient's vital signs. Watch for a decrease in blood pressure and an increase in pulse as an indication of hemorrhage.
- Inspect the stools for gross blood.
- Notify the physician if the patient develops increased pain or significant gastrointestinal bleeding.
- Allow the patient to eat when fully alert if there is no evidence of bowel perforation.
- Encourage the patient to drink a lot of fluids when intake is allowed. This will make up for the dehydration associated with the bowel preparation.

Abnormal findings

Colon cancer
Colon polyps
Inflammatory bowel disease (e.g., ulcerative or Crohn's colitis)
AV malformations
Hemorrhoids
Ischemic or postinflammatory strictures
Diverticulosis

Notes

colposcopy

Type of test Macroscopic examination

Normal findings Normal vagina and cervix

Test explanation and related physiology

Colposcopy provides an in situ macroscopic examination of the vagina and the cervix with a colposcope, which is a macroscope with a light source and a magnifying lens. With this procedure, tiny areas of dysplasia, carcinoma in situ, and invasive cancer that would be missed by the naked eye can be visualized, and biopsy specimens can be obtained. The study is performed on patients with abnormal vaginal epithelial patterns, cervical lesions, or suspicious Pap smear results and on those exposed to diethylstilbestrol (DES) in utero. It may be a sufficient substitute to cone biopsy (removal and examination of a cone of tissue from the cervix) in evaluating the cause of abnormal cervical cytologic findings.

Realizing that colposcopy is useful only in identifying a suspicious lesion is important. Definitive diagnosis requires biopsy of the tissue. One of the major advantages of this procedure is that of directing the biopsy to the area most likely to be truly representative of the lesion. A biopsy performed without colposcopy may not necessarily be representative of the lesion's true pathologic condition, resulting in a significant risk of missing a serious lesion.

The patient will need to have diagnostic conization if:

1. Colposcopy and endocervical curettage do not explain the problem or match the cytologic findings of the Pap smear within one grade.
2. The entire transformation zone is not seen.
3. The lesion extends up the cervical canal beyond the vision of the colposcope.

The need for up to 90% of cone biopsies is eliminated by an experienced colposcopist. Endocervical curettage may routinely accompany colposcopy to detect unknown lesions in the endocervical canal.

Contraindications

- Patients with heavy menstrual flow

Interfering factor

- Failure to cleanse the cervix of foreign materials (e.g., creams, medications) may impair visualization.

Procedure and patient care

Before

- Explain the procedure to the patient.
- Obtain a consent if required by the institution.

During

- Note the following procedural steps:
  1. The patient is placed in the lithotomy position, and a vaginal speculum is used to expose the vagina and cervix.
  2. After the cervix is sampled for cytologic findings, it is cleansed with a 3% acetic acid solution to remove excess mucus and cellular debris. The acetic acid also accentuates the difference between normal and abnormal epithelial tissues.
  3. The colposcope is focused on the cervix, which is then carefully examined.
  4. Usually the entire lesion can be outlined and the most atypical areas selected for biopsy specimen removal.
- Note that colposcopy is performed by a physician in approximately 5 to 10 minutes.
- Tell the patient that some women complain of pressure pains from the vaginal speculum and that momentary discomfort may be felt if biopsy specimens are obtained.

After

- Inform the patient that she may have vaginal bleeding if biopsy specimens were taken. Suggest that she wear a sanitary pad.
- Instruct the patient to abstain from intercourse and not to insert anything into the vagina (except a tampon) until healing of a biopsy is confirmed.
- Inform the patient when and how to obtain the results of this study.

Abnormal findings

Dysplasia   Invasive cancer
Carcinoma in situ   Cervical lesions

complement assay

Type of test Blood

Normal findings

Total complement: 41-90 hemolytic U
C3: 70-176 mg/dl
C4: 16-45 mg/dl

Test explanation and related physiology

Serum complements comprise a group of globulin proteins that act as enzymes. These enzymes facilitate the immunologic and inflammatory response. Complement increases vascular permeability, thereby allowing antibodies and white blood cells (WBCs) to be delivered to the area of inflammation. Complement also acts to increase chemotaxis (pulling of WBCs to the area of infection), phagocytosis, and immune adherence of the antibody to antigen. These processes are vitally important in the inflammatory response.

Serum complement levels are important in the detection of autoimmune diseases (e.g., lupus erythematosus, serum sickness). In these types of illnesses the complement assays are decreased secondary to consumption of the complement created by the development of the "autoimmune complexes" (i.e., antibody-antigen complexes). Two particular components (C3 and C4) are often assayed along with the total complement level. C3 and C4 are more accurate in detecting the previously described diseases and in following the course of the disease.

For this test, the blood is mixed with antibody-coated red blood cells (RBCs) of sheep. When complement is present in normal quantities, 50% of the RBCs are lysed. Decreased quantities of complement are associated with lower percentages of sheep RBC lyses.

Procedure and patient care

Before

- Explain the procedure to the patient.
- Tell the patient that no fasting or special preparations are required.

During

- Collect 7 to 10 ml of venous blood in a red-top tube.

After

- Apply pressure or a pressure dressing to the venipuncture site.
- Observe the venipuncture site for bleeding.

Abnormal findings

Increased levels

Rheumatic fever (acute)
Rheumatoid arthritis
Myocardial infarction (acute)
Ulcerative colitis
Cancer

Decreased levels

Cirrhosis
Autoimmune disease (e.g., systemic lupus erythematosus)
Serum sickness (immune complex diseases)
Glomerulonephritis
Lupus nephritis
Renal transplant rejection (acute)
Protein malnutrition
Anemias
Malnutrition
Hepatitis

Notes

complete blood count and differential count (CBC and diff)

The CBC and differential count are a series of tests of the peripheral blood that provide a tremendous amount of information about the hemotologic system and many other organ systems. They are inexpensively, easily, and rapidly performed as a screening test. The CBC and differential include automated measurement of the following studies, which are discussed separately.

Red blood cell count (RBC, see p. 617)
Hemoglobin (Hgb, see p. 402)
Hematocrit (Hct, see p. 400)
Red blood cell indices (RBC indices, see p. 620)
  Mean corpuscular volume (MCV)
  Mean corpuscular hemoglobin (MCH)
  Mean corpuscular hemoglobin concentration (MCHC)
White blood cell count (WBC) and differential count (see p. 787)
  Neutrophils (polynucleated cells or "polys," segmented cells or "segs," band cells, stab cells)
  Lymphocytes
  Monocytes
  Eosinophils
  Basophils
Blood smear (see p. 109)
Platelet count (see p. 563)

computed tomography of the abdomen
(CAT scan of the abdomen, CT scan of the abdomen)

Type of test X-ray with contrast dye

Normal findings No evidence of abnormality

Test explanation and related physiology

CT of the abdomen is a noninvasive yet very accurate x-ray procedure used to diagnose pathologic conditions such as tumors, cysts, abscesses, inflammation, perforation, bleeding, aneurysms, and calculi of the abdominal organs. The CT scan image results from passing x-rays through the abdominal organs at many angles. The variation in density of each tissue allows for a variable penetration of the x-rays. Each density is given a numeric value called a density coefficient, which is digitally computed into shades of gray. This is then displayed on a television screen as thousands of dots in various shades of gray. The final display appears as an actual photograph of the anatomic area sectioned by x-rays. The image can be enhanced by repeating the CT scan after IV administration of iodine containing contrast dye. These images can be recorded on a Polaroid or x-ray film.

Liver tumors, abscesses, trauma, cysts, and anatomic abnormalities can be seen. Pancreatic tumors, pseudocysts, inflammation, calcification, bleeding, and trauma can be detected. The kidneys and urinary outflow tract are well visualized (see CT of the kidney, p. 226). Although the bowel can be better visualized by an upper GI series, small bowel follow-through, or barium enema, large tumors and perforations of the bowel can be identified with the CT scan, especially when oral contrast is ingested. The spleen can be well visualized for hematoma, laceration, fracture, tumor infiltration, and splenic vein thrombosis with CT scanning. The retroperitoneal lymph nodes can be evaluated. These are usually present, but all nodes with a diameter greater than 2 cm are considered abnormal. The abdominal aorta and its major branches can be evaluated for aneurysmal dilation and intramural thrombi. The pelvic structures (including the uterus, ovaries, tubes, prostate, rectum) and musculature can be evaluated for tumors, abscesses, infection, or hypertrophy. Ascites can easily be demonstrated with the CT scan.

Contraindications

- Patients who are allergic to iodinated dye or shellfish
- Patients who are pregnant
- Patients whose vital signs are unstable
- Patients who are very obese, usually over 300 pounds
- Patients who are claustrophobic

Potential complications

- Allergic reaction to iodinated dye
  Allergic reactions vary from flushing, itching, and urticaria to severe, life-threatening anaphylaxis (evidenced by
  respiratory distress, drop in blood pressure, shock). In
  the unusual event of anaphylaxis the patient will be
  treated with diphenhydramine (Benadryl), steroids, and
  epinephrine. Oxygen and endotracheal equipment should
  be on hand for immediate use.
- Acute renal failure from dye infusion
  Adequate hydration beforehand may reduce this likelihood.

Interfering factors

The following can obscure visualization:

- Presence of metallic objects (e.g., hemostatis clips)
- Retained barium from previous studies
- Large amounts of fecal material or gas in the bowel

Procedure and patient care
Before

- Explain the procedure to the patient. The patient's cooperation is necessary because he or she must lie still during
  the procedure.
- Obtain informed consent if required by the institution.
- Assess the patient for allergies to iodinated dye or shellfish.
- Inform the radiologist if an allergy to iodinated contrast
  is suspected. The radiologist may prescribe a Benadryl
  and steroid preparation to be administered before testing.
  Usually a hypoallergenic, non-ionic contrast will be used
  during the test.
- Show the patient a picture of the CT machine and encourage the patient to verbalize his or her concerns, since
  some patients may have claustrophobia. Most patients

who are mildly claustrophobic can be scanned after appropriate premedication with antianxiety drugs.

- Keep the patient NPO for at least 4 hours before the test if oral contrast is to be administered. However, this test can be performed on an emergency basis on patients who have recently eaten.

During

- Note the following procedure for the abdominal CT scan:
  The patient is taken to the radiology department and placed on the CT scan table. The patient then is placed in an encircling camera (body scanner) that takes pictures of the various levels of the abdomen and pelvis. Any motion will cause blurring and streaking of the final picture. Therefore the patient is asked to remain motionless during x-ray exposure. Television equipment allows for immediate display of the CT scan image, which is then recorded on a Polaroid or x-ray film. In a separate room the technicians manipulate the CT scan table, thereby affecting the level of the abdomen that is scanned. Through audio communication the patient is instructed to hold his or her breath during x-ray exposure.
- Remember that oral and IV iodinated x-ray contrast dye provides better results for this test. One can accurately differentiate the gastrointestinal organs from the other abdominal organs with oral contrast. Likewise, the vessels and ureters are contrasted with the surrounding structures with use of IV dye.
- Note that this procedure is performed by a radiologist, usually in less than 30 minutes. If dye is administered, the procedure time may be doubled because the CT scan is done both with and without contrast dye.
- Tell the patient that the discomforts associated with this study include lying still on a hard table and the peripheral venipuncture. Mild nausea is a common sensation when contrast dye is used. An emesis basin should be readily available. Some patients may experience a salty taste, flushing, and warmth during the dye injection.

After

- Encourage the patient to drink fluids to avoid dye-induced renal failure and to promote dye excretion.

- Inform the patient that diarrhea may occur after ingestion of the oral contrast.
- Evaluate the patient for delayed reaction to dye (dyspnea, rashes, tachycardia, hives). This may occur 2 to 26 hours after the test. Treat with antihistamines or steroids.

Abnormal findings

Liver: tumor, abscess, bile duct dilation
Pancreas: tumor, pseudocyst, inflammation, bleeding
Spleen: hematoma, fracture, laceration, tumor, venous thrombosis
Gallbladder/biliary system: gallstones, tumor, bile duct dilation
Kidneys (see p. 228)
Uterus, tubes, ovary: tumor, abscess, infection, hydrosalpinx, cyst, fibroid
Prostrate: hypertrophy, tumor
Retroperitoneum: tumor, lymphadenopathy
Abdominal aneurysm
Ascites
Abscess
Appendicitis
Diverticulitis
Hemoperitoneum

Notes

computed tomography of the adrenals (CT scan of the adrenals)

Type of test X-ray with contrast dye

Normal findings No evidence of abnormality

Test explanation and related physiology

CT of the adrenal glands is a noninvasive yet very accurate method of detecting even small tumors (adenomas, carcinomas, pheochromocytomas) of the adrenal glands. Some radiologists believe they can diagnose even the type of adrenal tumor based on the density coefficients shown on the CT scan. Adrenal hemorrhage causing Addison's disease can also be detected with this study.

Contraindications

- Patients who are pregnant
- Patients who are allergic to iodinated dye or shellfish
- Patients who are claustrophobic
- Patients who are very obese, usually over 300 pounds
- Patients whose vital signs are unstable

Potential complications

- Allergic reaction to iodionated dye
  Allergic reactions may vary from mild flushing, itching, and urticaria to severe, life-threatening anaphylaxis (evidenced by respiratory distress, drop in blood pressure, shock). In the unusual event of anaphylaxis the patient may be treated with diphenhydramine (Benadryl), steroids, and epinephrine. Oxygen and endotracheal equipment should be on hand for immediate use.
- Acute renal failure from dye infusion
  Adequate hydration beforehand may reduce this likelihood

Interfering factors

The following can obscure visualization:

- Retained barium from previous studies
- Presence of metallic objects
- Large amounts of fecal material or gas in the bowel

Procedure and patient care

Before

- Explain the procedure to the patient. The patient's cooperation is necessary because he or she must lie still during the procedure.
- Obtain informed consent if required by the institution.
- Show the patient a picture of the CT machine and encourage him or her to verbalize concerns, since some patients may have claustrophobia. Patients who are mildly claustrophobic can be scanned after appropriate premedication with antianxiety drugs.
- Tell the patient that no fasting is required.
- Assess the patient for allergies to iodinated dye or shellfish.
- Inform the radiologist if an allergy to iodinated contrast is suspected. The radiologist may prescribe a Benadryl and steroid preparation to be administered before testing. Usually a hypoallergenic, non-ionic contrast will be used during the test.
- Keep the patient NPO at least 4 hours before the test.

During

- Note the following procedure for the adrenal CT scan: The patient is taken to the radiology department and asked to remain motionless because any motion will cause blurring and streaking of the final picture. An encircling x-ray camera (body scanner) takes pictures of various levels over the adrenal glands. Television equipment allows for immediate display, and the image is recorded by a Polaroid-type camera.
- Remember that a contrast agent may be administered orally to highlight the gut or intravenously to enhance visualization of the kidneys. This provides accurate localization of the suprarenal adrenal glands.
- Note that this procedure is performed by a radiologist in less than 30 minutes. If dye is administered, the procedure time is doubled because the CT scan is done with and without the contrast dye.
- Tell the patient that the discomforts associated with this study include lying still on a hard table and the peripheral venipuncture. Mild nausea is a common sensation when contrast dye is used. An emesis basin should be readily

available. Some patients may experience a salty taste, flushing, and warmth during the dye injection.

After

- Evaluate for delayed reaction to dye (dyspnea, rash, tachycardia, hives). This usually occurs 2 to 6 hours after the test. Treat with antihistamines or steroids.
- Encourage the patient to drink fluids to promote dye excretion.

Abnormal findings

Adenomas   Pheochromocytomas
Carcinomas   Adrenal hemorrhages

Notes

computed tomography of the brain (CT scan of the brain, Computerized axial transverse tomography [CATT])

Type of test X-ray with contrast dye

Normal findings No evidence of pathologic conditions

Test explanation and related physiology

CT of the brain consists of a computerized analysis of multiple tomographic x-ray films taken of the brain tissue at successive layers to provide a three-dimensional view of the cranial contents. The CT x-ray image provides a view of the head as if one were looking down through its top. The variation in density of each tissue allows for variable penetration of the x-ray beam. An attached computer calculates the amount of x-ray penetration of each tissue and displays this as shades of gray. The image is placed on a television screen and photographed. The final result is a series of actual anatomic pictures of coronal sections of the brain.

CT scanning is used in the differential diagnosis of intracranial neoplasms, cerebral infarctions, ventricular displacement or enlargement, cortical atrophy, cerebral aneurysms, intracranial hemorrhage and hematoma, and arteriovenous (AV) malformation.

Visualization of a neoplasm, previous infarction, or any pathologic process that destroys the blood-brain barrier may be enhanced by the IV injection of an iodinated contrast dye. CT scans may be repeated frequently to monitor the progress of any disease or to monitor the healing process. In many cases CT scanning has eliminated the need for more invasive procedures, such as cerebral arteriography and pneumoencephalography.

Contraindications

- Patients who are allergic to iodinated dye or shellfish
- Patients who are claustrophobic
- Patients who are pregnant
- Patients whose vital signs are unstable
- Patients who are very obese, usually over 300 pounds

Potential complications

- Allergic reaction to iodinated dye
  Allergic reactions vary from mild flushing, itching, and

urticaria to severe, life-threatening anaphylaxis (evidenced by respiratory distress, drop in blood pressure, shock). In the unusual event of anaphylaxis the patient may be treated with diphenhydramine (Benadryl), steroids, and epinephrine. Oxygen and endotracheal equipment should be on hand for immediate use.
- Acute renal failure from dye infusion
  Adequate hydration beforehand may reduce this likelihood.

Procedure and patient care

Before

- Explain the procedure to the patient. The patient's cooperation is necessary because he or she must lie still during the procedure.
- Obtain informed consent if required by the institution.
- Show the patient a picture of the CT machine and encourage the patient to verbalize his or her concerns, since some patients may have claustrophobia. Most patients who are mildly claustrophobic can be scanned after appropriate premedication with antianxiety drugs.
- Keep the patient NPO for 4 hours before the study because iodine may cause nausea. It is not usually known before the test if enhanced visualization by dye injection will be indicated. If contrast will not be used, food and fluids may be taken.
- Instruct the patient that wigs, hairpins, clips, or partial dental plates cannot be worn during the procedure because they hamper visualization of the brain.
- Assess the patient for allergies to iodinated dye or shellfish.
- Inform the radiologist if an allergy to iodinated contrast is suspected. The radiologist may prescribe a Benadryl and steroid preparation to be administered before testing. Usually a hypoallergenic, non-ionic contrast will be used during the test.
- Tell the patient that he or she may hear a "clicking" noise as the scanning machine moves around the head.

During

- Note the following procedure for the brain CT scan:
  The patient lies in the supine position on an examining table with the head resting on a snug-fitting rubber cap within a water-filled box. The patient's head is enclosed

only to the hairline (as in a hair dryer). The face is not covered, and the patient can see out of the machine at all times. Sponges are placed along the side of the head to ensure the patient's head does not move during the study. The scanner passes an x-ray beam through the brain from one side to the other. The machine then rotates 1 degree; the procedure is repeated at each degree through a 180-degree arc. The machine is then moved, and the entire procedure is repeated through a total of three to seven planes.

- Remember that usually an iodinated dye will then be used. A peripheral IV line is started, and the iodine dye is administered through it. The entire scanning process is repeated.
- Note that this procedure is performed by a radiologist in less than an hour. If dye is administered, the procedure time is doubled because the CT scan is done with and without the contrast dye.
- Tell the patient that the discomforts associated with this study include lying still on a hard table and the peripheral venipuncture. Mild nausea is a common sensation when contrast dye is used. An emesis basin should be readily available. Some patients may experience a salty taste, flushing, and warmth during the dye injection.

After

- Encourage the patient to drink fluids because dye is excreted by the kidneys and causes diuresis.
- Evaluate the patient for delayed reaction to dye (dyspnea, rash, tachycardia, hives). This usually occurs 2 to 6 hours after the test. Treat with antihistamines or steroids.

Abnormal findings

Intracranial neoplasms
Cerebral infarction
Ventricular displacement
Ventricular enlargement
Cortical atrophy
Cerebral aneurysms
Intracranial hemorrhage

Hematoma
AV malformation
Meningiomas
Multiple sclerosis
Hydrocephalus
Abscess

Notes

computed tomography of the chest (Chest CT scan)

Type of test X-ray with contrast dye

Normal findings No evidence of pathologic conditions

Test explanation and related physiology

CT scanning of the chest is a noninvasive yet very accurate x-ray procedure used to diagnose and evaluate pathologic conditions such as tumor, nodules, parenchymal coin lesion, cysts, abscess, pleural effusion, and enlarged lymph nodes. When an IV contrast material is given, vascular structures can be identified and a diagnosis of aortic aneurysm can be made. With oral contrast the esophagus and upper structures can be evaluated for tumor and other conditions. This procedure provides a cross-sectional view of the chest and is especially useful in detecting small differences in tissue densities, thus demonstrating lesions that cannot be seen on conventional radiology and tomography. The mediastinal structures can be visualized in a manner that cannot be equalled with conventional x-ray and tomographic scans.

The x-ray image results from using a body scanner machine to pass x-rays through the patient's chest at many different angles. The variation in density of each tissue allows for a variable penetration of the x-rays. Each density is given a numeric value called a coefficient, which is digitally computed into shades of gray. This is then displayed on a television screen as thousands of dots in various shades of gray. The final display appears as an actual photograph of the anatomic area sectioned by the x-rays.

Contraindications

- Patients who are pregnant
- Patients who are allergic to iodinated dye or shellfish
- Patients who are claustrophobic
- Patients who are very obese, usually over 300 pounds
- Patients whose vital signs are unstable

Potential complications

- Allergic reaction to iodinated dye
  Allergic reactions may vary from mild flushing, itching,

and urticaria to severe, life-threatening anaphylaxis (evidenced by respiratory distress, drop in blood pressure, shock). In the unusual event of anaphylaxis the patient may be treated with diphenhydramine (Benadryl), steroids, and epinephrine. Oxygen and endotracheal equipment should be on hand for immediate use.

- Acute renal failure from dye infusion
  Adequate hydration beforehand may reduce this likelihood.

Procedure and patient care

Before

- Explain the procedure to the patient. The patient's cooperation is necessary because he or she must lie still during the procedure.
- Obtain informed consent if required by the institution.
- Assess the patient for allergies to iodinated dye or shellfish.
- Inform the radiologist if an allergy to iodinated contrast is suspected. The radiologist may prescribe a Benadryl and steroid preparation to be administered before testing. Usually a hypoallergenic, non-ionic contrast will be used during the test.
- Show the patient a picture of the CT machine and encourage the patient to verbalize concerns regarding claustrophobia. Most patients who are mildly claustrophobic can tolerate this study after appropriate premedication with antianxiety drugs.
- Keep the patient NPO for 4 hours before the test in the event that contrast dye is administered.

During

- Note the following procedure for the chest CT scan:
  The patient is taken to the radiology department and asked to remain motionless in a supine position, since any motion will cause blurring and streaking of the final picture. An encircling x-ray camera (body scanner) takes pictures at varying intervals and levels over the chest area. Television equipment allows for immediate display, and the image is recorded by a Polaroid-type camera or on x-ray film. Occasionally, IV dye is administered to enhance the chest image, and the x-ray studies are repeated.

- Note that this procedure is performed by a radiologist in 30 to 45 minutes. If dye is administered, the procedure time may be doubled because the CT scan is done with and without contrast dye.
- Tell the patient that the discomforts associated with this study include lying still on a hard table and the peripheral venipuncture. Mild nausea is a common sensation when contrast dye is used. An emesis basin should be readily available. Some patients may experience a salty taste, flushing, and warmth during the dye injection.

After

- Encourage patients who received the dye injection to increase their fluid intake, since the dye is excreted by the kidneys and causes diuresis.
- Evaluate the patient for delayed reaction to the dye (dyspnea, rashes, tachycardia, hives). This usually occurs 2 to 6 hours after the test. Treat with antihistamines or steroids.

Abnormal findings

Pulmonary tumor
Inflammatory nodules
Granuloma
Cyst
Pleural effusion
Enlarged lymph nodes
Aortic aneurysm
Postpneumonitic scanning

Pneumonitis
Esophageal tumors
Hiatal hernia
Mediastinal tumors (e.g., lymphoma, thymoma)
Primary or metastatic chest wall tumors

Notes

computed tomography of the kidney (CT scan of the kidney)

Type of test X-ray with contrast dye

Normal findings No evidence of abnormality

Test explanation and physiology

CT of the kidney is a noninvasive yet very accurate x-ray procedure used to diagnose pathologic renal conditions such as tumors, cysts, ureteral obstructions, calculi, and congenital abnormalities. The CT image results from passing x-rays through the kidney at many angles. The variation and density of each tissue allows for variable penetration of the x-rays. Each density is given a numeric value called a coefficient, which is digitally computed into shades of gray. This is then displayed on a television screen as thousands of dots in various shades of gray. The final display appears as an actual photograph of the anatomic area sectioned by the x-rays. The image can be enhanced by repeating the CT scan after the IV administration of iodinated contrast dye.

Contraindications

- Patients who are allergic to iodinated dye or shellfish
- Patients who are pregnant
- Patients whose vital signs are unstable
- Patients who are very obese, usually over 300 pounds
- Patients who are claustrophobic

Potential complications

- Acute renal failure from the dye infusion
  Adequate hydration beforehand may reduce this likelihood.
- Allergic reaction to iodinated dye
  Allergic reactions may vary from mild flushing, itching, and urticaria to severe, life-threatening anaphylaxis (evidenced by respiratory distress, drop in blood pressure, shock). In the unusual event of anaphylaxis the patient may be treated with diphenhydramine (Benadryl), steroids, and epinephrine. Oxygen and endotracheal equipment should be on hand for immediate use.

Interfering factors

The following can obscure visualization:

- Presence of metallic objects (e.g., hemostasis clips)
- Retained barium from previous studies
- Fecal material or gas in the bowel

Procedure and patient care

Before

- Explain the procedure to the patient. The patient's cooperation is necessary because he or she must lie still during the procedure.
- Obtain informed consent if required by the institution.
- Show the patient a picture of the CT machine and encourage the patient to verbalize his or her concerns, since some patients may have claustrophobia. Most patients who are mildly claustrophic can be scanned after appropriate premedication with antianxiety drugs.
- Keep the patient NPO for 4 hours before the test if oral contrast dye is to be administered. Verify this with the radiology department.
- Assess the patient for allergies to iodinated dye or shellfish.
- Inform the radiologist if an allergy to iodine contrast is suspected. The radiologist may prescribe a Benadryl and steroid preparation to be administered before the test. Usually a hypoallergenic, non-ionic contrast material will be used during the test.

During

- Note the following procedure for the kidney CT scan: The patient is taken to the x-ray department and asked to remain motionless. Any motion will cause blurring and streaking of the final picture. An encircling x-ray camera (body scanner) takes pictures of various levels over the kidney area. The scanner makes loud, clicking sounds as it rotates. Television equipment allows for immediate display of the image, which is then recorded by a Polaroid-type camera or on x-ray film. Occasionally, IV contrast dye may be administered to enhance the kidney image.
- Note that this procedure is performed by a radiologist in less than 30 minutes. If dye is administered, the proce-

dure time may be doubled because the CT scan is done with and without contrast dye.

- Tell the patient that the discomforts associated with this study include lying still on a hard table and the peripheral venipuncture. Mild nausea is a common sensation when contrast dye is used. An emesis basin should be readily available. Some patients may experience a salty taste, flushing, and warmth during the dye injection.

After

- Encourage the patient to drink fluids to avoid dye-induced renal failure and to promote dye excretion.
- Evaluate the patient for delayed reaction to dye (dyspnea, rashes, tachycardia, hives). This usually occurs 2 to 6 hours after the test. Treat with antihistamines or steroids.

Abnormal findings

Tumors
Cysts
Obstructions of the collecting system
Calculi
Congenital kidney abnormalities

Notes

contraction stress test (CST, Oxytocin challenge test [OCT])

Type of test Manometric

Normal findings Negative

Test explanation and related physiology

The CST, frequently called the oxytocin challenge test (OCT), is a relatively noninvasive test of fetoplacental adequacy used in the assessment of high-risk pregnancy. For this study a temporary stress in the form of uterine contractions is applied to the fetus. The reaction of the fetus to the contractions is assessed by an external fetal heart monitor. Uterine contractions cause transient impediment of placental blood flow. If the placental reserve is adequate, the maternal-fetal oxygen transfer is not significantly compromised during the contractions and the fetal heart rate (FHR) remains normal (a *negative* test). The fetoplacental unit can then be considered adequate for the next 7 days.

If the placental reserve is inadequate, the fetus does not receive enough oxygen during the contraction. This results in intrauterine hypoxia and late deceleration of the FHR. The test is considered *positive* if consistent, persistent late decelerations of the FHR occur with two or more uterine contractions. False positive results caused by uterine hyperstimulation can occur in 10% to 30% of patients. Thus positive test results warrant a complete review of other studies (e.g., amniocentesis) before the pregnancy is terminated by delivery.

Results are considered *equivocal* if inconsistent, late decelerations occur. The test should be repeated 24 hours later. The concept of a "10-minute window"—a period of 10 minutes in which the criteria for either a positive or a negative test should be satisfied—has reduced the incidence of equivocal results. If an occasional late deceleration is followed by a 10-minute period of no decelerations during three contractions, the result is called a "negative window." The test is then negative rather than equivocal. A positive result can be ascertained from a 10-minute "positive window," in which during the 10-minute interval, criteria of a positive test are met.

The test is considered *unsatisfactory* if the results cannot be interpreted (e.g., because of hyperstimulation of the uterus or excessive movement of the mother), and it should be repeated.

Two advantages of the CST are that it can be done at any time and its results are available shortly afterward. Although this test can be performed reliably at 32 weeks of gestation, it usually is done after 34 weeks. CST can induce labor, and a fetus at 34 weeks is more likely to survive an unexpected induced delivery than a fetus at 32 weeks. Nonstress testing of the fetus is the preferred test in almost every instance and can be performed more safely at 32 weeks and then followed 2 weeks later by CST if necessary. The CST may be performed weekly until delivery terminates pregnancy.

The CST can be used clinically in any high-risk pregnancy where fetal well-being is threatened. These include pregnancies marked by diabetes, hypertensive disease of pregnancy (toxemia), intrauterine growth retardation, Rh-factor sensitization, history of stillbirth, postmaturity, or low estriol levels.

Contraindications

- Patients with multiple pregnancy because the myometrium is under greater tension and is more likely to be stimulated to premature labor
- Patients with premature ruptured membrane because labor may be stimulated by the CST
- Patients with placenta previa because vaginal delivery may be induced
- Patients with abruptio placentae because the placenta may separate from the uterus as a result of the oxytocin-induced uterine contractions
- Patients with previous hysterotomy because the strong uterine contractions may cause uterine rupture
- Patients with previous vertical or classic cesarean sections because the strong uterine contractions may cause uterine rupture (However, the test can be performed if it is carefully monitored and controlled.)
- Patients with pregnancies of less than 32 weeks because early delivery may be induced by the procedure

Potential complication

- Premature labor

Interfering factor

- Hypotension may cause false positive results.

Procedure and patient care

Before

- Explain the procedure to the patient.
- Obtain informed consent for the procedure.
- Teach the patient breathing and relaxation studies.
- Record the patient's blood pressure and the FHR before the test as baseline values.
- If the CST is performed on an elective basis, the patient may be kept NPO in case labor occurs.

During

- Note the following procedural steps:

  1. After the patient empties her bladder, place her in semi-Fowler's position and tilted slightly to one side to avoid vena caval compression by the enlarged uterus.
  2. Check her blood pressure every 10 minutes to avoid hypotension, which may cause diminished placental blood flow and a false positive test result.
  3. Place an external fetal monitor over the patient's abdomen to record the fetal heart tones, and attach an external tocodynamometer to the abdomen at the fundal region to monitor uterine contractions.
  4. Record the output of the fetal heart tones and uterine contractions on a two-channel strip recorder.
  5. Monitor baseline FHR and uterine activity for 20 minutes.
  6. If uterine contractions are detected during this pretest period, withhold oxytocin and monitor the response of the fetal heart tone to spontaneous uterine contractions.
  7. If no spontaneous uterine contractions occur, administer oxytocin (Pitocin) by IV infusion pump.
  8. Increase the rate of oxytocin infusion until the patient is having moderate contractions. Then record the FHR pattern.
  9. After the oxytocin infusion is discontinued, continue FHR monitoring for another 30 minutes until the uterine activity has returned to its preoxytocin state.

The body metabolizes oxytocin in approximately 20 to 25 minutes.

- Note that the CST is performed safely on an outpatient basis in the labor and delivery unit where qualified nurses and necessary equipment are available. The test is performed by a nurse with a physician available.
- Note that a new noninvasive method of performing the CST is called the *breast stimulation* or *nipple stimulation technique*. Stimulation of the nipple causes nerve impulses to the hypothalamus that trigger the release of oxytocin into the mother's bloodstream. This causes uterine contractions and may eliminate the need for IV administration of oxytocin. Uterine contractions are usually satisfactory after 15 minutes of nipple stimulation (gentle twisting of the nipples). Advantages of this technique include ease of performing the test, shorter duration of the study, and elimination of the need to start, monitor, and stop IV infusions. If sufficient contractions do not result from nipple stimulation, the standard CST procedure is followed.
- Note that the duration of this study is approximately 2 hours.
- Tell the patient that the discomfort associated with the CST may consist of mild labor contractions. Usually, breathing exercises are sufficient to control any discomfort. Administer analgesics if needed.

After

- Monitor the patient's blood pressure and the FHR.
- Discontinue the IV line and assess the sight for bleeding.

Abnormal finding

Fetoplacental inadequacy

Notes

Coombs' test, direct (Direct antiglobulin test)

Type of test Blood

Normal findings Negative; no agglutination

Test explanation and related physiology

The direct Coombs' test is used to detect autoantibodies against red blood cells (RBCs), which can cause cellular damage. Many diseases (e.g., erythroblastosis fetalis, lymphomas, lupus erythematosus, mycoplasmal infection, infectious mononucleosis) and drugs (e.g., quinidine) are associated with the production of these autoantibodies. These antibodies result in hemolytic anemia. Frequently the production of these autoantibodies against RBCs is not associated with any disease, and the resulting hemolytic anemia is therefore called *idiopathic.*

This test is performed by mixing the patient's RBCs, which are suspected of being covered with autoantibodies against RBCs, with Coombs' serum. Coombs' serum is a solution containing antibodies against human blood serum. If the patient's RBCs are coated with autoantibodies against RBCs, the Coombs' antibodies will react with the autoantibodies on the RBC and cause agglutination (clumping) of the RBCs. The greater the quantity of antibodies against RBCs present, the more clumping occurs. This test is read as positive with clumping on a scale of trace to +4. If the RBCs are not coated with autoantibodies against RBCs (immunoglobulins), agglutination will not occur. This is a negative test.

When a transfusion with incompatible blood is given, the Coombs' test can detect the antibodies coating the transfused RBCs. The Coombs' test is therefore very helpful in evaluating suspected transfusion reactions.

Interfering factors

- Drugs that may cause false positive results include ampicillin, captopril, cephalosporins, chlorpromazine (Thorazine), chlorpropamide, hydralazine, indomethacin (Indocin), insulin, isoniazid (INH), levodopa, methyldopa (Aldomet), penicillin, phenytoin (Dilantin), procainamide, quinidine, quinine, rifampin, streptomycin, sulfonamides, and tetracyclines.

Procedure and patient care
Before
- Explain the procedure to the patient.
- Tell the patient that no fasting is required.

During
- Collect approximately 5 to 7 ml of venous blood in a red-top or lavender-top tube.
- Use venous blood from the umbilical cord to detect the presence of antibodies in the newborn.
- List on the laboratory slip all medications that the patient has taken in the last few days.

After
- Apply pressure or a pressure dressing to the venipuncture site.
- Assess the venipuncture site for bleeding.

Abnormal findings
Autoimmune hemolytic anemia
Transfusion reaction
Erythroblastosis fetalis

Lymphomas
Lupus erythematosus
Mycoplasmal infection
Infectious mononucleosis

Notes

Coombs' test, indirect (Blood antibody screening)

Type of test Blood

Normal findings Negative; no agglutination

Test explanation and related physiology

The indirect Coombs' test detects circulating antibodies against RBCs. The major purpose of this test is to determine if the patient has serum antibodies (other than the major ABO system) to RBCs that he or she is about to receive by blood transfusion. Therefore this test is the "screening" portion of the "type and screen" routinely performed for blood compatibility testing (cross-matching).

In this test a small amount of the recipient's serum is added to the donor's RBCs. Then Coombs' serum is added to the mixture. Visible agglutination indicates that the recipient has antibodies to the donor's RBCs. If the recipient has no antibodies against the donor's RBCs, agglutination will not occur. Transfusion should then proceed safely and without any transfusion reaction.

Circulating antibodies against RBCs may also occur in a pregnant woman who is Rh-negative and is carrying an Rh-positive fetus.

Interfering factors

- Drugs that may cause false positive results include antiarrhythmics, antituberculins, cephalosporins, chlorpromazine (Thorazine), insulin, levodopa, methyldopa (Aldomet), penicillins, phenytoin (Dilantin), quinidine, sulfonamides, and tetracyclines.

Procedure and patient care

Before

- Explain the procedure to the patient.
- Tell the patient that no fasting is required.

During

- Collect approximately 7 ml of venous blood in a red-top tube.
- List on the laboratory slip all medications that the patient has taken in the last few days.

After

- Apply pressure or a pressure dressing to the venipuncture site.
- Assess the venipuncture site for bleeding.
- Remember that if this antibody screening test is positive, antibody identification is then done.

Abnormal findings

Incompatible cross-matched blood
Anti-Rh antibodies
Acquired hemolytic anemia
Presence of specific antibody
Erythroblastosis fetalis

Notes

cortisol, blood (Hydrocortisone, serum cortisol)

Type of test Blood

Normal findings

Adult/elderly: 8 AM—6-28 µg/dl or 170-625 nmol/L (SI units)

4 PM—2-12 µg/dl or 80-413 nmol/L (SI units)

Child: 8 AM— 15-25 µg/dl

4 PM—5-10 µg dl

Newborn: 1-24 µg/dl

Test explanation and related physiology

Cortisol is a potent glucocorticoid released from the adrenal cortex in response to adrenocorticotropic hormone (ACTH) stimulation. The best method of evaluating adrenal activity is by directly measuring plasma cortisol levels. Normally, cortisol levels rise and fall during the day. This is called the diurnal variation. Cortisol levels are highest around 6 to 8 AM and gradually fall during the day to their lowest point around midnight. Sometimes the earliest sign of adrenal hyperfunction is the loss of this diurnal variation, even though the cortisol levels are not yet elevated. For example, individuals with Cushing's syndrome often have top-normal plasma cortisol levels in the morning and do not exhibit a decline as the day proceeds. Low levels of plasma cortisol are suggestive of Addison's disease.

For this test, blood is usually collected at 8 AM and again at around 4 PM. One would expect that the 4 PM value to be one third to two thirds of the 8 AM value. Normal values may be transposed in individuals who have worked during the night and slept during the day for long periods of time.

Interfering factors

- Physical and emotional stress can artifically elevate cortisol levels.
- Recent radioisotope scans can affect test results.
- Drugs that may cause increased levels include estrogen, oral contraceptives, and spironolactone (Aldactone).
- Drugs that may cause decreased levels include androgens and phenytoin (Dilantin).

Procedure and patient care
Before
- Explain the procedure to the patient to minimize anxiety.
- Assess the patient for signs of physical stress (e.g., infection, acute illness) or emotional stress and report these to the physician.

During
- Collect approximately 7 to 10 ml of venous blood in a red-top or green-top tube in the morning after the patient has had a good night's sleep.
- Collect another blood sample at about 4 PM.
- Indicate on the laboratory slip the time of the venipuncture and any drugs that can affect test results.

After
- Apply pressure or a pressure dressing to the venipuncture site.
- Observe the venipuncture site for bleeding.

Abnormal findings

Increased levels	Decreased levels
Cushing's syndrome	Addison's disease
Adrenal adenoma	Hypopituitarism
Ectopic ACTH-producing tumors	Hypothyroidism
Hyperthyroidism	Liver disease
Obesity	
Stress	

Notes

cortisol, urine (Hydrocortisone, urine cortisol)

Type of test Urine (24 hour)

Normal findings

Adult/elderly: 10-100 µg/24 hr
Adolescent: 5-55 µg/24 hr
Child: 2-27 µg/24 hr

Test explanation and related physiology

Cortisol is a potent glucocorticoid released from the adrenal cortex in response to adrenocorticotropic hormone (ACTH) stimulation. This test is used in the evaluation of adrenocortical function, especially hyperfunction. An elevated cortisol level in a properly collected urine specimen supports the diagnosis of Cushing's syndrome in an unstressed patient.

Interfering factors

- Pregnancy causes increased cortisol levels.
- Recent radioisotope scans can interfere with test results.
- Stress can increase cortisol levels.
- Drugs that may affect test results include oral contraceptives and spironolactone (Aldactone).

Procedure and patient care

Before

- Explain the procedure to the patient.
- Assess the patient for signs of physical stress (e.g., infection, acute illness) or emotional stress and report these to the physician.

During

- Begin the 24-hour collection after the patient urinates. Discard this specimen.
- Collect all urine passed by the patient during the next 24 hours.
- Post the hours for urine collection in a prominent spot.
- Note that it is not necessary to measure each urine specimen.
- Remind the patient to void before defecating so that the urine is not contaminated by feces.

- Tell the patient not to put toilet paper in the collection container.
- Encourage the patient to drink fluids during the 24 hours unless this is contraindicated for medical purposes.
- Collect the last specimen as close as possible to the end of the 24-hour period. Add this to the collection.
- Place the 24-hour urine collection in a plastic container and keep on ice. Use a preservative.
- Note on the laboratory slip the date and time that the specimen collection began and ended.
- Indicate on the laboratory slip any medications that can affect test results.

After

- Send the specimen to the laboratory promptly.

Abnormal findings

Increased levels

Cushing's syndrome
Stress
Pregnancy

Decreased levels

Addisons's disease
Hypopituitarism

Notes

cortisone administration test (Dent test)

Type of test Blood

Normal findings Depend on baseline values

Test explanation and related physiology

The cortisone administration test is used in differentiating the causes of hypercalcemia. Oral administration of cortisone for 10 days lowers the serum calcium level in patients who have hypercalcemia resulting from causes other than hyperparathyroidism (e.g., sarcoidosis, vitamin D intoxication, bone metastasis). At the doses given, cortisone does not lower calcium levels in hyperparathyroid patients. A decreased serum calcium level indicates that the hypercalcemia is caused by sarcoidosis or some other disorder. This fact helps differentiate the hyperparathyroid patient from the patient with hypercalcemia resulting from other causes.

This study is rarely used today, since serum parathyroid hormone (PTH) assays are so easily performed and are more helpful than the Dent test in determining the cause of hypercalcemia.

Interfering factors

- Increase or decrease in dietary calcium

Procedure and patient care

Before

- Explain the procedure to the patient.
- Inform the patient about the 10-day administration of cortisone.
- Instruct the patient to take the cortisone acetate orally with milk or with an antacid to protect against gastric irritation.
- Obtain a baseline calcium level determination before the test.

During

- Collect approximately 7 to 10 ml of venous blood in a red-top tube.

After

- Apply pressure or a pressure dressing to the venipuncture site.
- Assess the venipuncture site for bleeding.

Abnormal findings

Hyperparathyroidism
Hypercalcemia from causes other than hyperparathyroidism

Notes

creatinine, blood (Serum creatinine)

Type of test Blood

Normal findings

Adult: female, 0.5-1.1 mg/dl or 44-97 μmol/L (SI units)
      male, 0.6-1.2 mg/dl
Elderly: decrease in muscle mass may cause decreased values
Adolescent: 0.5-1.0 mg/dl
Child: 0.3-0.7 mg/dl
Infant: 0.2-0.4 mg/dl
Newborn: 0.3-1.2 mg/dl

Possible critical values >4 mg/dl (indicates serious impairment in renal function)

Test explanation and related physiology

This test measures the amount of creatinine in the blood. Creatinine is a catabolic product of creatine, which is used in skeletal muscle contraction. The daily production of creatine, and subsequently creatinine, depends on muscle mass, which fluctuates very little. Creatinine, as with blood urea nitrogen (BUN), is excreted entirely by the kidneys and is therefore directly proportional to renal excretory function. Thus, with normal renal excretory function, the serum creatinine level should remain constant and normal. Only renal disorders, such as glomerulonephritis, pyelonephritis, acute tubular necrosis, and urinary obstruction, will cause an abnormal elevation in creatinine.

The serum creatinine test, as with BUN, is used to diagnose impaired renal function. However, unlike BUN, the creatinine level is affected very little by dehydration, malnutrition, or hepatic function. The creatinine level is interpreted in conjunction with the BUN. These tests are referred to as *renal function studies*.

Interfering factors

- Drugs that may increase creatinine values include aminoglycosides (e.g., gentamicin), cimetidine, heavy metal chemotherapeutic agents (e.g., cisplatin), and nephrotoxic drugs such as cephalosporins (e.g., cefoxitin).

Procedure and patient care

Before

- Explain the procedure to the patient.
- Tell the patient that no fasting is required.

During

- Collect approximately 5 ml of blood in a red-top tube.
- For pediatric patients, usually draw blood from a heel stick.

After

- Apply pressure or a pressure dressing to the venipuncture site.
- Observe the venipuncture site for bleeding.

Abnormal findings

Increased levels

Glomerulonephritis
Pyelonephritis
Acute tubular necrosis
Urinary tract obstruction
Reduced renal blood flow
   (e.g., shock, dehydration,
   congestive heart failure,
   atherosclerosis)
Diabetes
Nephritis
Rhabdomyolysis
Acromegaly
Gigantism

Decreased levels

Debilitation
Decreased muscle mass
   (e.g., muscular dystrophy, myasthenia gravis)

Notes

creatinine clearance

Type of test Urine (24 hour); blood

Normal findings

Adult (<40 years): male, 97-137 ml/min
female, 88-128 ml/min
Values decrease 6.5 ml/min/decade because of decline in glomerular filtration rate (GFR).
Newborn: 40-65 ml/min

Test explanation and related physiology

The creatinine clearance is a measure of the glomerular filtration rate (GFR), that is, the number of milliliters of filtrate made by the kidneys per minute. Urine and serum creatinine levels are assessed, and the clearance rate is calculated.

The amount of filtrate made in the kidney depends on the amount of blood present to be filtered and on the ability of the glomeruli to act as a filter. The amount of blood present for filtration is decreased in renal artery atherosclerosis, dehydration, or shock. The ability of the glomeruli to act as a filter is decreased by diseases such as glomerulonephritis, acute tubular necrosis, and most other primary renal diseases. Significant bilateral obstruction to urinary outflow affects glomerular filtration (creatinine clearance) only after it is longstanding.

When one kidney alone becomes diseased, the opposite kidney, if normal, has the ability to compensate by increasing its filtration rate. Therefore, with unilateral kidney disease or nephrectomy, a decrease in creatinine clearance is not expected if the other kidney is normal.

The creatinine clearance test requires a 24-hour urine collection and a serum creatinine level. Creatinine clearance is then computed using the following formula:

$$\text{Creatinine clearance} = \frac{UV}{P}$$

U = Number of milligrams per deciliter of creatinine excreted in the urine over 24 hours

V = Volume of urine in milliliters per minute

P = Serum creatinine in milligrams per deciliter

A 24-hour urine collection for creatinine is often measured along with other urine collections to assess the completeness of other 24-hour collections.

Interfering factors

- Exercise may cause increased creatinine values.
- Incomplete urine collection may give a falsely lowered value.
- Drugs that may cause increased levels include aminoglycosides (e.g., gentamicin), cimetidine, heavy metal chemotherapeutic agents (e.g., cisplatin), and nephrotoxic drugs such as cephalosporins (e.g., cefoxitin).

Procedure and patient care

Before

- Explain the procedure to the patient.
- Tell the patient that no special diet is usually required.
- Note that some laboratories instruct the patient to avoid cooked meat, tea, coffee, or drugs on the day of the test. Check with the laboratory.

During

- Instruct the patient to begin the 24-hour urine collection. Discard the initial specimen and start the 24-hour timing as of that point.
- Collect all the urine passed during the next 24 hours.
- Show the patient where to store the urine specimen.
- Keep the specimen on ice or refrigerated during the 24 hours.
- Indicate the starting time on the urine container and laboratory slip.
- Post the hours for the urine collection in a noticeable place to prevent accidental discarding of a specimen.
- Instruct the patient to void before defecating so that urine is not contaminated by feces.
- Remind the patient not to put toilet paper in the collection container.
- Encourage the patient to drink fluids during the 24 hours unless this is contraindicated for medical purposes.
- Instruct the patient to avoid vigorous exercise during the 24 hours because exercise may cause an increased creatinine clearance.

- Collect the last specimen as close as possible to the end of the 24-hour period. Add this urine to the container.
- Make sure a venous blood sample is drawn in a red-top tube during the 24-hour collection.
- Mark the patient's age, weight, and height on the requisition sheet.

After

- Transport the urine specimen promptly to the laboratory.
- Apply pressure or a pressure dressing to the venipuncture site.
- Observe the venipuncture site for bleeding.

Abnormal findings
Increased levels

Exercise
Pregnancy

Decreased levels

Impaired kidney function (e.g., renal artery atherosclerosis, glomerulonephritis, acute tubular necrosis)
Conditions causing decreased GFR (congestive heart failure, cirrhosis with ascites, shock, dehydration)

Notes

creatinine phosphokinase (CPK, CP, Creatinine kinase [CK])

Type of test Blood

Normal findings

Total CPK
Adult/elderly: male, 12-70 U/ml or 55-170 U/L (SI units)
               female, 10-55 U/ml or 30-135 U/L (SI units)
Values are higher after exercise.
Newborn: 68-580 U/L (SI units)
Isoenzymes
CPK-MM: 100%
CPK-MB: 0%
CPK-BB: 0%

Test explanation and related physiology

CPK is found predominantly in the heart muscle, skeletal muscle, and brain. Serum CPK levels are elevated whenever injury occurs to these muscle cells. CPK levels can rise within 6 hours after damage to these cells. If damage is not persistent, the levels peak at 18 hours after injury and will return to normal in 2 to 3 days.

To test specifically for myocardial muscle injury, electrophoresis on the total CPK is performed to detect the three CPK isoenzymes: CPK-BB (CPK_1), CPK-MB (CPK_2), and CPK-MM (CPK_3). The CPK-MB isoenzyme portion appears to be specific for myocardial cells. These serum CPK levels rise 3 to 6 hours after infarction occurs. Assuming no further myocardial damage, the level peaks at 12 to 24 hours and returns to normal 12 to 48 hours after infarction. CPK-MB levels do not usually rise with chest pain caused by angina, pulmonary embolism, or congestive heart failure.

The CPK-MB isoenzyme level is helpful in both quantifying the degree of myocardial infarction and also in timing the onset of infarction. With the more frequent use of thrombolytic therapy for myocardial infarction, the CPK-MB isoenzyme is often used to determine appropriateness of thrombolytic therapy. High levels of CPK-MB would suggest that significant infarction has already occurred, thereby precluding the benefit of thrombolytic therapy.

Because the CPK-BB isoenzyme is predominantly found in the brain and lung, injury to either of these organs (e.g., cerebrovascular accident, pulmonary infarction) will be associated with elevated levels of this isoenzyme.

The CPK-MM isoenzyme normally comprises almost all the circulatory CPK enzymes in healthy people. When the total CPK level is elevated as a result of increases in CPK-MM, there is injury or stress to the skeletal muscle. Examples of this include myopathies, vigorous exercise, multiple IM injections, electroconvulsive therapy, cardioversion, chronic alcoholism, or surgery.

CPK is the main cardiac enzyme studied in patients with heart disease. Because its blood clearance and metabolism are well known, its frequent determination can accurately reflect timing, quantity, and resolution of a myocardial infarction. Lactic dehydrogenase (LDH, see p. 450) and aspartate aminotransferase (AST, see p. 78) are also important enzymes used to confirm a myocardial infarction.

Interfering factors

- IM injections can cause elevated CPK levels.
- Drugs that may cause increased levels include amphotericin B, ampicillin, some anesthetics, anticoagulants, aspirin, clofibrate, dexamethasone (Decadron), furosemide (Lasix), and morphine.
- Strenuous exercise and recent surgery may cause increased levels.
- Early pregnancy may produce decreased levels.

Procedure and patient care
Before

- Explain the procedure to the patient.
- Discuss with the patient the need and reason for frequent venipuncture in diagnosing myocardial infarction.
- Avoid IM injections in patients with cardiac disease.
  These injections may falsely elevate the total CPK level.
- Tell the patient that no food or fluid restrictions are necessary.

During

- Collect a venous blood sample in a red-top tube. This is usually done daily for 3 days and then at 1 week.

- Rotate the venipuncture sites.
- Avoid hemolysis.
- Record the time and date of any IM injection that has been administered.
- Record the exact time and date of venipuncture on each laboratory slip. This aids in the interpretation of the temporal pattern of enzyme elevations.

After
- Apply pressure or a pressure dressing to the venipuncture site.
- Observe the venipuncture site for bleeding.

Abnormal findings

Increased levels of total CPK

Acute myocardial infarction
Acute cerebrovascular disease
Electric shock
Convulsions
Muscular dystrophy
Delirium tremens
Chronic alcoholism
Polymyositis
Hypokalemia
Central nervous system trauma
Pulmonary infarction
Dermatomyositis

Increased levels of CPK-MB isoenzyme

Acute myocardial infarction
Cardiac aneurysm surgery
Cardiac defibrillation
Malignant hyperthermia
Reye's syndrome
Muscular dystrophy
Cardiac ischemia
Myocarditis
Rhabdomyolysis

Increased levels of CPK-BB isoenzyme

Pulmonary infarction
Electroconvulsive therapy
Brain injury
Cerebrovascular accident (stroke)
Shock
Adenocarcinoma
Intestinal ischemia
Pulmonary embolism
Subarachnoid hemorrhage
Seizures
Brain cancer

Increased levels of CPK-MM isoenzyme

Muscular dystrophy
Myositis
Delirium tremens
Recent convulsions
Electroconvulsive therapy
Recent surgery
Electromyography
Hypokalemia
Hypothyroidism
IM injections
Crush injuries
Hemophilia

cryoglobulin

Type of test Blood

Normal findings No cryoglobulins detected

Test explanation and related physiology

Cryoglobulins are abnormal globulin protein complexes that exist within the blood of patients with various diseases. These proteins will precipitate at low temperatures and will redissolve with rewarming. These cryoglobulins can precipitate within the blood vessel of the fingers when exposed to cold temperatures. This precipitation causes sludging of the blood within those blood vessels. These patients may have symptoms of Raynaud's phenomenon (pain, cyanosis, coldness of the fingers).

These proteins exist in varying degrees depending on the disease entity with which they are associated. Serum levels greater than 5 mm are associated with multiple myeloma, macroglobulinemia, and leukemia. Globulin levels between 1 and 5 mm are associated with rheumatoid arthritis. Levels less than 1 mm can be associated with systemic lupus erythematosus, rheumatoid arthritis, infectious mononucleosis, viral hepatitis, endocarditis, cirrhosis, and glomerulonephritis.

For this test the blood sample is taken to the chemistry laboratory, where it is refrigerated for 72 hours. After that time the specimen is evaluated for precipitation. If precipitation is identified, it is measured and recorded. The tube is then rewarmed and the specimen reexamined for dissolution of that precipitation. If precipitation of the refrigerated specimen is identified and dissolved on rewarming, cryoglobulins are present.

Procedure and patient care

Before

- Explain the procedure to the patient.
- Inform the patient that an 8-hour fast may be required. This will minimize turbity of the serum caused by ingestion of a recent (especially fatty) meal. Turbity may make the detection of precipitation rather difficult.

During

- Collect 10 ml of venous blood in a red-top tube that has been prewarmed to body temperature.

After

- Apply pressure or a pressure dressing to the venipuncture site.
- Observe the venipuncture site for bleeding.
- If cyroglobulins are found to be present, warn the patient to avoid cold temperatures and contact with cold objects in order to minimize Raynaud's symptoms. Tell the patient to wear gloves in cold weather.

Abnormal findings

Multiple myeloma
Leukemia
Macroglobulinemia
Various connective tissue
  diseases (e.g., lupus ery-
  thematosus)

Infectious mononucleosis
Hepatitis
Endocarditis
Lymphomas and other ma-
  lignancies
Glomerulonephritis

Notes

crystals (Urinary crystals)

Type of test Urine

Normal findings Negative

Test explanation and physiology

Crystals found in the urine sediment on microscopic examination indicate that renal stone formation is imminent, if not already present. Urate crystals occur in patients with high serum uric acid levels (gout). Phosphate and calcium oxalate crystals occur in the urine of patients with hyperparathyroidism or malabsorption states. The type of crystal found varies with the disease and pH of the urine. For example, urate crystals form in acidic urine, and calcium oxalate crystals form in alkaline urine.

Interfering factors

- Radiographic dyes may cause precipitation of urinary crystals.
- Drugs that may cause increased levels of crystals include ampicillin and sulfonamides.

Procedure and patient care

Before

- Explain the procedure to the patient.

During

- Collect a fresh specimen of urine.

After

- Send the urine specimen immediately to the laboratory. Crystals are more likely to develop in urine that has been refrigerated or standing at room temperature.

Abnormal findings

Renal stone formation
Drug therapy
Urinary tract infection

Notes

culdoscopy

Type of test Endoscopy

Normal findings Normal-appearing female reproductive organs

Test explanation and related physiology

The pelvic organs can be directly visualized by placing a culdoscope (a lighted instrument similar to a cystoscope) through a small incision in the posterior vaginal vault and into the perineal space between the rectum and the uterus (cul-de-sac of Douglas). This procedure affords direct visualization of the uterus, fallopian tubes, ovaries, broad ligaments, uterosacral ligaments, rectal wall, and the sigmoid colon.

Culdoscopy is used in the evaluation of infertility because it can determine tubal abnormalities. It is also used in the detection of suspected ectopic pregnancy and in the study of unexplained pelvic pain or masses.

Culdoscopy has fallen out of favor since the introduction of laparoscopy. However, it may still be indicated for very obese women who desire tubal sterilization.

Contraindications

- Patients who are unable to assume the knee-chest position
- Patients with acute vulvar or vaginal infections
- Patients with acute peritonitis
- Patients with palpable masses in the cul-de-sac
- Patients with previous pelvic surgery causing adhesion of the bowel to the cul-de-sac

Potential complications

- Pelvic infection
- Pelvic hemorrhage
- Perforation of the rectum, bladder, or small intestines

Procedure and patient care

Before

- Explain the procedure to the patient.
- Ensure that an informed consent has been obtained.

- Keep the patient NPO after midnight on the day of the test.
- Depending on the physician's preference, prepare the patient for a possible enema, partial perineal shave, and/or vaginal douche.

C

During

- Note the following procedural steps:

    1. Culdoscopy is performed in the operating room with the patient in the knee-chest position.
    2. The head of the table is tilted downward to displace the bowel from the pelvis.
    3. Spinal or local anesthesia is used.
    4. A small incision is made in the posterior vaginal vault, and a culdoscope is passed into the cul-de-sac.
    5. The pelvic and abdominal organs are visualized and examined. After the study the scope is removed.
    6. No sutures are used to close the incision in the vaginal cuff.

- Note that this procedure is performed by a physician in approximately 1 hour.
- Tell the patient that women are usually very uncomfortable in the required knee-chest position for this procedure.

After

- Inform the patient that douching or intercourse is not permitted until the vaginal septum has healed. This takes approximately 1 to 2 weeks.
- Encourage the patient to take sitz baths for several days after the procedure.
- Inform the patient that mild oral analgesics may be taken for discomfort.
- Observe for signs and symptoms of infection (elevated temperature, flush, chills). Report these to the physician.
- Check the patient's vital signs for any indication of hemorrhage (e.g., a decrease in blood pressure, an increase in pulse).

Abnormal findings

Tubal abnormalities
Ectopic pregnancy
Pelvic mass

cystography (Cystourethrography, Voiding cystography, Voiding cystourethrography)

Type of test X-ray with contrast dye

Normal findings Normal bladder structure and function

Test explanation and related physiology

Filling the bladder with radiopaque contrast material provides visualization of the bladder for radiographic study. Either fluoroscopic or x-ray films demonstrate bladder filling and collapse after emptying. Filling defects or shadows within the bladder indicate primary bladder tumors. Extrinsic compression or distortion of the bladder is seen with pelvic tumor (e.g., rectal, cervical) or hematoma (secondary to pelvic bone fractures). Extravasation of the dye is seen with traumatic rupture or perforation of the bladder. Vesicoureteral reflux (abnormal backflow of urine from bladder to ureters), which can cause persistent or recurrent pyelonephritis, may also be demonstrated during cystography. Although the bladder is visualized during an intravenous pyelogram (IVP, see p. 432), primary pathologic bladder conditions are best studied by cystography.

Contraindications

■ Patients with urethral or bladder infection or injury

Potential complications

■ Urinary tract infection
  This may result from catheter placement or from the instillation of contaminated contrast material.
■ Allergic reaction to iodinated dye
  This rarely occurs because the dye is not administered intravenously.

Procedure and patient care

Before

■ Explain the procedure to the patient.
■ Obtain informed consent if required by the institution.
■ Give clear liquids for breakfast on the morning of the test.

- Assure the patient that he or she will be draped to prevent unnecessary exposure.
- Insert a Foley catheter if ordered.

During

- Note the following procedural steps:
    1. The patient is taken to the radiology department and placed in a supine or lithotomy position.
    2. Unless the catheter is already present, one is placed.
    3. Through the catheter, approximately 300 ml of air or radiopaque dye (much less for children) is injected into the bladder.
    4. The catheter is clamped.
    5. X-ray films are taken.
    6. If the patient is able to void, the catheter is removed and the patient is asked to urinate while films are taken of the bladder and urethra (voiding cystourethrogram).

- Ensure that males wear a lead shield over the testes to prevent irradiation of the gonads.
- Remember that female patients cannot be shielded without blocking bladder visualization.
- Note that a radiologist performs the study in approximately 15 to 30 minutes.
- Tell the patient that this test is moderately uncomfortable if bladder catheterization is required.

After

- Assess the patient for signs of urinary tract infection.
- Encourage the patient to drink fluids to eliminate the dye and to prevent accumulation of bacteria.

Abnormal findings

Bladder tumors
Pelvic tumors
Hematomas

Bladder trauma
Vesicoureteral reflux

Notes

cystometry (Cystometrogram [CMG])

Type of test Manometric

Normal findings

Normal sensations of fullness and temperature
Normal pressures and volumes
Maximal cystometric capacity: male, 350-750 ml
female, 250-550 ml
Intravesical pressure when bladder is empty: usually <40 cm H_2O
Detrusor pressure: <10 cm H_2O

Test explanation and related physiology

The purpose of cystometry is to evaluate the motor and sensory function of the bladder when incontinence is present or when neurologic bladder dysfunction is suspected. A graphic recording of pressure exerted at varying phases of the filling of the urinary bladder is produced. A pressure/volume relationship of the bladder is made. This urodynamic study assesses the neuromuscular function of the bladder by measuring the efficiency of the detrusor muscle, intravesical pressure and capacity, and the bladder's response to thermal stimulation.

Cystometry can determine whether bladder pathology is caused by neurologic, infectious, or obstructive diseases. Cystometry is indicated to elucidate the causes for frequency and urgency, especially before surgery on the urologic outflow tract. Cystometry is also part of the evaluation for the following: incontinence, persistent residual urine, vesicoureteral reflux, neurologic disorders, sensory disorders, and the effect of certain drugs on bladder function.

Contraindications

- Urinary tract infections, because of the possibility of false results and the potential for the spread of infection

Procedure and patient care

Before

- Explain the purpose and the procedure to the patient.
- Tell the patient that no fluid or food restrictions are needed.

- Assure the patient that he or she will be draped to prevent unnecessary exposure.
- Assess the patient for signs and symptoms of urinary tract infection.
- Instruct the patient not to strain while voiding because the results can be skewed.
- If the patient has a spinal cord injury, transport him or her on a stretcher. The test will then be performed with the patient on the stretcher.

During

- Note the following procedural steps:

  1. Cystometry, usually performed in a urologist's office or in a special procedure room, begins with the patient being asked to void.
  2. The amount of time required to initiate voiding and the size, force, and continuity of the urinary stream are recorded. The amount of urine, the time of voiding, and the presence of any straining, hesitancy, and terminal urine dribbling are also recorded.
  3. The patient is placed in a lithotomy or supine position.
  4. A retention catheter is inserted through the urethra and into the bladder.
  5. Residual urine volume is measured and recorded.
  6. Thermal sensation is evaluated by the instillation of approximately 30 ml of room-temperature saline solution into the bladder, followed by an equal amount of warm water. The patient reports any sensations.
  7. This fluid is withdrawn from the bladder.
  8. The urethral catheter is connected to a cystometer (a tube used to monitor bladder pressure).
  9. Sterile water, normal saline solution, or carbon dioxide gas is slowly introduced into the bladder at a controlled rate, usually with the patient in a sitting position.
  10. Patients are asked to indicate the first urge to void and then when they have the feeling that they must void. The bladder is full at this point.
  11. The pressures and volumes are plotted on a graph.
  12. The patient is asked to void, and a maximal intravesical voiding pressure is recorded.
  13. The bladder is drained for any residual urine.

14. If no additional studies are to be done, the urethral catheter is removed.

- Throughout the study, ask the patient to report any sensations, such as pain, flushing, sweating, nausea, bladder filling, and an urgency to void.
- Note that certain drugs may be administered during the cystometric examination to distinguish between underactivity of the bladder because of muscle failure and underactivity associated with denervation. Cholinergic drugs (e.g., bethanechol [Urecholine]) may be given to enhance the tone of a flaccid bladder. Anticholinergic drugs (e.g., atropine) may be given to promote relaxation of a hyperactive bladder. If these drugs are to be given, the catheter is left in place. The drugs are given, and the examination is repeated 20 to 30 minutes later, using the first test as a control value.
- Note that this test is performed by a urologist in approximately 45 minutes.
- Explain to the patient that the discomfort is that associated with the urethral catheterization.

After

- Observe the patient for any manifestations of infection (e.g., elevated temperature, chills).
- Examine the urine for hematuria. Notify the physician if the hematuria persists after several voidings.
- Provide a warm sitz bath or tub bath for the patient's comfort, if desired.

Abnormal findings

Neurogenic bladder
Bladder obstruction
Bladder infections

Bladder hypertonicity
Diminished bladder capacity

Notes

cystoscopy (Endourology)

Type of test Endoscopy

Normal findings Normal structure and function of the urethra, bladder, ureters, and prostate (in males)

Test explanation and related physiology

Cystoscopy provides direct visualization of the urethra and bladder through the transurethral insertion of a cystoscope into the bladder. Cystoscopy is used *diagnostically* to allow:

1. Direct inspection and biopsy of the prostate, bladder, and urethra
2. Collection of a separate urine specimen directly from each kidney by the placement of ureteral catheters
3. Measurement of bladder capacity and determination of ureteral reflux
4. Identification of bladder and ureteral calculi
5. Placement of ureteral catheters for retrograde pyelography (see p. 646)
6. Identification of the source of hematuria

Cystoscopy is used *therapeutically* to provide:

1. Resection of small, superficial bladder tumors
2. Removal of foreign bodies and stones
3. Dilation of the urethra and ureters
4. Placement of catheters to drain urine from the renal pelvis
5. Coagulation of bleeding areas
6. Implantation of radium seeds into a tumor
7. Resection of hypertrophied or malignant prostate gland overgrowth

The cystoscope consists primarily of an obturator and a telescope. The obturator is used to insert the cystoscope atraumatically. After the cystoscope is within the bladder, the obturator is removed and the telescope is passed through the cystoscope. The lens and lighting system of the telescope permit adequate visualization of the lower genitourinary tract. Transcopic instruments, such as forceps, scissors, needles, and electrodes, are used when appropriate.

Endourology is an endoscopic procedure that allows for visualization of the bladder and urethra. It is more comprehensive than cystoscopy because it includes a detailed visualization of the urethra. This test is important in the evaluation of hematuria, chronic infection, suspected stones, and radiographic filling defects. On inspection the urethra may show inflammation or structural causes of obstruction (e.g., stricture, neoplasia, prostatic hypertrophy). If the obstruction is functional rather than structural (e.g., detrusor–bladder neck dyssynergia), no site of obstruction will be demonstrated by endoscopy.

Potential complications

- Perforation of the bladder
- Sepsis by seeding the bloodstream with bacteria from infected urine
- Hematuria
- Urinary retention

Procedure and patient care

Before

- Explain the procedure to the patient.
- Ensure that an informed consent is obtained.
- If enemas are ordered to clear the bowel, assist the patient as needed and record the results.
- Encourage the patient to drink fluids several hours before the procedure to maintain a continuous flow of urine for collection and to prevent multiplication of bacteria that may be introduced during this technique.
- If the procedure will be done with the patient under local anesthesia, allow a liquid breakfast.
- If the procedure will be performed with the patient under general anesthesia, follow the routine precautions. Keep the patient NPO after midnight on the day of the test. Fluids may be given intravenously.
- Administer the preprocedural medications as ordered, 1 hour before the study. Sedatives decrease the spasm of the bladder sphincter, thus decreasing the patient's discomfort.

During

- Note the following procedural steps:

  1. Cytoscopy is usually performed in the operating room but can also be done in the urologist's office.
  2. The patient is placed in the lithotomy position with his or her feet in stirrups.
  3. The external genitalia are cleansed with an antiseptic solution such as providone-iodine (Betadine).
  4. A local anesthetic is instilled into the urethra, if general anesthesia has not been used.
  5. The cystoscope is inserted, and the desired diagnostic or therapeutic studies are performed.

- Instruct the patient to lie very still during the entire procedure to prevent trauma to the urinary tract.
- Tell the patient that he or she will have the desire to void as the cystoscope passes the bladder neck.
- When the procedure is completed, keep the patient on bed rest for a short time.
- Note that if *endourology* is performed, the urethra will also be evaluated.
- Note that this procedure is performed by a urologist in approximately 25 minutes.
- When local anesthesia is used, inform the patient of the associated discomfort (much more than with urethral catheterization).

After

- Instruct the patient not to walk or stand alone immediately after the legs have been removed from the stirrups. The orthostasis that may result from standing erect may cause dizziness and fainting.
- Assess the patient's ability to void for at least 24 hours after the procedure. Urinary retention may be secondary to edema caused by instrumentation.
- Note the urine color. Pink-tinged urine is common. The presence of bright-red blood or clots should be reported to the physician.
- Monitor for complaints of back pain, bladder spasms, urinary frequency, and burning on urination. Warm sitz baths and mild analgesics may be ordered and given. Sometimes belladonna and opium (B&O) suppositories are given to relieve bladder spasms. Warm, moist heat to

the lower abdomen may help relieve pain and promote muscle relaxation.

- Encourage increased intake of fluids. A dilute urine decreases dysuria. Fluids also maintain a constant flow of urine to prevent stasis and the accumulation of bacteria in the bladder.
- Check and record the patient's vital signs as ordered. Watch for a decrease in blood pressure and an increase in pulse as an indication of hemorrhage.
- Observe for signs and symptoms of sepsis (elevated temperature, flush, chills, decreased blood pressure, increased pulse).
- Note that occasionally, antibiotics are ordered 1 day before and 3 days following the procedure to reduce the incidence of bacteremia that may occur with instrumentation of the urethra and bladder.
- Encourage the patient to use cathartics, especially after cystoscopic surgery. Increases in intraabdominal pressure caused by constipation may initiate severe lower urologic bleeding.

Abnormal findings

Tumors
Stones
Prostatic hyperplasia
Inflammation
Urethral/ureteral stricture
Prostatitis
Vesical neck contracture

Notes

cytomegalovirus (CMV)

Type of test Blood

Normal findings No virus isolated

Test explanation and related physiology

CMV is the most common of the congenital infections. Approximately 10% of infected newborns exhibit permanent damage, usually mental retardation and auditory damage. Fetal infection can cause microcephaly, hydrocephaly, cerebral palsy, mental retardation, or death. No specific therapy is known for this infection. If the diagnosis is established early by viral culture or serology, abortion may be an option. A fourfold increase in CMV titer in paired sera drawn 10 to 14 days apart is usually indicative of an acute infection.

Procedure and patient care

Before

- Explain the procedure to the patient.

During

- Collect a specimen from the mother with suspected acute infection as early as possible.
- Collect the convalescent specimen 2 to 4 weeks later.
- Collect the blood in a vacutainer indicated by the specific laboratory.

After

- Apply pressure or a pressure dressing to the venipuncture site.
- Assess the venipuncture site for bleeding.

Abnormal finding

CMV infection

Notes

delta-aminolevulinic acid (Delta-ALA, Aminolevulinic acid [ALA])

Type of test Urine (24 hour)

Normal findings 1-7 mg/24 hr or 11.1-57.2 μmol/24 hr (SI units)

Possible critical values >20 mg/24 hr

Test explanation and related physiology

Delta-ALA, the basic precursor for the porphyrins (see p. 573), is an enzyme needed for the normal conversion to porphobilinogen during heme synthesis. Impaired conversion, which causes abnormal red blood cell (RBC) formation, occurs in lead intoxication and in porphyrias. These conditions cause the urine levels of ALA to rise before other chemical or hematologic changes.

Urine levels of ALA are obtained to screen for lead poisoning and to aid in the diagnosis of certain types of genetic deficiencies of porphyrin metabolism. Elevated levels may also be seen in patients with hepatitis and hepatic carcinoma.

Healthy people usually do not have ALA present in their urine. However, increased values may be seen in patients taking some medications (e.g., penicillin, barbiturates, griseofulvin).

Interfering factors

- Drugs that may cause increased ALA levels include penicillin, barbiturates, and griseofulvin.

Procedure and patient care

Before

- Explain the procedure to the patient.

During

- Instruct the patient to begin a 24-hour urine collection after voiding. Discard the initial specimen and start the 24-hour timing at that point.
- Collect all urine passed during the next 24 hours.
- Show the patient where to store the urine container.

- Keep the specimen on ice or refrigerated during the 24 hours.
- Keep the urine in a light-resistant container with a preservative.
- Indicate the starting time on the urine container and on the laboratory slip.
- Post the hours for the urine collection in a noticeable place to prevent accidental discarding of the specimen.
- Instruct the patient to void before defecating so that urine is not contaminated by feces.
- Remind the patient not to put toilet paper in the collection container.
- Encourage the patient to drink fluids during the 24 hours unless this is contraindicated for medical purposes.
- Collect the last specimen as close as possible to the end of the 24-hour period. Add this to the urine collection.
- If the patient has a Foley catheter in place, cover the drainage bag to prevent exposure to light.
- Indicate on the laboratory slip any drugs that can affect test results.

After

- Transport the urine specimen promptly to the laboratory.

Abnormal findings
Increased levels

Porphyrias
Lead intoxication

Hepatitis
Hepatic carcinoma

Notes

dexamethasone suppression test (DST, Prolonged/rapid DST, Cortisol suppression test, ACTH suppression test)

Type of test   Blood; urine (24 hour)

Normal findings

Prolonged method
Expected values (normal)
   Low dose: >50% reduction of plasma cortisol and 17-
      hydroxycorticosteroid (17-OCHS) levels
   High dose: >50% reduction of plasma cortisol and 17-
      OCHS levels
Cushing's syndrome caused by:
   Bilateral adrenal hyperplasia
      Low dose: no change
      High dose: >50% reduction of plasma cortisol and
         17-OCHS levels
   Adrenal adenoma or carcinoma
      Low dose: no change
      High dose: no change
   Ectopic ACTH-producing tumor
      Low dose: no change
      High dose: no change
Rapid method
Normal: nearly 0 cortisol levels

Test explanation and related physiology

The DST is an important test for diagnosing adrenal hyperfunction (Cushing's syndrome) and distinguishing its
cause. This test is based on pituitary adrenocorticotropic
hormone (ACTH) secretion being dependent on plasma
cortisol levels. As plasma cortisol levels increase, ACTH secretion is suppressed; as cortisol levels decrease, ACTH secretion is stimulated. Dexamethasone is a synthetic steroid
(similar to cortisol) that will suppress ACTH secretion. Under normal circumstances this will result in reduced stimulation to the adrenal glands and ultimately a drop of 50% or
more in plasma cortisol and 17-OCHS levels. This important feedback system does not function properly in patients
with Cushing's syndrome.

In Cushing's syndrome caused by bilateral adrenal hyperplasia, the pituitary gland is reset upward and responds only to high plasma levels of cortisone and steroids. Also, in Cushing's syndrome caused by adrenal adenoma or cancer, which acts autonomously, cortisol secretion will continue despite a decrease in ACTH. Finally, when Cushing's syndrome is caused by an ectopic ACTH-producing tumor (as in lung cancer), that tumor is also considered autonomous and will continue to secrete ACTH despite high cortisol levels. Again, no decrease occurs in plasma cortisol. Knowledge of these defects in the normal cortisol-ACTH feedback system is the basis for understanding the DST.

The DST may also identify depressed persons likely to respond to electroconvulsive therapy or antidepressants rather than to psychological or social interventions. ACTH production will not be suppressed after administration of low-dose dexamethasone in these patients.

The *prolonged* DST can be performed over a 6-day period on an outpatient basis. The *rapid* DST is easily and quickly performed and is used primarily as a screening test to diagnose Cushing's syndrome. It is less accurate and less informative than the prolonged DST, but when its results are normal, the diagnosis of Cushing's syndrome can safely be excluded. The ease with which the rapid DST can be performed makes it useful in clinical medicine.

Interfering factors

- Stress can cause ACTH release and obscure interpretation of test results.
- Drugs that can affect test results include barbiturates, estrogens, oral contraceptives, phenytoin (Dilantin), spironolactone (Aldactone), steroids, and tetracyclines.

Procedure and patient care

Before

- Explain the procedure (prolonged or rapid test) to the patient.
- Obtain the patient's weight as a baseline for evaluating side effects of steroids.

During

Prolonged test

- Obtain a baseline 24-hour urine collection for corticosteroids (urine 17-OCHS [see p. 419] or urinary cortisol[see p. 239]).

- Collect blood for determination of baseline plasma cortisol levels (see p. 237), if indicated.
- Collect 24-hour urine specimens daily over a 6-day period. Since 6 continuous days of urine collections are needed, no urine specimens are discarded except for the first voided specimen on day 1, after which the collection begins.
- On day 3, administer a low dose (0.5 mg) of dexamethasone by mouth every 6 hours for a total of 2 mg.
- On day 5, administer a high dose (2.0 mg) of dexamethasone by mouth every 6 hours for a total of 8 mg.
- Administer the dexamethasone with milk or an antacid to prevent gastric irritation.
- Remember that the urine samples for cortisol and 17-OCHS do not need a preservative.
- Note that the creatinine content is measured in all the 24-hour urine collections to demonstrate their accuracy and adequacy.
- Keep the urine specimens refrigerated or on ice during the collection period.

Rapid test
- Give the patient 1 mg of dexamethasone by mouth at 11 PM.
- Administer the dexamethasone with milk or an antacid to prevent gastric irritation.
- If ordered, administer a barbiturate to sedate the patient and to ensure a good night's sleep.
- At 8 AM the next morning, draw blood for determination of plasma cortisol level before the patient arises.
- If no cortisol suppression occurs after 1 mg of dexamethasone, administer a higher dose (8 mg) to suppress ACTH production. This is referred to as the *overnight 8 mg dexamethasone suppression test*.

After
- Evaluate the patient for evidence of gastric irritation.
- Assess the patient for steroid-induced side effects by monitoring weight, glucose levels, and potassium levels.
- Send specimens to the laboratory promptly.

Abnormal findings

Adrenal hyperfunction (Cushing's syndrome)
Hyperthyroidism
Mental depression

Notes

digital subtraction angiography (DSA, Digital venous subtraction angiography [DVSA], Digital radiography)

Type of test   X-ray with contrast dye

Normal findings   Normal arterial vasculature

Test explanation and related physiology

DSA is a sophisticated type of computerized fluoroscopy that can use venous or arterial catheterization to visualize the arteries of the body, especially the carotid and cerebral arteries. This procedure enables small differences in x-ray absorption between an artery and the surrounding tissue to be converted to digital information and stored. DSA is especially useful when adjacent bone inhibits visualization of the blood vessel to be evaluated. This study is particularly valuable in the preoperative and postoperative evaluation of patients with obliterative vascular disease or a central nervous system tumor. It is also used to identify suspected arterial aneurysms and other vascular malformations.

For DSA an image "mask" is made of the area of clinical interest and then stored in the computer. After the IV or intraarterial injection of the contrast material, subsequent images are made. The computer than subtracts the preinjection "mask" image from the postinjection image. This removes all undesired images (e.g., bone) and leaves an arterial image of high contrast and quality. If venous injection of dye is used rather than arterial injection for this procedure, the complications and risks associated with conventional arteriography are avoided. However, DSA is more often performed via an arterial injection of contrast material.

Contraindications

- Patients with allergies to shellfish or iodinated dye
- Patients who are uncooperative or agitated
- Patients who are pregnant
- Patients with renal disorders
- Patients with bleeding disorders
- Patients with unstable cardiac disorders

Potential complications

- Allergic reaction to iodinated dye
  Allergic reactions may vary from mild flushing, itching,

and urticaria to severe, life-threatening anaphylaxis (evidenced by respiratory distress, drop in blood pressure, shock). In the unusual event of anaphylaxis the patient may be treated with diphenhydramine (Benadryl), steroids, and epinephrine. Oxygen and endotracheal equipment should be on hand for immediate use.

- Thrombosis
- Infection

Procedure and patient care
Before

- Explain the procedure to the patient.
- Ensure that written and informed consent for this procedure is in the patient's chart.
- Instruct patients that they must be able to hold their breath and remain very still during the test. Movement, including swallowing, may cause blurred images.
- Inform the patient that a warm flush may be felt when the dye is injected.
- Assess the patient for allergies to iodinated dye.
- Inform the radiologist if an allergy to iodinated contrast is suspected. The radiologist may prescribe a Benadryl and steroid preparation to be administered before testing. Usually a hypoallergenic, non-ionic contrast will be used during the test.
- Determine if the patient has been taking anticoagulants.
- Keep the patient NPO for the designated time before the test, usually 2 hours.

During

- In the angiography room, place the patient on an x-ray table in a supine position.
- Note the following procedural steps:

  1. The area over the desired vein (e.g., basilic, femoral) or artery (e.g., brachial, femoral) is prepared and draped in a sterile manner.
  2. A local anesthetic is used, and a catheter is inserted.
  3. The contrast medium is administered by mechanized injector at a controlled rate.
  4. The process is observed by fluoroscopy and displayed by the computer after converting the image to a digital form.

5. As soon as the vessel being studied has been defined, the catheter is removed.
6. A bandage is placed over the vascular insertion site. Pressure is applied for several minutes (longer for arterial punctures).

- Note that this procedure is usually performed by an angiographer in less than 1 hour.
- During the dye injection, remind the patient that a burning flush may be felt.
- Tell the patient that the only other discomfort associated with this study is the puncture for vascular access.

After

- Monitor the patient's vital signs for the designated interval.
- Observe the puncture site for hematoma, hemorrhage, or infection.
- Encourage the patient to drink fluids to aid excretion of the iodine contrast material. The contrast dye also acts as a diuretic.
- Evaluate the patient for delayed reaction to the dye (dyspnea, rashes, tachycardia, hives). This usually occurs 2 to 6 hours after the test. Treat with antihistamines and steroids.

Abnormal findings

Arterial stenosis
Aneurysm
Tumor and other masses
Arterial occlusion
Cerebrovascular accident
  (stroke)

Meningioma
Pheochromocytoma
Emboli

Notes

disseminated intravascular coagulation screening (DIC screening)

Type of test Refer to specific tests in Table 7.

Normal findings No evidence of DIC

Text explanation and related physiology

DIC screening is a group of tests used to detect disseminated intravascular coagulation. Many pathologic conditions can instigate or are associated with DIC. The more common ones include bacterial septicemia, amniotic fluid embolism, retention of a dead fetus, malignant neoplasia, liver cirrhosis, extensive surgery (especially on the liver), postextracorporeal heart bypass, extensive trauma, severe burns, and transfusion reactions.

In DIC the entire clotting mechanism is triggered inappropriately. This results in significant systemic or localized intravascular formation of fibrin clots. Consequences of this futile clotting are intravascular sludging and excessive bleed-

TABLE 7 Disseminated intravascular coagulation (DIC) screening tests

Test	Positive result
Bleeding time (p. 98)	Prolonged
Platelet count (p. 563)	Decreased
Prothrombin time (p. 600)	Prolonged
Activated partial thromboplastin time (p. 544)	Prolonged
Fibrinogen (factor I concentration) (p. 351)	Decreased
Fibrin degradation products (p. 349)	Present
RBC smear (p. 109)	Damaged RBCs and decreased number of platelets
Euglobulin lysis time (p. 328)	Normal or prolonged

ing caused by consumption of the platelets and clotting factors that have been used in intravascular clotting. The fibrinolytic system is also activated to break down the fibrin involved in the intravascular coagulation. This results in fibrin degradation products (FDPs), which by themselves act as anticoagulants. These FDPs only serve to enhance the bleeding tendency.

Organ injury can occur as a result of the intravascular clots, which cause microvascular occlusion in various organs. This may cause serious anoxic injury in affected organs. Also, red blood cells (RBCs) passing through partly plugged vessels are injured and subsequently hemolyzed. The result may be ongoing hemolytic anemia. Figure 5 provides a summary of DIC pathophysiology and effects. Heparin is sometimes used to treat DIC because it inhibits the ongoing futile

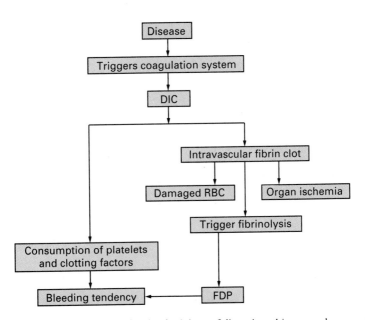

Figure 5 Illustration of pathophysiology of disseminated intravascular coagulation (DIC), which may result in bleeding tendency, organ ischemia, and hemolytic anemia. **RBC**, Red blood cell; **FDP**, fibrin degradation product.

thrombin formation. This decreases the use of clotting factors and platelets, and bleeding ceases.

When a patient with a bleeding tendency is suspected to have DIC, a series of readily performed laboratory tests should be performed (Table 7). With these tests the hematologist can make the appropriate diagnosis confidently. All these tests are discussed separately.

Notes

Doppler studies

Type of test Ultrasound

Normal findings

Venous

A normal Doppler venous signal with spontaneous respiration

Normal venous system without evidence of occlusion

Arterial

Normal arterial Doppler signal with systolic and diastolic components

No reduction in blood pressure in excess of 20 mm Hg compared to the normal extremity

A normal ankle-to-brachial arterial blood pressure index of 0.85 or greater

No evidence of arterial occlusion

Test explanation and related physiology

Doppler studies are used to identify occlusion of the veins or arteries. *Venous* patency is demonstrated through Doppler ultrasound by detecting moving red blood cells (RBCs) within the vein. The Doppler transducer directs an ultrasound beam at the vein. Moving RBCs reflect the beam back to the transducer, which then transforms the flow velocity into a "swishing" noise that is augmented by an audio speaker. If the vein is occluded, no swishing sounds are detected.

With *arterial* Doppler studies, one can identify and locate peripheral arteriosclerotic occlusive disease. By slowly deflating blood pressure cuffs placed on the calf and ankle, the systolic pressure in the various arteries of the extremities can be accurately measured by detecting the first evidence of blood flow with the Doppler transducer. The extremely sensitive Doppler ultrasound detector can recognize the "swishing" sound of even the most minimal blood flow. Normally, there is a minimal drop in systolic blood pressure from the arteries of the arms to those of the legs. If the drop of blood pressure exceeds 20 mm Hg, occlusive disease is believed to exist immediately proximal to the area tested.

Interfering factors

- Venous or arterial occlusive disease proximal to the site of testing
- Cigarette smoking, because nicotine can cause constriction of the peripheral arteries and alter the results

Procedure and patient care

Before

- Explain the procedure to the patient.
- Inform the patient that this is a painless procedure.
- Remove all clothing from the extremity to be examined.
- Instruct the patient to abstain from cigarette smoking for at least 30 minutes before the test.

During

- Note the following procedural steps:

Venous Doppler studies

1. A conductive gel is applied to the skin overlaying the venous system of the extremity in multiple areas.
2. Usually, for the lower extremity, the deep venous system is identified in the ankle, calf, thigh, and groin.
3. The characteristic "swishing" sound of the Doppler indicates a patent venous system. Failure to detect this signal indicates venous occlusion.
4. Usually, both the superficial and venous systems are evaluated.

Arterial Doppler studies

1. These are performed with the use of blood pressure cuffs, which are placed around the thigh, calf, and ankle.
2. A conductive paste is applied to the skin overlying the artery distal to the cuffs.
3. The proximal cuff is inflated to a level above systolic blood pressure in the normal extremity.
4. The Doppler ultrasound transducer is placed immediately distal to the inflated cuff.
5. The pressure in the cuff is slowly released.
6. The highest pressure at which the blood flow is detected by the characteristic "swishing" Doppler signal is recorded as the blood pressure of that artery.
7. The test is repeated at each successive level.
8. The ankle pressure is divided by the arm (brachial artery) pressure. This is known as the *AB index*. If the

AB index is less than 0.85, significant arterial occlusive disease exists within the extremity.

- Note that these studies are usually performed in the vascular laboratory or the radiology department and take approximately 30 minutes.

After
- Encourage the patient to verbalize his or her fears in terms of test results.
- Remove the transducer gel from the extremity.
- Inform the patient that the physician must interpret the studies and that results will be available in a few hours.

Abnormal findings

Venous occlusion, secondary to thrombosis or thrombo-phlebitis

Small or large vessel arterial occlusive disease

Spastic arterial disease (e.g., Raynaud's phenomenon)

Small vessel arterial occlusive disease (as in diabetes)

Embolic arterial occlusion

Notes

echocardiography (Cardiac echo and heart sonogram)

Type of test Ultrasound

Normal findings

Normal position, size, and movement of the cardiac valves and heart muscle wall

Normal directional flow of blood within the heart chambers

Test explanation and related physiology

Echocardiography is a noninvasive ultrasound procedure used to evaluate the structure and function of the heart. In diagnostic ultrasonography a harmless high-frequency sound wave emitted from a transducer penetrates the heart. Sound waves are bounced off the heart structures and reflected back to the transducer as a series of echoes. These echoes are amplified and displayed on an oscilloscope. Tracings can also be recorded on moving graph paper or on videotape. The study usually includes M-mode recordings, two-dimensional (2-D) recordings, and a Doppler study.

The *M-mode echocardiography* is a linear tracing of the motion of the heart structures over time. This allows the various cardiac structures to be located and studied as to their movement during a cardiac cycle.

Two-D echocardiography angles a beam within one sector of the heart. This produces a picture of the spatial anatomic relationships within the heart.

A recent addition has been *color Doppler echocardiography*. This test detects the pattern of the blood flow and measures changes in velocity of blood flow within the heart and great vessels. These variations in blood flow and velocity alter the ultrasound frequency. By assigning computerized weighted numbers to these altered frequencies, one is able to map and determine origins of velocity changes and blood turbulence. Turbulent blood or altered velocity and direction of blood flow can then be identified by changes in color. This is seen in a photograph. In most Doppler ultrasound color flow imaging, the colors blue and red represent the direction of a given stream of blood. The various hues from dull to bright represent varying blood velocities. The most useful application of the color flow imaging is in determining the direction and turbulence of blood flow across regurgitant or narrowed valves. Doppler color flow imaging may also be helpful in assessing proper functioning of prosthetic valves.

Echocardiography, in general, is used in the diagnosis of a pericardial effusion, valvular heart disease (e.g., mitral valve prolapse, stenosis, regurgitation), subaortic stenosis, myocardial wall abnormalities (e.g., cardiomyopathy), infarction, and aneurysm. Cardiac tumors (e.g., myxomas) are easily diagnosed with ultrasound. Atrial and ventricular septal defects and other congenital heart diseases are also recognized by ultrasound. Finally, postinfarction mural thrombi are readily apparent with this testing.

Contraindications

- Patients who are uncooperative

Interfering factors

- Chronic obstructive pulmonary disease (COPD)
  Patients who have severe COPD have a significant amount of air and space between the heart and the chest cavity. Air space does not conduct ultrasound waves well.
- Obesity
  In obese patients the space between the heart and the transducer is greatly enlarged, and therefore accuracy of the test is decreased.

Procedure and patient care

Before

- Assure the patient that this is a painless study.
- Complete the request for the echocardiogram, including the pertinent patient history.

During

- Note the following procedural steps:
  1. The patient is placed in the supine position.
  2. Electrocardiographic (EKG) leads are placed (see EKG study).
  3. A gel, which allows better transmission of sound waves, is placed on the chest wall immediately under the transducer.
  4. Ultrasound is directed to the heart, and appropriate tracings are obtained.

- Note that this procedure usually takes approximately 45 minutes and is performed by an ultrasound technician in a darkened room within the cardiac laboratory or radiology department.
- Tell the patient that no discomfort is associated with this study but that the transmission gel is usually cooler than body temperature.

After

- Remove the gel from the patient's chest wall.
- Inform the patient that the physician must interpret the study and that the results will be available in a few hours.

Abnormal findings

Valvular stenosis
Valvular regurgitation
Mitral valve prolapse
Pericardial effusion
Ventricular or atrial mural
   thrombi

Myxoma
Poor ventricular muscle
   motion
Septal defects

Notes

electrocardiography (Electrocardiogram [ECG, EKG])

Type of test Electrodiagnostic

Normal findings Normal heart rate (60-100 beats/min), rhythm, and wave deflections

Test explanation and related physiology

The EKG is a graphic representation of the electrical impulses that the heart generates during the cardiac cycle. The electrical impulses are conducted to the body's surface, where they are detected by electrodes placed on the patient's limbs and chest. These monitoring electrodes detect the electrical activity of the heart from a variety of spatial perspectives. The EKG lead system is composed of several electrodes, which are placed on each of the four extremities and at varying sites on the chest. Each combination of electrodes is called a *lead*.

A *12-lead EKG* provides a comprehensive view of the flow of the heart's electrical currents in two different planes. There are six limb leads (combination of electrodes on the extremities) and six chest leads (corresponding to six sites on the chest). Leads I, II, and III are considered the *standard* limb leads. Lead I records the difference in electrical potential between the left arm (LA) and the right arm (RA). Lead II records the electrical potential between the RA and the left leg (LL). Lead III reflects the difference between the LA and the LL. The right leg (RL) electrode is an inactive ground in all leads. There are three *augmented* limb leads: aV_R, aV_L, and aV_F (a, augmented; V, vector [unipolar]; R, right arm; L, left arm; F, left foot or leg). The augmented leads measure the electrode potential between the center of the heart and the right arm (aV_R), the left arm (aV_L), and the left leg (aV_F). The six standard chest, or "precordial," leads (V_1, V_2, V_3, V_4, V_5, V_6) are recorded by placing electrodes at six different positions on the chest, surrounding the heart.

EKGs are recorded on special paper with a graphic background of horizontal and vertical lines for rapid measurement of time intervals (X coordinate) and voltages (Y coordinate). Time duration is measured by vertical lines 1 mm apart, each representing 0.04 second. Voltage is measured by horizontal lines 1 mm apart. Five 1 mm squares are equal to 0.5 mV.

The normal EKG pattern is composed of waves arbitrarily designated by the letters P, Q, R, S, and T. The Q, R, and S waves are grouped together and described as the QRS complex. The significance of the waves and time intervals is as follows:

P wave. This represents atrial electrical depolarization associated with atrial contraction. It represents electrical activity associated with the spread of the original impulse from the sinoatrial (SA) node through the atria. If the P waves are absent or altered, the cardiac impulse originates outside the SA node.

P-R interval. This represents the time required for the impulse to travel from the SA node to the atrioventricular (AV) node. If this interval is prolonged, a conduction delay exists in the AV node (e.g., a first-degree heart block). If the P-R interval is shortened, the impulse must have reached the ventricle through a "shortcut" (as in Wolff-Parkinson-White syndrome).

QRS complex. This represents ventricular electrical depolarization associated with ventricular contraction. This complex consists of an initial downward (negative) deflection (Q wave), a large upward (positive) deflection (R wave), and a small downward deflection (S wave). A widened QRS complex indicates a abnormal or prolonged ventricular depolarization time (as in a bundle branch block).

ST segment. This represents the period between the completion of depolarization and the beginning of repolarization of the ventricular muscle. This segment may be elevated or depressed in transient muscle ischemia (e.g., angina) or in muscle injury (as in the early stages of myocardial infarction).

T wave. This represents ventricular repolarization (i.e., return to neutral electrical activity).

Through the analysis of these waveforms and time intervals, valuable information about the heart may be obtained. The EKG is used primarily to identify abnormal heart rhythms (arrhythmias, or dysrhythmias) and to diagnose acute myocardial infarction, conduction defects, and ventricular hypertrophy. It is important to note that the EKG may be normal, even in the presence of heart disease, if the heart disorder does not affect the electrical activity of the heart.

Interfering factors

- Inaccurate placement of the electrodes
- Electrolyte imbalances
- Poor contact between the skin and the electrodes
- Movement or muscle twitching during the test
- Drugs that can affect results include digitalis, quinidine, and barbiturates

Procedure and patient care

Before

- Explain the procedure to the patient.
- Tell the patient that no food or fluid restriction is necessary.
- Assure the patient that the flow of electric current is *from* the patient. He or she will feel nothing during this procedure.
- Expose only the patient's chest and arms. Keep the abdomen and thighs adequately covered.

During

- Note the following procedural steps:

  1. The skin areas designated for electrode placement are prepared by using alcohol swabs or sandpaper to remove skin oil or debris. Sometimes the skin is shaved if the patient has large amount of hair.
  2. Electrode paste is applied to ensure electrical conduction between the skin and the electrodes.
  3. The four limb leads are usually held in place by straps that encircle the extremity. Newer machines have clamps that can easily be opened and applied to the extremity.
  4. Many cardiologists recommend that arm electrodes be placed on the upper arm because fewer muscle tremors are detected there.
  5. The chest leads are applied either one at a time, three at a time, or six at a time, depending on the type of EKG machine.
     These leads are positioned as follows:
     V_1: in the fourth intercostal space (4ICS) at the right sternal border
     V_2: in 4ICS at the left sternal border
     V_3: midway between V_2 and V_4

V_4: in 5ICS at the midclavicular line

V_5: at the left anterior axillary line at the level of V_4 horizontally

V_6: at the left midaxillary line on the level of V_4 horizontally

- List medications the patient is taking on the EKG request form.
- Note that cardiac technicians, nurses, or physicians perform this procedure in less than 5 minutes at the bedside or in the cardiology clinic.
- Tell the patient that although this procedure carries no discomfort, he or she must lie still in the supine position without talking while the EKG is recorded.

After

- Remove the electrodes from the patient's skin and wipe off the electrode gel.
- Indicate on the EKG strip or request slip if the patient was experiencing chest pain during the study. The pain may be correlated to an arrhythmia on the EKG.

Abnormal findings

Arrhythmias (dysrhythmias)
Acute myocardial infarction
Conduction defects
Ventricular hypertrophy
Wolff-Parkinson-White
  syndrome

Conduction system diseases
Myocardial ischemia
Hypertrophy of the heart
Pulmonary infarction
Electrolyte imbalances
Pericarditis

Notes

electroencephalography (Electroencephalogram [EEG])

Type of test Electrodiagnostic

Normal findings Normal frequency, amplitude, and characteristics of brain waves

Test explanation and related physiology

The EEG is a graphic recording of the electrical activity of the brain. EEG electrodes are placed on the scalp over multiple areas of the brain to detect and record electrical impulses within the brain. This study is invaluable in the investigation of epileptic states, where the focus of seizure activity is characterized by rapid, spiking waves seen on the graph. Patients with cerebral lesions (e.g., tumors, infarctions) will have abnormally slow EEG waves, depending on the size and location of the lesion. Because this study determines the overall activity of the brain, it can be used to evaluate trauma and drug intoxication and also to determine cerebral death in comatose patients.

The EEG can also be used to monitor cerebral blood flow during surgical procedures. For example, during carotid endarterectomy, the carotid vessel must be temporarily occluded. When this surgery is performed with the patient under general anesthesia, the EEG can be used for the early detection of cerebral tissue ischemia, which would indicate that continued carotid occlusion will result in a cerebrovascular accident (CVA, stroke) syndrome. Temporary shunting of the blood during the surgery is then required.

Interfering factors

- Fasting may cause hypoglycemia, which could modify the EEG pattern.
- Drinks containing caffeine (e.g., coffee, tea, cocoa, cola) interfere with the test results.
- Body and eye movements during the test can cause changes in the brain wave patterns.
- Drugs that may affect test results include sedatives.

Procedure and patient care

Before

- Explain the procedure to the patient.
- Assure the patient that this test cannot "read the mind" or detect senility.
- Assure the patient that the flow of electrical activity is *from* the patient. He or she will not feel anything during the test.
- Instruct the patient to wash his or her hair the night before the test. No oils, sprays, or lotion should be used.
- Check if the physician wants to discontinue any medications before the study. (Anticonvulsants should be taken unless contraindicated by the physician.)
- Instruct the patient if sleep time should be shortened the night before the test. Adults may not be allowed to sleep more than 4 or 5 hours and children not more than 5 to 7 hours if a sleep EEG will be done.
- Do *not* administer any sedatives or hypnotics before the test because they will cause abnormal waves on the EEG.
- Inform the patient not to fast before the study. Fasting may cause hypoglycemia, which could alter test results.
- Instruct the patient not to drink any coffee, tea, cocoa, or cola on the morning of the test because of their stimulating effect.
- Tell the patient that he or she needs to remain still during the test. Any movement, including opening the eyes, will create interference and alter the EEG recording.

During

- Note the following procedural steps:

    1. The EEG is usually performed in a specially constructed room that is shielded from outside disturbances.
    2. The patient is placed in a supine position on a bed or reclining on a chair.
    3. Sixteen or more electrodes are applied to the scalp with electrode paste in a uniform pattern over both sides of the head, covering the prefrontal, frontal, temporal, parietal, and occipital areas.
    4. One electrode may be applied to each earlobe for grounding.

5. After the electrodes are applied, the patient is instructed to lie still with his or her eyes closed.
6. The technician continuously observes the patient during the EEG recording for any movements that could alter results.
7. Approximately every 5 minutes the recording is interrupted to permit the client to move if desired.

- In addition to the resting EEG, note that the following *activating procedures* can be performed:

  1. Patient is *hyperventilated* (asked to breathe deeply 20 times a minute for 3 minutes) to induce alkalosis and cerebral vasoconstriction, which can activate abnormalities.
  2. *Photostimulation* is performed by flashing a light over the patient's face with the eyes opened or closed. Photostimulated seizure activity may be seen on the EEG.
  3. A *sleep EEG* may be performed to aid in the detection of some abnormal brain waves that are seen only if the patient is sleeping (e.g., frontal lobe epilepsy). The sleep EEG is performed after orally administering methyprylon (Noludar) or chloral hydrate (Noctec). A recording is performed while the patient is falling asleep, while the patient is asleep, and while the patient is waking.

- Note that this study is performed by an EEG technician in approximately 45 minutes to 2 hours.
- Tell the patient that no discomfort is associated with this study, other than possibly missing sleep.

After

- Help the patient remove the electrode paste. The paste may be removed with acetone or witch hazel.
- Instruct the patient to shampoo the hair.
- Ensure safety precautions until the effects of any sedatives have worn off. Keep the bed's siderails up.
- Tell the patient that one who has had a sleep EEG should not drive home alone.

Abnormal findings

Seizure disorders (e.g., epilepsy)
Brain tumor
Brain abscess
Head injury
Cerebral death

Encephalitis
Intracranial hemorrhage
Cerebral infarct
Narcolepsy
Alzheimer's disease

Notes

electromyography (EMG)

Type of test Electrodiagnostic

Normal findings No evidence of neuromuscular abnormalities

Test explanation and related physiology

By placing a recording electrode into a skeletal muscle, one can monitor the electrical activity of the muscle in a way very similar to electrocardiography. The electrical activity is displayed on an oscilloscope as an electrical waveform. An audioelectrical amplifier can be added to the system so that both the appearance and the sound of the electrical potentials can be analyzed and compared simultaneously. EMG is used to detect primary muscular disorders along with muscular abnormalities caused by other system diseases (e.g., nerve dyfunction, sarcoidosis, paraneoplastic syndrome).

Spontaneous muscle movement, such as fibrillation and fasciculation, can be detected during EMG. When seen, these waves indicate injury or disease of the nerve innervating that muscle or spastic myotonic muscle disease. Reduced amplitude size of the electrical waveform is indicative of a primary muscle disorder (e.g., polymyositis, muscular dystrophies, various myopathies). A progressive decrease in amplitude of the electrical waveform is a classic sign of myasthenia gravis. A decrease in the number of muscle fibers able to contract is seen with peripheral nerve damage. This study is usually done in conjunction with nerve conduction studies (see p. 295) and may be also called *electromyoneurography*.

Contraindications

- Patients receiving anticoagulant therapy
- Patients with extensive skin infection

Potential complication

- Rarely, hematoma at the needle insertion site

Interfering factors

- Edema, hemorrhage, or thick subcutaneous fat can interfere with test results.
- Patients with excessive pain may have false results.

Procedure and patient care

Before

- Explain the procedure to the patient. Allay any fears and allow the patient to express concerns.
- Obtain informed consent if required by the institution.
- Tell the patient that fasting is not usually required. However, some facilities may restrict stimulants (coffee, tea, cocoa, cola, cigarettes) for 2 to 3 hours before the test.
- If serum enzyme tests (e.g., AST [SGOT], CPK, LDH) are ordered, the specimen should be drawn before EMG or 5 to 10 days after the test because the EMG may cause misleading elevations of these enzymes.
- Premedication or sedation is usually avoided because of the need for patient cooperation.

During

- Note the following procedural steps:
  1. This study is usually done in an EMG laboratory.
  2. The patient's position depends on the muscle being studied.
  3. A needle that acts as a recording electrode is inserted into the muscle being examined.
  4. A reference electrode is placed nearby on the skin surface.
  5. The patient is asked to keep the muscle at rest.
  6. The oscilloscope display is viewed for any evidence of spontaneous electrical activity, such as fasciculation or fibrillation.
  7. The patient is asked to contract the muscle slowly and progressively.
  8. The electrical waves produced are examined for their number, form, and amplitude.

  - Note that the EMG is performed by a physical therapist, physiatrist, or neurologist in approximately 20 minutes.
  - Tell the patient that this test is moderately uncomfortable; slight pain may occur with the insertion of the needle electrode.

After

- Observe the needle site for hematoma or inflammation.
- Provide pain medication if needed.

Abnormal findings

Polymyositis
Muscular dystropy
Multiple sclerosis
Myopathies
Amyotrophic lateral
   sclerosis (ALS)
Muscle denervation
Muscular abnormalities
   caused by other system
   diseases (e.g., nerve
   dysfunction, sarcoidosis,
   paraneoplastic syndrome)

Traumatic injury
Myasthenia gravis
Guillain-Barré syndrome
Diabetic neuropathy
Anterior poliomyelitis

Notes

electroneurography (ENG, Nerve conduction studies)

Type of test Electrodiagnostic

Normal findings

No evidence of peripheral nerve injury or disease
(Conduction velocity is usually decreased in the elderly.)

Test explanation and related physiology

ENG, or nerve conduction studies, allow for the detection
and location of peripheral nerve injury or disease. By initiating an electrical impulse at one site (proximal) of a nerve and
recording the time required for that impulse to travel to
a second site (distal) of the same nerve, the conduction
velocity of any impulse in that nerve can be determined.
This study is usually done in conjunction with electromyography (see p. 292) and may be also called *electromyoneurography.*

The normal value for conduction velocity varies from one
nerve to another. Individual variation also exists. For these
reasons, it is always best to compare the conduction velocity
of the suspected side with the contralateral nerve conduction
velocity. In general a range of normal conduction velocity
will be approximately 50 to 60 meters per second.

Traumatic transection or contusion of a nerve will usually
cause maximal slowing of conduction velocity in the affected
side as compared with the normal side. Neuropathies, both
local and generalized, also will cause a slowing of conduction velocity. A velocity greater than normal does not indicate a pathologic condition.

Because conduction velocity requires contraction of a
muscle as an indication of an impulse arriving at the recording electrode, primary muscular disorders may cause a falsely
slow nerve conduction velocity. This "muscular" variable is
eliminated if one evaluates the suspected pathologic muscle
group before performing nerve conduction studies. This
evaluation can be done by measuring distal latency, that is,
the time required for stimulation of the distal end of the
nerve to cause muscular contraction. The nerve conduction
study is then performed normally by stimulating the proxi-

mal portion of the nerve bundle. Conduction velocity is determined by the following equation:

Conduction velocity (in meters/second) =

$$\frac{\text{Distance (in meters)}}{\text{Total latency} - \text{Distal latency}}$$

Interfering factors

- Patients in severe pain may have false results.

Procedure and patient care
Before

- Explain the procedure to the patient. Allay any fears and allow the patient to express concerns.
- Obtain informed consent if required by the institution.
- Tell the patient that no fasting or sedation is usually required.

During

- Note the following procedural steps:

  1. This test can be performed in a nerve conduction laboratory or at the patient's bedside.
  2. The patient's position depends on the area of suspected peripheral nerve injury or disease.
  3. A recording electrode is placed on the skin overlying a muscle innervated solely by the relevant nerve.
  4. A reference electrode is placed nearby.
  5. All skin-to-electrode connections are ensured by using electrical paste.
  6. The nerve is stimulated by a shock-emitting device at an adjacent location.
  7. The time between nerve impulse and muscular contraction (distal latency) is measured in milliseconds on an EMG machine.
  8. The nerve is similarly stimulated at a location proximal to the area of suspected injury or disease.
  9. The time required for the impulse to travel from the site of initiation to muscle contraction (total latency) is recorded in milliseconds.
  10. The distance between the site of stimulation and the recording electrode is measured in centimeters.
  11. Conduction velocity is converted to meters per second and is computed as in the above equation.

- Note that this test takes approximately 15 minutes and is performed by a physiatrist or a neurologist.
- Tell the patient that this test is uncomfortable in that a mild shock is required for nerve impulse stimulation.

After

- Remove the electrode gel from the patient's skin.

Abnormal findings

Peripheral nerve injury or disease
Myasthenia gravis
Muscular dystrophy

Tumor
Guillain-Barré syndrome
Carpal tunnel syndrome
Diabetic neuropathy

Notes

electronystagmography

Type of test Electrodiagnostic

Normal findings

Normal nystagmus response
Normal oculovestibular reflex

Test explanation and related physiology

Electronystagmography is used to evaluate nystagmus (involuntary rapid eye movement) and the muscles controlling eye movement. By measuring changes in the electrical field around the eye, this study can make a permanent recording of eye movement at rest and in response to various stimuli. It delineates the presence or absence of nystagmus, which is caused by the initiation of the oculovestibular reflex. This test is used in the differential diagnosis of lesions in the vestibular system, the brainstem, and the cerebellum. It may also help evaluate unilateral hearing loss and vertigo.

Contraindications

- Patients with perforated eardrums, who should not have water irrigation
- Patients with pacemakers

Interfering factors

- Blinking of the eyes can alter test results.
- Drugs that can alter results include sedatives, stimulants, and antivertigo agents.

Procedure and patient care

Before

- Explain the procedure to the patient.
- Instruct the patient not to apply face makeup before the test because electrodes will be taped to the skin around the eyes.
- Hold solid food before the test to reduce the likelihood of vomiting.
- Instruct the patient not to drink caffeine or alcoholic beverages for approximately 24 to 48 hours (as ordered) before the test.
- Check with the physician regarding withholding any medications that could interfere with the test results.

During

- Note the following procedural steps:

    1. This procedure is usually performed in a darkened room with the patient seated or lying down on an examining table.
    2. If there is any wax in the ear, it is removed.
    3. Electrodes are taped to the skin around the eyes.
    4. Various procedures are used to stimulate nystagmus, such as pendulum tracking, changing head position, changing gaze position, and caloric tests.
    5. Several recordings are made with the patient at rest and also to demonstrate patient response to various procedures (e.g., blowing air into the ear, irrigating the ear with water).
    6. Nystagmus response is compared to the expected ranges, and the results are recorded as normal, border-line, or abnormal.

- Note that this this procedure is performed by a physician in approximately 1 hour.
- Tell the patient that nausea and vomiting may occur during the test.

After

- Consider prescribing bed rest until nausea, vertigo, or weakness subsides.

Abnormal findings

Brainstem lesions
Vestibular system lesions
Cerebellum lesions

Congenital disorders
Demyelinating disease

Notes

electrophysiologic study (EPS, Cardiac mapping)

Type of test Electrodiagnostic

Normal findings Normal conduction intervals, refractive periods, and recovery times

Test explanation and related physiology

In this invasive procedure, electrode catheters are fluoroscopically placed through a peripheral vein and into the right atrium and/or ventricle. With close cardiac monitoring the electrode catheters are used to pace the heart and potentially induce arrhythmias (dysrhythmias). Defects in the heart conduction system can then be identified. Also, arrhythmias that are otherwise unapparent can be induced, identified, and treated. The effectiveness of the antiarrhythmic drugs (e.g., lidocaine, phenytoin, quinidine) can be assessed by determining the electrical threshold required to induce arrhythmias.

Contraindications

- Patients who are uncooperative
- Patients with acute myocardial infarction

Potential complications

- Cardiac arrhythmias (dysrhythmias) leading to ventricular tachycardia or fibrillation
- Perforation of the myocardium
- Catheter-induced embolic cerebrovascular accident (CVA, stroke) or myocardial infarction
- Peripheral vascular problems
- Hemorrhage
- Phlebitis at the venipuncture site

Interfering factors

- Drugs that can interfere with test results include analgesics, sedatives, and tranquilizers.

Procedure and patient care

Before

- Instruct the patient to fast 6 to 8 hours before the procedure. Usually, fluids are permitted up until 3 hours before the test.

- Obtain an informed consent from the patient.
- Encourage the patient to verbalize his or her fears regarding this test.
- Shave and prepare the catheter insertion site.
- Collect a blood sample for potassium or drug levels, if indicated.
- Obtain peripheral IV access for the administration of drugs.

During

- Note the following procedural steps:

  1. After being transported to the cardiac catheterization laboratory, the patient has electrocardiographic (EKG) leads attached.
  2. The catheter insertion site, usually the femoral vein, is prepared and draped in a sterile manner.
  3. Under fluoroscopic guidance the catheter is passed to the atrium and ventricle.
  4. Baseline surface intracardiac EKGs are recorded.
  5. Various parts of the cardiac electroconduction system are stimulated by atrial or ventricular pacing.
  6. Mapping of the electroconduction system and its defects is performed.
  7. Arrhythmias (dysrhythmias) are identified.
  8. Drugs may be administered to assess their efficacy in preventing EPS-induced arrhythmias.

- Note that this procedure is performed by a cardiologist within a darkened cardiac catheterization laboratory in approximately 1 to 4 hours.
- Tell the patient that he or she may experience palpatations, lightheadedness, or dizziness when arrhythmias are induced. For most patients, this is an anxiety-producing experience. Report these sensations to the physician.
- Inform the patient that discomfort from catheter insertion is minimal.

After

- Keep the patient on bed rest for approximately 6 to 8 hours.
- Evaluate the venous access site for swelling and bleeding.
- Monitor the patient's vital signs for at least 2 to 4 hours for hypotension and arrhythmias (dysrhythmias). Additional monitoring is especially important for certain medi-

cations that the patient received during the test. For example, if the patient received quinidine, he or she should be monitored for hypotension and abdominal cramping.
- Continue cardiac monitoring to identify arrhythmias. Transfer arrangements to a monitored unit may be necessary.
- Cover the area with sterile dressings if the electrical catheter is left in place for subsequent studies.

Abnormal findings

Electroconduction defects
Cardiac arrhythmias (dysrhythmias)
Sinoatrial (SA) node defects (e.g., sick sinus syndrome)
Atrioventricular (AV) node defects and heart blocks

Notes

endometrial biopsy

Type of test Microscopic examination of tissue

Normal findings
No pathologic conditions
Presence of a "secretory-type" endometrium 3 to 5 days
  before normal menses

Test explanation and related physiology
   Performing an endometrial biopsy can determine whether
ovulation has occurred. A biopsy specimen taken 3 to 5 days
before normal menses should demonstrate a "secretory-type"
endometrium on histologic examination if ovulation and
corpus luteum formation have occurred. If not, only a pre-
ovulatory "proliferative-type" endometrium will be seen.
   Occasionally an endometrial biopsy is performed to indicate estrogen's effect in patients with suspected ovarian dysfunction or absence. Similarly, adequate circulating progesterone levels can be determined by identifying secretory endometrium. Another major use of endometrial biopsy is to
diagnose endometrial cancer, tuberculosis, polyps, or inflammatory conditions and to evaluate uterine bleeding.

Contraindications
- Patients with infections (e.g., trichomonal, candidal, suspected gonococcal) of the cervix or vagina
- Patients in whom the cervix cannot be visualized (e.g.,
  because of abnormal position or previous surgery)

Potential complications
- Perforation of the uterus
- Uterine bleeding
- Interference with early pregnancy
- Infection

Procedure and patient care
Before
- Explain the procedure to the patient.
- Ensure that written and informed consent for this proce-
  dure is obtained from the patient.
- Tell the patient that no fasting or sedation is usually re-
  quired.

During

- Note the following procedural steps:

  1. The patient is placed in the lithotomy position, and a pelvic examination is performed to determine the position of the uterus.
  2. The cervix is exposed and cleansed.
  3. A biopsy instrument is inserted into the uterus, and specimens are obtained from the anterior, posterior, and lateral walls.
  4. The specimens are placed in a solution containing 10% formalin solution and sent to the pathologist for histologic examination.

- Note that this procedure is performed by an obstetrician/gynecologist in approximately 10 to 30 minutes.
- Tell the patient that this procedure may cause momentary discomfort (menstrual-type cramping).

After

- Assess the patient's vital signs at regular intervals for the next 48 hours. Any temperature elevation should be reported to the physician because this procedure may activate pelvic inflammatory disease (PID).
- Advise the patient to wear a pad because some vaginal bleeding is to be expected. Instruct the patient to call her physician if excessive bleeding (requiring more than one pad per hour) occurs.
- Inform the patient that douching and intercourse are not permitted for 72 hours after the biopsy specimen removal.
- Instruct the patient to rest during the next 24 hours and to avoid heavy lifting to prevent uterine hemorrhage.

Abnormal findings

Anovulation
Tumor
Tuberculosis

Polyps
Inflammatory conditions

Notes

endoscopic retrograde cholangiopancreatography (ERCP, ERCP of the biliary and pancreatic ducts)

E

Type of test Endoscopy

Normal findings

Normal size of biliary and pancreatic ducts
No obstruction or filling defects within the biliary or pancreatic ducts

Test explanation and related physiology

ERCP, with the use of a fiberoptic endoscope, provides for radiographic visualization of the bile and pancreatic ducts. This is especially useful in jaundiced patients. If a partial or total obstruction of those ducts exists, the characteristics of the obstructing lesion can be demonstrated. Stones, benign strictures, cysts, ampullary stenosis, anatomic variations, and malignant tumors can be identified. Only ERCP and percutaneous transhepatic cholangiography (PTHC) can provide direct visualization of the biliary and pancreatic ducts. PTHC (see p. 551) is an invasive procedure with significant morbidity. ERCP, on the other hand, is associated with much less morbidity but must be performed by an experienced endoscopist.

In contrast to an oral cholecystogram or an IV cholangiogram, which does not visualize (display) the biliary tree when high levels of bilirubin are present, the biliary ducts can be visualized by ERCP. As a result, this test is extremely important in the evaluation of jaundiced patients.

Contraindications

- Patients who are uncooperative
  Cannulation of the ampulla of Vater requires that the patient lie very still.
- Patients whose ampulla of Vater is not accessible endoscopically because of previous upper gastrointestinal surgery (e.g., gastrectomy patients whose duodenum containing the ampulla is surgically separated from the stomach)
- Patients with esophageal diverticula

The scope can fall into a diverticulum and perforate its wall.

- Patients with known acute pancreatitis

Potential complications

- Perforation of the esophagus, stomach, or duodenum
- Gram-negative sepsis
  This is a result of introducing bacteria through the biliary system and into the blood. Usually this occurs in patients who have obstructive jaundice.
- Pancreatitis
  This results from pressure of the dye injection.
- Aspiration of gastric contents into the lungs
- Respiratory arrest as a result of oversedation

Interfering factors

- Barium within the abdomen as a result of a previous upper GI series or barium enema x-ray precludes adequate visualization of the biliary and pancreatic ducts.

Procedure and patient care

Before

- Explain the procedure to the patient.
- Obtain informed consent from the patient.
- Inform the patient that breathing will not be compromised by the insertion of the endoscope.
- Keep the patient NPO as of midnight the day of the test.
- Administer appropriate premedication (e.g. midazolam [Versed] and atropine) if ordered.

During

- Note the following procedural steps:

  1. A flat plate of the abdomen is done to ensure that any barium from previous studies will not obscure visualization of the bile duct.
  2. The patient is placed in the supine position or on the left side.
  3. The patient is usually sedated with a narcotic and a sedative-hypnotic.
  4. The pharynx is sprayed with a local anesthetic (lidocaine [Xylocaine]) to inactivate the gag reflex and to lessen the discomfort caused by the passage of the scope.

5. A side-viewing fiberoptic duodenoscope is inserted through the oral pharynx and passed through the esophagus, stomach, and into the duodenum (Figure 6)
6. Glucagon is often administered intravenously to minimize the spasm of the duodenum and improve visualization of the ampulla of Vater.
7. Through the accessory lumen within the scope, a small catheter is passed through the ampulla and into the common bile or pancreatic ducts.
8. Radiographic dye is injected, and x-ray films are taken.

- Note that the test usually takes about 1 hour and is performed by a physician trained in endoscopy. The x-ray films are interpreted by the radiologist.
- Tell the patient that no discomfort is associated with the dye injection but that minimal gagging may occur with initial introduction of the scope into the oral pharynx.

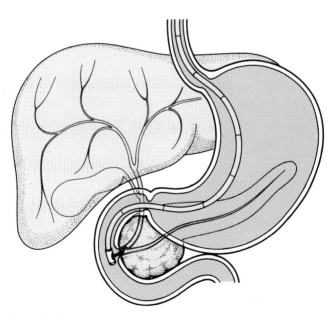

Figure 6 Endoscopic retrograde cholangiopancreatography (ERCP). The fiberoptic scope is passed into the duodenum. Note a small catheter being advanced into the biliary duct.

After

- Do *not* allow the patient to eat or drink until the gag reflex returns.
- Observe the patient closely for development of abdominal pain, nausea, and vomiting. This may herald the onset of ERCP-induced pancreatitis.
- Observe safety precautions until the effects of the sedatives have worn off.
- Monitor the patient for signs of respiratory depression. Medication (e.g., naloxone [Narcan]) should be available to counteract serious respiratory depression. Resuscitative equipment should also be present.
- Assess the patient for signs and symptoms of septicemia, which may indicate the onset of ERCP-induced cholangitis.
- Inform the patient that he or she may be hoarse and complain of a sore throat for several days. Drinking cool fluids and gargling will help relieve some of this soreness.

Abnormal findings

Tumors, strictures, and gallstones of the common bile duct
Sclerosing cholangitis
Biliary sclerosis
Cysts of the common bile duct
Tumor, strictures, inflammation, or pseudocyst of the pancreatic duct
Anatomic biliary or pancreatic duct variations

Notes

epithelial casts (Renal tubular casts)

Type of test Urine

Normal findings No or occasional epithelial cells

Test explanation and related physiology

Casts are clumps of material or cells. They are formed in the renal collecting tubule and have the shape of the tubule, thus the term *cast*. Epithelial casts are formed from tubular epithelial cells. The presence of occasional epithelial cells is not remarkable. Tubular (epithelial) casts are most suggestive of glomerulonephritis.

Procedure and patient care

Before

- Explain the procedure to the patient.

During

- Collect a fresh urine specimen in a urine container.
- If the specimen is contaminated by vaginal discharge or bleeding, a "clean-catch" or "midstream" specimen will be needed. This requires meticulous cleansing of the urinary meatus with an iodine preparation to reduce contamination of the specimen by external organisms. Then the cleansing agent must be completely removed, or it will contaminate the specimen. The midstream collection is obtained by:
  1. Having the patient begin to urinate in a bedpan, urinal, or toilet and then stop urinating (This washes the urine out of the distal urethra.)
  2. Correctly positioning a sterile urine container, into which the patient voids 3 to 4 ounces of urine
  3. Capping the container
  4. Allowing the patient to finish voiding

After

- Send the specimen immediately to the laboratory.
- Note that the urine specimen should be checked for casts when it is fresh because the casts break up when the urine specimen sits.

Abnormal findings
Increased levels

Glomerulonephritis
Eclampsia
Heavy metal poisoning

Ethylene glycol intoxication
Acute renal allograph
  rejection

Notes

Epstein-Barr virus titer (EBV)

Type of test Blood

Normal findings

Titers $\leq 1:10$ are nondiagnostic.

Titers of $1:10$-$1:60$ indicate infection at some undetermined time.

Titers of $1:320$ or greater suggest active infection.

Fourfold increase in titer in paired sera drawn 10 to 14 days apart is usually indicative of an acute infection.

Test explanation and related physiology

EBV is the most common agent associated with infectious mononucleosis syndrome (see mononucleosis spot test, p. 511). It is seen most often in children, adolescents, and young adults. Clinical features include those of acute fatigue, fever, sore throat, lymphadenopathy, and splenomegaly. Laboratory findings of lymphocytosis, atypical lymphocytes, and the development of transient serum heterophil antibodies are found in patients with acute EBV infection. Most patients with infectious mononucleosis recover uneventfully and return to normal activity within 4 to 6 weeks.

After recovery from primary EBV infection, a lifelong latent EBV carrier status is established. In the last several years, specific immunologic tests to identify EBV activity indicate that latent EBV can reactivate and become associated with a constellation of chronic signs and symptoms resembling infectious mononucleosis. Clinical manifestations of chronic EBV are variable and include nonspecific symptoms such as profound fatigue, pharyngitis, myalgias, arthralgias, low-grade fever, headache, paresthesias, and loss of abstract thinking. The routine laboratory workup is of no diagnostic value. Atypical lymphocytes occasionally are found, but the heterophil tests (see monospot test, p. 511) are almost always negative. Diagnosis is best established by demonstrating immunologic evidence of antibodies to the *diffuse* (D) and *restricted* (R) components of *early antigen* (EA) complex and/or by the presence of *Epstein-Barr nuclear antigen* (EBNA) measured 6 months after primary EBV infection.

EBV antibody titers are tests indicating the body's response to EBV antigens, which are complex substances produced by the EBV during various phases of replication. Although laboratories performing these tests present the results in slightly different units, the titers are recorded in four parts:

VCA (viral capsid antigen)
EAD (early antigen diffuse component)
EAR (early antigen restricted component)
EBNA (Epstein-Barr nuclear antigen)

The interpretation of EBV antibody tests is based on the following assumptions.

1. Once the person becomes infected with EBV, the anti-VCA antibodies appear first.
2. Anti-EA (EAD or EAR) antibodies appear next or are present with anti-VCA antibodies early in the course of illness. An anti-EA antibody titer greater than 80 in a patient 2 years after acute infectious mononucleosis indicates chronic EBV syndrome.
3. As the patient recovers, anti-VCA and anti-EA antibodies decrease and anti-EBNA antibodies appear. Anti-EBNA antibody persists for life and reflects a past infection.
4. After the patient is well, anti-VCA and anti-EBNA antibodies are always present but at lower ranges. Occasionally, anti-EA antibody may also be present after recovery.

Procedure and patient care

Before

- Explain the procedure to the patient.
- Tell the patient that no fasting or special preparation is required.

During

- Collect 5 to 10 ml of venous blood in a red-top tube.
- Record the day of onset of illness on the laboratory slip.
- Obtain serum samples as soon as possible after the onset of the illness.
- Obtain a second blood specimen 14 to 21 days later.

After

- Apply pressure or a pressure dressing to the venipuncture site.
- Observe the venipuncture site for bleeding.

Abnormal findings

Infectious mononucleosis   Chronic EBV carrier state
Chronic fatigue syndrome   Burkitt's lymphoma

Notes

E

erythrocyte sedimentation rate (ESR, Sed rate test)

Type of test Blood

Normal findings

Westergren method

> Male: up to 15 mm/hr
> Female: up to 20 mm/hr
> Child: up to 10 mm/hr
> Newborn: 0-2 mm/hr

Test explanation and related physiology

The ESR is a nonspecific test used to detect inflammatory, neoplastic, infectious, and necrotic processes. Since the ESR is a nonspecific test, it is not diagnostic for any specific organ disease or injury. The test is performed by measuring the distance (in millimeters) that red blood cells (RBCs) descend (or settle) in normal saline in 1 hour. Because the pathologic conditions just mentioned increase the protein content of plasma, RBCs have a tendency to stack up on one another, thereby increasing their weight and causing them to descend faster. Therefore in these diseases the ESR will be increased.

The test can be used to detect disease that is otherwise not suspected. Many physicians use the ESR test in this way for routine patient evaluation. Other physicians regard this test as so nonspecific that it is useless as a routine study. The ESR test can occasionally be helpful in differentiating disease entities or complaints. For example, in the patient with chest pain the ESR will be increased with myocardial infarction but will be normal with angina.

ESR is a fairly reliable indicator of the course of disease and can therefore be used to monitor disease therapy, especially for inflammatory autoimmune diseases. In general, as the disease worsens, the ESR increases; as the disease improves, the ESR decreases. If the results of the ESR are equivocal or inconsistent with the clinical impressions, the C-reactive protein test is often done.

Interfering factors

- Artificially low results can occur when the collected specimen is allowed to stand longer than 3 hours before the testing.
- Pregnancy (second and third trimester) can cause elevated levels.
- Menstruation can cause elevated levels.
- Drugs that may cause increased ESR levels include dextran, methyldopa (Aldomet), oral contraceptives, penicillamine, procainamide, theophylline, and vitamin A.
- Drugs that may cause decreased levels include aspirin, cortisone, and quinine.

Procedure and patient care

Before

- Explain the procedure to the patient.
- Hold medications that can affect test results (if indicated).

During

- Collect approximately 5 to 10 ml of venous blood in a lavender-top tube.

After

- Transport the specimen immediately to the laboratory.
- Apply pressure or a pressure dressing to the venipuncture site.
- Assess the venipuncture site for bleeding.

Abnormal findings

Increased levels

Toxemia
Syphilis
Nephritis
Multiple myeloma
Bacterial infections
Acute pelvic inflammatory disease
Pneumonia
Rheumatoid arthritis
Rheumatic fever
Acute myocardial infarction
Hyperfibrinogenemia

Decreased levels

Congestive heart failure
Sickle cell anemia
Hypofibrinogenemia
Polycythemia vera
Infectious mononucleosis
Degenerative arthritis
Angina pectoris

Systemic lupus erythem-
  atosus
Severe anemia
Hodgkin's disease
Carcinoma

Notes

esophageal function studies (Esophageal manometry, Esophageal motility studies)

Type of test Manometric

Normal findings

Lower esophageal sphincter pressure: 10-20 mm Hg
Swallowing pattern: normal peristaltic waves
Acid reflux: negative
Acid clearing: less than 10 swallows
Bernstein test: negative

Test explanation and related physiology

Esophageal function studies include the following: (1) determination of the *lower esophageal sphincter (LES) pressure* (manometry); (2) graphic recording of esophageal swallowing waves, or *swallowing pattern* (manometry); (3) detection of reflux of gastric acid back into the esophagus (acid reflux); (4) detection of the ability of the esophagus to clear acid (acid clearing); and (5) an attempt to reproduce symptoms of heartburn (Bernstein test). Each is discussed separately.

Manometry studies. Two manometry studies are used in assessing esophageal function: measurement of LES pressure and graphic recording of swallowing waves (motility). The LES is a sphincter muscle that acts as a valve to prevent reflux of gastric acid into the esophagus. Free reflux of gastric acid occurs when the sphincter pressures are low. An example of such a disorder in the adult is gastroesophageal reflux. In children, it is called chalasia (incompetent or relaxed LES).

With increased sphincter pressure, as found in patients with achalasia (failure of the LES to relax normally with swallowing) and with diffuse esophageal spasms, food cannot pass from the esophagus into the stomach. Increased LES pressures are noted on manometry. In achalasia, few, if any, swallowing waves are detected. In contrast, diffuse esophageal spasm is characterized by strong, frequent, asynchronous, and nonpropulsive waves.

Acid reflux with pH probe. Acid reflux is the primary component of gastroesophageal reflux. Patients who have an incompetent LES will regurgitate gastric acid into the esophagus. This will then cause a drop in pH testing done by the pH probe.

Acid clearing. Patients with normal esophageal function can completely clear hydrochloric acid from the esophagus in less than 10 swallows. Patients with decreased esophageal motility (frequently caused by severe esophagitis) require a greater number of swallows to clear the acid.

Bernstein test (acid perfusion). The Bernstein test is simply an attempt to reproduce the symptoms of gastroesophageal reflux. If the patient suffers pain with the instillation of hydrochloric acid into the esophagus, the test is positive and proves the patient's symptoms are caused by reflux esophagitis. If the patient has no discomfort, a cause other than esophageal reflux must be sought to explain the patient's discomfort.

Contraindications

- Patients who cannot cooperate
- Patients who are medically unstable

Potential complication

- Aspiration of gastric contents

Interfering factors

- Eating shortly before the test can affect results.
- Drugs such as sedatives can alter test results.

Procedure and patient care

Before

- Explain the procedure to the patient.
- Instruct the patient not to eat or drink anything for at least 8 hours before the test.
- Allay any fears and allow the patient to verbalize concerns. Be sensitive to the patient's fears about choking during the procedure.

During

- Note the following procedural steps:
    1. Esophageal studies are usually performed in the endoscopy laboratory.
    2. The fasting, unsedated patient is asked to swallow two or three very tiny tubes. The tubes are equipped

so that pressure measurements can be taken at 5 cm (in length) intervals.

3. The outer ends of the tubes are attached to a pressure transducer.
4. First, all tubes are passed through the stomach. Then three tubes are slowly pulled back into the esophagus. A rapid and extreme increase in the pressure readings indicates the high-pressure zone of the LES.
5. The *LES pressure* is recorded.
6. With all tubes in the esophagus, the patient is asked to *swallow*. Motility wave patterns are recorded.
7. The pH indicator probe is placed in the esophagus.
8. The stomach is filled with approximately 100 ml of 0.1 N hydrochloric acid. A decrease in the pH of the esophageal pH probe indicates gastroesophageal *reflux*.
9. Hydrochloric acid is instilled into the esophagus, and the patient is asked to swallow. The number of swallows are counted to determine *acid clearing*. Greater than 10 swallows to clear the acid, as determined by the pH probe, indicates decreased esophageal motility.
10. Finally, 0.1 N hydrochloric acid and saline solution are alternately instilled into the esophagus for the *Bernstein test*. The patient is not told which solution is being infused. If the patient volunteers symptoms of discomfort while the acid is running, the test is considered positive. If no discomfort is recognized, the test is negative.

- Note that these tests are performed by an esophageal technician in approximately 30 minutes.
- Inform the patient that the test results are interpreted by a physician and are available in a few hours.
- Tell the patient that, except for some initial gagging when swallowing the tubes, these tests are not uncomfortable.

After

- Inform the patient that it is not unusual to have a mild sore throat after placement of the small tubes.

Abnormal findings

Presbyesophagus
Diffuse esophageal spasm
Chalasia

Achalasia
Gastroesophageal reflux
Reflux esophagitis

Notes

esophagogastroduodenoscopy (EGD, Upper gastrointestinal [UGI] endoscopy, Gastroscopy)

Type of test Endoscopy

Normal findings Normal esophagus, stomach, and duodenum

Test explanation and related physiology

Endoscopy enables direct visualization of the upper gastrointestinal (GI) tract by means of a long, flexible, fiberoptic lighted scope. The esophagus, stomach, and duodenum are examined for tumors, varices, mucosal inflammations, hiatal hernias, polyps, ulcers, and obstructions. The endoscope has one to three channels. The first channel is used for viewing, the second for insufflation of air and aspiration of fluid, and the third for passing cable-activated instruments to biopsy suspected pathologic conditions. Also, probes can be passed through the third channel to allow for coagulation or injection of sclerosing agents to areas of active GI bleeding. A laser beam can pass through the endoscope to perform endoscopic surgery (e.g., obliteration of tumors or polyps, control of bleeding). The fiberoptics of endoscopy are so refined that video images and "still pictures" can be taken.

Endoscopy can not only evaluate the esophagus, stomach, and duodenum, but with the use of an extra-long fiberoptic endoscope, can visualize and biopsy the upper small intestinal tract. This procedure is referred to as *enteroscopy*. Abnormalities of the small intestine, such as arteriovenous (AV) malformations, tumors, enteropathies (e.g., celiac disease), and ulcerations, can be diagnosed with enteroscopy.

Besides being much more sensitive and specific than an upper GI series in diagnosing diseases of the esophagus, stomach, and duodenum, the EGD also can be used therapeutically. An experienced endoscopist can often control active GI bleeding by electrocoagulation, laser coagulation, or the injection of sclerosing agents such as alcohol. Also, with the endoscope, benign and malignant strictures can be dilated to reestablish patency of the upper GI tract. Biliary stents and a percutaneous gastrostomy can be placed with the use of EGD. The role of endoscopic surgery is expanding in light of its dramatic success and minimal morbidity.

Contraindications

- Patients who cannot cooperate fully
  As in all studies that require technical finesse, patient co-operation is essential for successful, safe, and accurate test completion.
- Patients with severe upper GI bleeding
  The viewing lens will become covered with blood clots, thereby preventing adequate visualization. However, if the stomach can be lavaged and aspirated to clear the blood clots, EGD can be performed.
- Patients with esophageal diverticula
  The scope can easily fall into the diverticulum and perforate the wall of the esophagus.
- Patients with suspected perforation
  The perforation can be worsened by the insufflation of pressurized air into the GI tract.
- Patients who have recently had GI surgery
  The anastomosis may not be able to withstand the pressure of the required air insufflation. This may lead to anastomotic disruption.

Potential complications

- Perforation of the esophagus, stomach, and duodenum
- Bleeding from a biopsy site
- Pulmonary aspiration of gastric contents
- Oversedation from the medication administered during the test
- Hypotension induced by the sedative medication
  Usually, however, the patient already has some significant element of hypovolemia or dehydration.
- Local IV phlebitic reaction to the injection of sclerosing sedative medication

Interfering factors

- Food in the stomach
- Excessive GI bleeding

Procedure and patient care

Before

- Explain the procedure to the patient.
- Obtain informed consent if required by the institution.
- Instruct the patient to abstain from eating as of midnight the day of the test.

- Reassure the patient that this test is not painful. Tell the patient the throat will be anesthetized with a spray to depress the gag reflex.
- Encourage the patient to verbalize fears. Provide support.
- Remove the patient's dentures and eyewear before testing.
- Remind the patient that he or she will not be able to speak during the test but that respiration will not be affected.
- Instruct the patient not to bite down on the endoscope.
- Instruct the patient as to appropriate oral hygiene, since the tube will be passed through the mouth.

During

- Note the following procedural steps:

   1. The patient is placed on the endoscopy table in the left lateral decubitus position.
   2. The throat is topically anesthetized with viscous naloxone (Xylocaine) or another anesthetic spray. This is to decrease the gag reflex caused by passage of the endoscope.
   3. The patient is usually heavily sedated. This minimizes anxiety and allows the patient to experience a "light" sleep.
   4. The endoscope is gently passed through the mouth and finally into the esophagus. Once in the esophagus, visualization can be carried out.
   5. Air is insufflated to distend the upper GI tract for adequate visualization.
   6. The esophagus, stomach, and duodenum are evaluated.
   7. During *enteroscopy* the upper small bowel is visualized and biopsied if needed.
   8. Biopsies or any endoscopic surgery is performed with direct visualization.
   9. At the completion of direct inspection and surgery, the excess air and GI secretions are aspirated through the scope.

- Note that the test is performed in the endoscopy laboratory by a physician trained in GI endoscopy and takes approximately 20 to 30 minutes.
- Tell the patient that the test is mildly uncomfortable.

After

- Inform the patient that he or she may have hoarseness or a sore throat after the test.
- Withhold any fluids until the patient is completely alert and the swallowing reflex returns to normal, usually in about 2 to 4 hours.
- Observe the patient's vital signs. Evaluate the patient for bleeding, fever, abdominal pain, dyspnea, or dysphagia.
- Inform patients that they may experience some postendoscopic bloating, belching, and flatulence.
- Observe safety precautions until the effects of the sedatives have worn off.
- Inform the patient that the sedation may cause some retrograde and antegrade amnesia for a few hours.

Abnormal findings

Tumors (benign and malignant) of the esophagus, stomach, and duodenum
Esophageal diverticula
Hiatal hernia
Esophagitis, gastritis, duodenitis
Gastroesophageal varices
Peptic ulcers
Peptic stricture and subsequent scarring
Extrinsic compression by cysts and tumors outside the upper GI tract
Sources of upper GI bleeding

Notes

estriol excretion (Estrogen fractions)

Type of test Urine (24 hour); blood

Normal findings Rising estriol levels, indicating normal fetal growth

Possible critical values Values 40% below the average of two previous values demand immediate evaluation of fetal well-being.

Test explanation and related physiology

Serial urine and blood studies for estriol excretion provide an objective means of assessing placental function and fetal normality in high-risk pregnancies. Excretion of estriol (the type of estrogen present in blood and urine in the largest amounts) increases around the eighth week of gestation and continues to rise until shortly before delivery. Because the fetal contribution to the esteriol value is considerable, the measurement of excreted estriol has become an important index of fetal well-being. Rising values indicate an adequately functioning fetoplacental unit. Decreasing values suggest fetoplacental deterioration (failing pregnancy, dysmaturity, preeclampsia/eclampsia, complicated diabetes mellitus, encephaly, fetal death) and require prompt reassessment of the pregnancy. If the estriol levels fall, early delivery of the fetus may be indicated.

Serial studies are usually begun at approximately 28 to 30 weeks of gestation and are repeated weekly. The frequency of these estriol determinations can be increased as needed to evaluate a high-risk pregnancy. Collection may be done daily. Although the first collection is the baseline value, all collection results are compared with previous ones because decreasing values suggest fetal deterioration. Some physicians suggest using an average of three previous values as a control value.

Estriol excretion studies can be done using 24-hour urine tests or blood studies. Because urinary creatinine excretion is relatively constant, its determination can be used to assess the adequacy of the 24-hour urine collection for estriol. A serially increasing estriol/creatinine ratio is a favorable sign in pregnancy. Plasma estriol determinations can also be used to evaluate the fetoplacental unit. These tests have been developed more recently than the urinary studies, and their use is still limited and controversial. These studies can conveniently and rapidly assess the quantity of free estriol in the plasma by radioimmunoassay. The plasma collected by venipuncture is an accurate reflection of the current status of the placenta and fetus. The advantage of the plasma estriol determination is that it is more easily obtained than a 24-hour urine specimen and is less affected by medications.

Interfering factors

- Recent administration of radioisotopes can alter test results.
- Glycosuria and urinary tract infections can increase urine estriol levels.
- Drugs that may elevate levels include adrenocorticosteroids, ampicillin, estrogen-containing drugs, phenothiazines, and tetracyclines.
- Drugs that may decrease levels include clomiphene.

Procedure and patient care
Before

- Explain the procedure to the patient.
- If the woman is going to collect the 24-hour urine specimen at home, give her the collection bottle (with a preservative) and instruct her to keep the urine refrigerated.
- Tell the patient that no food or fluid restrictions are needed.

During

Blood
- Collect approximately 5 ml of venous blood in a red-top tube.

24-hour urine
- Instruct the patient to begin the 24-hour urine collection after voiding. Discard the initial specimen and start the 24-hour timing at that point.
- Collect all the urine passed during the next 24 hours. Make sure the patient knows where to store the urine container.
- Keep the specimen on ice or refrigerated during the 24 hours.

- Indicate the starting time on the urine container and laboratory slip.
- Post the hours for the urine collection in a prominent place to prevent accidental discarding of the specimen.
- Instruct the patient to void before defecating so that the urine is not contaminated by feces.
- Remind the patient not to put toilet paper in the collection container.
- Encourage the patient to drink fluids during the 24 hours.
- Collect the last specimen as close as possible to the end of the 24-hour period. Add this urine to the collection.
- List any drugs that can affect test results on the laboratory slip.

After

- Apply pressure or a pressure dressing to the venipuncture site.
- Observe the venipuncture site for bleeding.
- Transport the 24-hour urine specimen promptly to the laboratory.
- Inform the patient how and when to obtain the results of this study.

Abnormal findings

Increased levels

Ovarian tumors
Testicular tumors
Adrenal tumors
Multiple pregnancy
Urinary tract infections
Glucosuria

Decreased levels

Failing pregnancy
Fetal distress
Dysmaturity
Preeclampsia/eclampsia
Complicated diabetes
  mellitus
Anencephaly
Congenital anomalies
Fetal death
Turner's syndrome
Hypopituitarism
Adrenogenital syndrome
Stein-Leventhal syndrome
Anorexia nervosa
Menopause
Placental insufficiency
Rh isoimmunization

euglobulin lysis time (Euglobulin clot lysis, Fibrinolysis/euglobulin lysis)

Type of test Blood

Normal findings 90 minutes-6 hours

Possible critical values <1 hour, indicating excessive fibrinolytic activity (danger of bleeding)

Test explanation and related physiology

The euglobulin lysis test is used to evaluate systemic fibrinolysis. The fibrinolytic system normally breaks down small fibrin deposits. When this system is abnormally overactive, as in primary fibrinolysis, any fibrin clot that is formed will be dissolved immediately, thereby resulting in a bleeding tendency. This system is only minimally overactive in disseminated intravascular coagulation (DIC, secondary fibrinolysis).

The euglobulin lysis time is a measure of the activity of this fibrinolytic system. Fibrin formed in the euglobulin fraction of plasma is normally very rapidly dissolved by plasmin (fibrinolysin). The time measured from clot formation to clot lysis is referred to as the euglobulin lysis time. In primary fibrinolysis (caused by streptokinase administration, cancer of the prostate, shock, other conditions) the euglobulin lysis time is rapid (short). In DIC the euglobulin lysis time is usually normal. However, if all the plasmin has been consumed, the time may be prolonged.

This is one of the best tests used to differentiate primary fibrinolysis from DIC. This differentiation is important in considering appropriate therapy for the patient with a bleeding tendency. Epsilon-aminocaproic acid may be required to treat primary fibrinolysis; heparin may be indicated for DIC.

This test also may be used to monitor streptokinase or urokinase therapy in patients with acute myocardial infarction.

Interfering factors

- Vigorous exercise, increasing age, and hyperventilation may cause increased fibrinolysis.

- Postmenopausal females and normal newborns may have decreased fibrinolysis.
- Decreased fibrinogen levels may result in a falsely shortened lysis time because of the reduced amount of fibrin to be lysed.
- Patients who are obese may have decreased fibrinolysis.
- Drugs that may cause increased fibrinolysis include steroids and adrenocorticotropic hormone (ACTH).

Procedure and patient care

Before

- Explain the procedure to the patient.
- Instruct the patient not to exercise before the blood sample is collected.
- Tell the patient that no fasting is required.

During

- Collect approximately 5 ml of blood in a blue-top tube.
- Avoid excessive agitation of the blood sample.
- Deliver the blood specimen to the laboratory immediately on ice.

After

- Apply pressure or a pressure dressing to the venipuncture site.
- Assess the venipuncture site for bleeding.

Abnormal findings

Increased fibrinolysis (shortened lysis time)

Incompatible blood transfusion
Cirrhosis
Thrombocytopenia purpura
Leukemia
Obstetric complications (e.g., antepartum hemorrhage, septic abortion, hydatidiform mole, amniotic embolism)
Primary fibrinolysis (e.g., caused by streptokinase or urokinase administration, cancer of the prostate, shock)
Prostatic cancer
Shock
Extensive vascular trauma or surgery

Decreased fibrinolysis (increased lysis time)

Prematurity
Diabetes

evoked potential studies (EP studies, Evoked brain potentials, Evoked responses)

Type of test Electrodiagnostic

Normal findings No neural conduction delay

Test explanation and related physiology

EP studies focus on changes and responses in brain waves that are evoked from stimulation of a sensory pathway. Clinical abnormalities are usually detected by an increase in *latency*, which refers to the delay between the stimulus and the wave response. Latency depends on factors such as body size, position of the body where the stimulus is applied, conduction velocity of axons in the neural pathways, number of synapses in the system, location of nerve generators of EP components (brainstem or cortex), and the presence of central nervous system pathology. Conduction delays indicate damage to the nerve fibers of the sensory system being evaluated. EPs are divided by sensory modality into visual, auditory, and somatosensory responses.

Visual evoked responses (VERs) are usually stimulated by a strobe light flash, reversible checkerboard pattern, or retinal stimuli. A visual stimulus to the eye causes an electrical response in the occipital area that can be recorded with electrodes placed along the vertex and on the occipital lobes. Ninety percent of patients with multiple sclerosis show abnormal latencies in VERs, a phenomenon attributed to demyelination of nerve fibers. In addition to multiple sclerosis, patients with other neurologic disorders (e.g., Parkinson's disease) show an abnormal latency with VERs. The degree of latency seems to correlate with the disease severity. Abnormal results may also be seen in patients with lesions of the optic nerve, optic tract, visual center, and eye. Absence of binocularity, which is a neurologic developmental disorder in infants, can be detected and evaluated by VERs.

Auditory brainstem evoked potentials (ABEPs) are usually stimulated by clicking sounds to evaluate the central auditory pathways of the brainstem. Either ear can be evoked to detect lesions in the brainstem that involve the auditory pathway without affecting hearing. One of the most successful applications of ABEPs has been screening low-birth-weight newborns for auditory disorders. This enables infants with poor hearing to be fitted with corrective devices as soon as possible before learning to speak. ABEPs also have great therapeutic implications in the early detection of posterior fossa tumors.

Somatosensory evoked responses (SERs) usually are stimulated by sensory stimulus to an area of the body. The time is then measured for the stimulus' current to travel along the nerve to the cortex of the brain. SERs are used to evaluate patients with spinal cord injuries, to monitor spinal cord functioning during surgery and during treatment of diseases (e.g., multiple sclerosis), to evaluate the location and extent of areas of brain dysfunction after head injury, and to pinpoint tumors at an early stage.

One of the main benefits of EPs is their objectivity, since voluntary patient response is not needed. This makes EPs useful with nonverbal and uncooperative patients. This objectivity permits the distinction of organic from psychogenic problems. This is invaluable in settling lawsuits concerning workmen's compensation insurance. The projected future of EPs will aid in diagnosing and monitoring mental disorders and child learning disabilities and in detecting adult mental disorders (e.g., alcoholic brain damage).

Procedure and patient care

Before

- Explain the procedure to the patient.
- Instruct the patient to shampoo his or her hair before the test.
- Tell the patient that no fasting or sedation is required.

During

- Note that the position of the electrode depends on the type of EP study to be done:

  1. For *VERs,* electrodes are placed on the scalp along the vertex and the cortex lobes. Stimulation occurs by using a strobe light, checkerboard pattern, or retinal stimuli.
  2. *ABEPs* are stimulated with clicking noises or tone bursts delivered via earphones. The responses are detected by scalp electrodes placed along the vertex and on each earlobe.
  3. *SERs* are stimulated using electrical stimuli applied to

nerves at the wrist (medial nerve) or the knee (peroneal nerve). The response is detected by electrodes placed over the sensory cortex of the opposite hemisphere on the scalp.

- Note that this study is performed by a physician in less than a half hour.
- Tell the patient that little discomfort is associated with this study.

After

- Remove the gel used for the adherence of the electrodes.

Abnormal findings

Multiple sclerosis
Parkinson's disease
Tumors
Absence of binocularity
Auditory disorders
Spinal cord injury

Spinal cord dysfunction
Optic tract lesions
Eye lesions
Visual field defects
Cerebrovascular accident
   (CVA, stroke)

Notes

exercise stress testing (Stress testing, Exercise testing, Electrocardiograph [EKG] stress testing, Graded exercise testing)

Type of test Electrodiagnostic

Normal findings Patient able to obtain and maintain maximal heart rate of 85% for predicted age and sex with no cardiac symptoms or EKG change

Test explanation and related physiology

Exercise stress testing is a noninvasive study that provides information about the patient's cardiac function. During stress testing the EKG, heart rate, and blood pressure are monitored while the patient engages in some type of physical activity (stress). Three common methods of stress testing include climbing stair steps (Master's two-step test), pedaling a stationary bike, or walking on a treadmill. With the stationary bicycle the pedaling tension is slowly increased to increase the heart rate. With the treadmill test the speed and grade of incline are increased. The treadmill test is the most frequently used because it is most easily standardized and reproducible.

The usual goal of the testing is to increase the heart rate to just below maximal levels or to the "target heart rate." Usually this target heart rate is 80% to 90% of the maximal heart rate. The test is usually discontinued if the patient reaches that target heart rate or if the patient develops any symptoms or EKG changes. The maximal heart rate is determined by a chart that takes into account the patient's age and sex. The normal maximal heart rate for adults varies from 150 to 200 beats per minute. Patients taking calcium channel blockers and sympathetic blockers have a lower-than-expected maximal heart rate.

Exercise stress testing is based on the principle that occluded arteries will be unable to meet the heart's increased demand for oxygen during the testing. This may become obvious with symptoms (e.g., chest pain, fatigue, dyspnea, tachycardia, cardiac arrhythmias [dysrhythmias], fall in blood pressure) or EKG changes (e.g., ST segment variance greater than 1 mm, increasing premature ventricular contractions [PVCs] or other rhythm disturbances).

The indications for stress testing are:

1. To evaluate chest pain in a patient suspected of having coronary disease. Occasionally a person may have significant coronary stenosis that is not apparent during normal physical activity. If, however, the pain can be reproduced with exercise, one may infer that coronary occlusion is present.
2. To determine the limits of safe exercise during a cardiac rehabilitation program or to assist patients with cardiac disease in maintaining good physical fitness
3. To detect labile or exercise-related hypertension
4. To detect intermittent claudication in patients with suspected vascular occlusive disease in the extremities. In this situation the patient may experience leg muscle cramping while performing the exercise.
5. To evaluate the effectiveness of treatment in patients who take antianginal or antiarrhythmic medications

Contraindications

- Patients who have unstable angina
- Patients who have severe aortic valvular heart disease
- Patients who cannot participate in an exercise program because of their impaired lung or motor function
- Patients who have recently had a myocardial infarction In this case, however, limited stress testing can be done.

Potential complications

- Fatal cardiac arrhythmias
- Severe angina
- Myocardial infarction
- Fainting

Interfering factors

- Heavy meals before testing can divert blood to the gastrointestinal tract.
- Nicotine from smoking can cause coronary artery spasm.
- Medical problems such as left ventricular hypertrophy, hypertension, valvular heart disease (especially of the aortic valve), left bundle branch block, severe anemia, hypoxemia, and chronic pulmonary disease can affect results.
- Drugs that can affect test results include beta blockers (e.g., propranolol [Inderal]), calcium channel blockers, digoxin, and nitroglycerine.

Procedure and patient care
Before

- Explain the procedure to the patient.
- Instruct the patient to abstain from eating, drinking, and smoking for 4 hours.
- Inform the patient about the risks of the test and obtain informed consent.
- Instruct the patient to bring comfortable clothing and shoes in which to exercise. Slippers are not acceptable.
- Inform the patient if any medications should be discontinued before testing.
- Obtain a pretest EKG.
- Record the patient's vital signs for baseline values.
- Apply and secure appropriate EKG electrodes.

During

- Note that a physician is present during stress testing.
- After the patient begins to exercise, adjust the treadmill machine settings to apply increasing levels of stress at specific intervals. It is helpful to encourage and support the patient at each level of increased stress.
- Encourage patients to verbalize any symptoms.
- Note that during the test the EKG tracing and vital signs are monitored continuously.
- Terminate the test if the patient complains of chest pain, exhaustion, dyspnea, fatique, or dizziness.
- Note that the testing usually takes approximately 45 minutes.
- Inform the patient that the physician in attendence usually interprets the results and will explain them subsequently to the patient.

After

- Place the patient in the supine position to rest after the test.
- Monitor the EKG tracing and record vital signs at poststress intervals, usually 3 and 30 minutes.
- Remove electrodes and paste.

Abnormal finding

Coronary artery occlusive disease

Notes

fatty casts

Type of test   Urine

Normal findings   No casts present

Test explanation and related physiology

Casts are clumps of materials or cells. They are formed in the renal collecting tubule and have the shape of the tubule, thus the term *cast*. Fatty casts are usually composed of individual fat droplets. The presence of fatty casts occurs most often in patients with nephrotic syndrome.

Procedure and patient care

Before

- Explain the procedure to the patient.

During

- Collect a fresh urine specimen in a urine container.
- Note that if the specimen is contaminated by vaginal discharge or bleeding, a "clean-catch" or "midstream" specimen will be needed. This requires meticulous cleansing of the urinary meatus with an iodine preparation to reduce contamination of the specimen by external organisms. Then the cleansing agent must be completely removed, or it will contaminate the specimen. The midstream collection is obtained by:

  1. Having the patient begin to urinate in a bedpan, urinal, or toilet and then stop urinating (This washes the urine out of the distal urethra.)
  2. Correctly positioning a sterile urine container, into which the patient voids 3 to 4 ounces of urine
  3. Capping the container
  4. Allowing the patient to finish voiding

After

- Send the specimen immediately to the laboratory.
- Do *not* allow the specimen to sit, since the casts will break up.

Abnormal findings

Nephrotic syndrome
Diabetic nephropathy
Glomerulonephritis
Chronic renal disease

Notes

F

febrile/cold agglutinins

Type of test   Blood

Normal findings

Febrile (warm) agglutinins: no agglutination in titers
≤1:80
Cold agglutinins: no agglutination in titers ≤1:16

Test explanation and related physiology

Febrile agglutinins serologic studies are used to diagnose infectious diseases such as salmonellosis, rickettsial diseases, brucellosis, and tularemia. Appropriate antibiotic treatment of the infectious agent is associated with a drop in the titer activity of febrile agglutinins.

Cold agglutinins occur in patients who are infected by other agents, most notably *Mycoplasma pneumoniae*.

The febrile and cold agglutinins are antibodies that cause red blood cells (RBCs) to aggregate at high or low temperatures, respectively. Normally, agglutination may occur in concentrated serum (less than 1:32 dilution). Agglutination occurring at titers greater than 1:16 for cold agglutinins and 1:80 for febrile agglutinins is considered abnormal and diagnostic of the infectious agent the agglutinins represent.

Temperature regulation is important for the performance of these tests. For *cold agglutinins* the red-top tube is previously warmed to above 37° C. For *febrile agglutinins* the red-top tube is cooled. The specimen is immediately taken to the laboratory so that no hemolysis will occur. Under no circumstances should the cold agglutinin specimen be refrigerated or the febrile agglutinin be heated. At the laboratory the cold agglutinin specimen is chilled and evaluated for agglutination of RBCs. The febrile agglutinin specimen is heated and also inspected for agglutination of RBCs. Serial dilutions are performed to detect the dilution at which agglutination occurs.

Procedure and patient care

Before

- Explain the procedure to the patient.
- Tell the patient that no fasting is required.

During

- Collect approximately 7 ml of venous blood in a red-top tube (warmed or cooled; see previous discussion).

After

- Apply pressure or a pressure dressing to the venipuncture site.
- Observe the venipuncture site for bleeding.
- Transport the specimen immediately to the laboratory.

Abnormal findings

Increased febrile agglutinins

Salmonellosis infections
Rickettsial diseases
Brucellosis
Tularemia

Increased cold agglutinins

Mycoplasma pneumoniae infection
Viral illness
Infectious mononucleosis
Multiple myeloma
Scleroderma
Cirrhosis
Staphylococcemia
Thymic tumors

Notes

fecal fat (Fat absorption, Quantitative stool fat determination)

Type of test Stool

Normal findings

5 g/24 hr of fat
Retention coefficient ≥95%

Test explanation and related physiology

The fecal fat test measures the fat content in the stool. The total output of fecal fat per 24 hours in a 3-day stool collection provides the most reliable measurement.

Children with cystic fibrosis have mucous plugs that obstruct the pancreatic ducts. The pancreatic enzymes (amylase, lipase, trypsin, chymotrypsin) cannot be expelled into the duodenum and are therefore either completely absent or present only in diminished quantities within the gastrointestinal tract. Lipase and bicarbonate are lipolytic, and without them fat is not digested for absorption. This results in impaired fat absorption (malabsorption). These patients have large, greasy, and foul-smelling stools; this is known as *steatorrhea.*

Analysis of fecal fat, although reliable, is not specific to cystic fibrosis. Any condition that may cause malabsorption (e.g., sprue, Crohn's disease, Whipple's disease) or maldigestion (e.g., bile duct obstruction, pancreatic duct obstruction secondary to tumor or gallstones) is also associated with increased fecal fat. Short gut syndrome is also associated with high fecal fat output.

Interfering factors

- Drugs that can alter test results include enemas and laxatives, especially mineral oil.

Procedure and patient care

Before

- Explain the procedure to the patient.
- Give the patient instructions regarding the appropriate diet (a diet diary may be requested by the laboratory):
  1. For adults, usually 100 g of fat per day is suggested

for 3 days before and throughout the collection period.

2. Children, and especially infants, cannot ingest 100 g of fat. Therefore a *fat retention coefficient* is determined by measuring the difference between the ingested fat and fecal fat and then expressing that difference (the amount of fat retained) as a percentage of the ingested fat:

$$\frac{\text{Ingested fat} - \text{Fecal fat}}{\text{Ingested fat}} \times 100\% = \text{Fat coefficient}$$

- Note that the fat retention coefficient in normal children and adults is 95% or greater. A low value indicates steatorrhea.
- Instruct the patient to defecate in a dry, clean container. Occasionally a tongue blade is required to transfer the stool to the specimen container.
- Tell the patient not to urinate in the stool container.
- Inform the patient that even diarrhea stools should be collected.
- Instruct the patient that toilet paper should not be placed in the stool container.
- Tell the patient not to take any laxatives or enemas during this test because they will interfere with intestinal motility and alter test results.

During

- Collect each stool specimen and send immediately to the laboratory during the 24- to 72-hour testing period.
- Label each specimen and include the time and date of collection.
- If the specimen is collected at home, give the patient a large stool container to keep in the freezer.

After

- Inform the patient that a normal diet can be resumed.

Abnormal findings
Increased levels

Cystic fibrosis

Malabsorption secondary to sprue, celiac disease, Whipple's disease, Crohn's disease (regional enteritis), or radiation enteritis

Maldigestion secondary to obstruction of the pancreatobiliary tree (e.g., cancer, stricture, gallstones)

Short gut syndrome secondary to surgical resection, surgical bypass, or congenital anomaly

Notes

ferritin

Type of test Blood

Normal findings

Male: 12-300 ng/ml or 12-300 µg/L (SI units)
Female: 10-150 ng/ml or 10-150 µg/L (SI units)

Test explanation and related physiology

The serum ferritin study is a good indicator of available iron stores. Ferritin, the major iron storage protein, is normally present in the serum in concentrations directly related to iron storage. In normal patients, 1 ng/ml of serum ferritin corresponds to approximately 8 mg of stored iron. Ferritin levels in adult men and postmenopausal women are generally significantly higher than in younger adult females. Decreases are associated with iron deficiency anemia and are also seen in patients with severe protein depletion. Increased levels are a sign of iron excess, as seen in hemochromatosis, hemosiderosis, megaloblastic anemia, hemolytic anemia, and certain liver disorders.

A limitation of this study is that ferritin levels can also be elevated in conditions not reflecting iron stores (e.g., acute inflammatory diseases, infections, metastatic cancer, lymphomas).

When combined with the serum iron level and total iron-binding capacity (Fe and TIBC, see p. 437), this test is useful in differentiating and classifying anemias. For example, in patients with iron deficiency anemia the ferritin, iron, and saturation levels are low, whereas the TIBC and transferrin levels are high. Ferritin levels are normal or high in patients with thalassemia.

Interfering factors

- Recent transfusions and recent ingestion of a meal containing high iron content can cause elevated ferritin levels.
- Hemolytic diseases may be associated with an artificially high iron content.
- Disorders of excessive iron storage (e.g., hemochromatosis, hemosiderosis) are associated with high ferritin levels.

- Menstruating women may have decreased ferritin levels.
- Drugs that may increase ferritin levels include iron preparations.

Procedure and patient care

Before

- Explain the procedure to the patient.
- Tell the patient that no fasting is required.

During

- Collect approximately 5 to 7 ml of venous blood in a red-top tube.

After

- Apply pressure or a pressure dressing to the venipuncture site.
- Assess the venipuncture site for bleeding.

Abnormal findings

Increased levels

Hemochromatosis
Hemosiderosis
Megaloblastic anemia
Hemolytic anemia
Alcoholic/inflammatory
  hepatocellular disease
Inflammatory diseases
Hodgkin's disease
Breast cancer

Decreased levels

Iron deficiency anemia
Severe protein deficiency

Notes

fetal scalp blood pH

Type of test Blood

Normal findings

pH: 7.25-7.35
O_2 saturation: 30%-50%
Po_2: 18-22 mm Hg
Pco_2: 40-50 mm Hg
Base excess: 0 to -10 mEq/L

Test explanation and related physiology

Measurement of the pH of fetal scalp blood provides valuable information on fetal acid-base status. This screening test is useful clinically for diagnosing fetal distress.

Although the oxygen partial pressure (Po_2), carbon dioxide partial pressure (Pco_2), and bicarbonate ion concentration can be measured with the fetal scalp blood sample, the pH is the most useful clinically. The pH normally ranges from 7.25 to 7.35 during labor. A mild decline of pH within the normal range is noted with contractions and as labor progresses.

Fetal hypoxia causes anaerobic glycolysis, resulting in excess production of lactic acid. This causes an increase in hydrogen ion concentration (acidosis) and a decrease in pH. Acidosis reflects the effect of hypoxia on cellular metabolism. A high correlation exists between low pH levels and low Apgar scores.

Contraindications

- Patients with premature membrane rupture
- Patients with active cervical infection (e.g., gonorrhea)

Potential complications

- Continued bleeding from the puncture site
- Hematoma
- Ecchymosis
- Infection

Procedure and patient care

Before

- Explain the procedure to the patient.
- Obtain informed consent for this procedure.
- Tell the patient that no fasting or sedation is required.

During

- Note the following procedural steps:

   1. Amnioscopy is performed with the mother in the lithotomy position.
   2. The cervix is dilated, and the endoscope (amnioscope) is introduced into the cervical canal.
   3. The fetal scalp is cleansed with an antiseptic and dried with a sterile cotton ball.
   4. A small amount of petroleum jelly is applied to the fetal scalp to cause droplets of fetal blood to bead.
   5. After the skin on the scalp is pierced with a small metal blade, beaded droplets of blood are collected in long, heparinized capillary tubes.
   6. The tube is sealed with wax and placed on ice to retard cellular respiration, which can alter the pH.
   7. The physician performing the procedure applies firm pressure to the puncture site to retard bleeding.
   8. Scalp blood sampling can be repeated as necessary.

- Note that this study is performed by a physician in approximately 10 to 15 minutes.
- Tell the patient that she may be uncomfortable during the cervical dilation.

After

- Inform the patient that she may have vaginal discomfort and menstrual-type cramping.

After delivery
- Assess the newborn and identify and document the puncture site (sites).
- Cleanse the fetal scalp puncture site with an antiseptic solution and apply an antibiotic ointment.

Abnormal finding

Fetal distress

Notes

fetoscopy

Type of test Endoscopy

Normal findings No fetal distress

Test explanation and related physiology

Fetoscopy is an endoscopic procedure that allows direct visualization of the fetus via the insertion of a tiny, telescope-like instrument through the abdominal wall and into the uterine cavity. Direct visualization may lead to diagnosis of a severe malformation, such as a neural tube defect (NTD). During the procedure, fetal blood samples to detect congenital blood disorders (e.g., hemophilia, sickle cell anemia) can be drawn from a blood vessel in the umbilical cord for biochemical analysis. Fetal skin biopsies can also be done to detect primary skin disorders.

Fetoscopy is performed at approximately 18 weeks' gestation. At this time the vessels of the placental surface are of adequate size and the fetal parts are readily identifiable. A therapeutic abortion would not be as hazardous at this time than if done later in the pregnancy.

Potential complications

- Spontaneous abortion
- Premature delivery
- Amniotic fluid leak
- Intrauterine fetal death
- Amnionitis

Procedure and patient care

Before

- Explain the procedure to the patient.
- Obtain informed consent for this procedure.
- Assess the fetal heart rate (FHR) before the test to serve as a baseline value.
- Administer meperidine (Demerol), if ordered, before the test because it crosses the placenta and quiets the fetus. This prevents excessive fetal movement, which would make the procedure more difficult.

During

- Note the following procedural steps:

    1. The woman is placed in the supine position on an examining table.
    2. The abdominal wall is anesthetized locally.
    3. Ultrasonograpy is done to locate the fetus and the placenta.
    4. The endoscope is inserted.
    5. Biopsies and blood samples may be obtained.

- Note that this procedure is performed by a physician in 1 to 2 hours.
- Tell the patient that the only discomfort associated with this study is the injection of the local anesthetic.

After

- Assess the FHR and compare with the baseline value to detect any side effects related to the procedure.
- Monitor the mother and fetus carefully for alterations in blood pressure, pulse, uterine activity, fetal activity, vaginal bleeding, and loss of amniotic fluid.
- Administer RhoGAM to Rh-negative mothers unless the fetal blood is found to be Rh negative.
- Note that a repeat ultrasound is usually performed the day after the procedure to confirm the adequacy of the amniotic fluid and fetal viability.
- Instruct the mother to avoid strenuous activity for 1 to 2 weeks following the procedure and to report any pain, bleeding, amniotic fluid loss, or fever.
- At times, if ordered, administer antibiotics prophylactically after the test to prevent amnionitis.

Abnormal findings

Developmental defects (e.g., neural tube defects)
Congenital blood disorders (e.g., hemophilia, sickle cell anemia)
Primary skin disorders

Notes

fibrin degradation products (FDPs, Fibrin split products [FSPs], Fibrin breakdown products)

Type of test Blood

Normal findings <10 μg/ml or dilution <1:20

Possible critical values >40 μg/ml

Test explanation and related physiology

The measurement of FDPs provides a direct indication of the activity of the fibrinolytic system. When plasma acts to dissolve fibrin blood clots, FDPs (X, D, E, and Y) are formed. These degradation products, which have an anticoagulant effect and inhibit clotting, can be measured. When they are present in large amounts, they indicate increased fibrinolysis, as occurs in disseminated intravascular coagulation (DIC) and primary fibrinolytic disorders. This test is one of the DIC screening tests.

Interfering factors

- Traumatic venipunctures may alter test results.
- Drugs that may cause elevated levels include barbiturates, heparin, streptokinase, and urokinase.

Procedure and patient care

Before

- Explain the procedure to the patient.
- Tell the patient that no fasting is required.

During

- Draw the sample before initiating heparin therapy.
- Collect a venous blood sample (usually only 2 ml) in a small blue-top tube or the colored tube designated by the laboratory.
- Avoid excessive agitation of the blood sample.
- Note that it is best to place the blood on ice and take it immediately to the hematology laboratory.
- List on the laboratory slip any drugs that may cause elevated levels.

After

- Apply pressure or a pressure dressing to the venipuncture site.
- Assess the venipuncture site for bleeding.

Abnormal findings
Increased levels

Liver disease
Congenital heart disease
Leukemia
Thromboembolic states
Transplant rejection
Renal disease
Obstetric complications (e.g., preeclampsia, abruptio placentae, intrauterine fetal death)

Following massive blood transfusion
Disseminated intravascular coagulation (DIC)
Hypoxia
Portacaval shunt
Infections
Burns
Septicemia
Following cardiopulmonary pump surgery

Notes

fibrinogen uptake test with ^{125}I (Fibrinogen uptake test [FUT], Radioactive fibrinogen scanning)

Type of test Nuclear scan

Normal findings No area of increased radionuclide uptake within the venous system of the lower extremity

Test explanation and related physiology

The iodine-125 fibrinogen uptake test (^{125}I FUT) is a noninvasive radionuclear study used to identify thrombi in the veins of the lower extremities. When thrombi formation occurs, large amounts of fibrinogen are present at the site of clot formation. Fibrinogen is an important hemostatic factor (factor II). When fibrinogen is tagged with ^{125}I and given intravenously, it can be detected in the bloodstream by a gamma ray detector. At areas where clot formation is occurring (e.g., venous thromboses), the ^{125}I count will be greatly increased. The test is approximately 80% to 90% accurate in the diagnosis of deep vein thrombophlebitis (DVT).

Although clinicians previously thought that the test could recognize only clots being formed, it is now known that the ^{125}I FUT can detect established clots. This test is also useful in the early detection of subclinical deep vein thrombosis. Therefore immobilized patients at great risk for DVT can be identified early. However, the ^{125}I FUT has several disadvantages:

1. This test cannot detect deep vein thrombosis in the proximal thigh. Normally, high quantities of fibrinogen exist in that area, and the background counts are too high to detect minimal degrees of increased uptake.
2. It is necessary to wait at least 24 hours between administering ^{125}I and detecting increased fibrinogen uptake. This is a major disadvantage when one needs to know immediately if thrombosis exists.
3. Because the fibrinogen used in this test is obtained from donated blood, the inherent risks of blood transfusion exist.

Initially, this test was used to evaluate medical-surgical or obstetric patients at high risk for the formation of deep vein thrombosis. These patients were studied over 1 to 2 weeks to detect extremely early deep vein thrombosis. In the present study, patients can be studied daily for 7 to 14 days after administration of ^{125}I.

Contraindications

- Patients for whom the diagnosis of deep vein thrombosis is needed in less than 24 hours
- Patients with ongoing inflammation in the leg (e.g., superficial phlebitis, cellulitis, active arthritis)
  Fibrinogen exists in increased levels at these areas and will give a false positive result.
- Patients with lymphedema, because the fibrinogen level is high in the extremities
- Patients who are allergic to iodine or shellfish
  A steroid and diphenhydramine (Benadryl) preparation may be used for these patients.

Interfering factors

- Other areas of inflammation within the suspected extremity
- Lymphedema

Procedure and patient care

Before

- Explain the procedure to the patient.
- Determine whether the patient is allergic to iodine or shellfish.
- Assess the patient's extremity for signs of inflammation or lymphedema.
- Tell the patient that no fasting or sedation is required.

During

- Note the following procedural steps:
  1. The patient is transferred to the nuclear medicine department, where ^{125}I fibrinogen is administered.
  2. The extremity is marked in multiple areas for subsequent examination.
  3. Countered readings are obtained 10 minutes after ^{125}I administration over the premarked sites.
  4. The patient is returned to his or her room.
  5. Twenty-four hours later, either at the patient's bedside or on his or her return to the nuclear medicine de-

partment, the Geigerlike detector is placed over the previously marked areas for counter readings.

6. The amount of ^{125}I identified at the premarked sites is recorded and compared with the amount present in the opposite leg or in the precordium.

7. If the amount of ^{125}I detected at any area is 15 times greater than normal extremity, heart, or baseline pre-injection levels, the test is considered positive for deep vein thrombosis.

- To avoid uptake of ^{125}I by the thyroid gland, provide Lugol's solution or potassium iodine, if ordered, for the patient before and during the scanning procedure.
- Note that a nuclear medicine technologist performs this procedure in less than 1 hour daily.
- Tell the patient that no discomfort is associated with this test other than the fibrinogen injection.

After

- Caution all nursing mothers to refrain from breastfeeding for 24 to 48 hours after injection of ^{125}I.

Abnormal finding

Deep vein thrombophlebitis (DVT)

Notes

folic acid (Folate)

Type of test Blood

Normal findings 5-20 μg/ml or 14-34 mmol/L (SI units)

Test explanation and related physiology

Folic acid, one of the B vitamins, is necessary for normal function of red and white blood cells (RBCs, WBCs) and for the adequate synthesis of certain purines and pyrimidines, which are precursors for deoxyribonucleic acid (DNA). As with vitamin B_{12} (see Schilling test, p. 653), folate depends on normal function of the intestinal mucosa.

Folic acid blood levels are done to evaluate hemolytic disorders and to detect anemia caused by folic acid deficiency (in which the RBCs are abnormally large, causing a megaloblastic anemia). These RBCs have a shortened life span and impaired oxygen-carrying capacity.

The main causes of folic acid deficiency include dietary deficiency, malabsorption syndrome, pregnancy, and certain anticonvulsant drugs. Decreased folic acid levels are seen in patients with folic acid deficiency anemia (megaloblastic anemia), hemolytic anemia, malnutrition, malabsorption syndrome, malignancy, liver disease, sprue, and celiac disease. Some drugs (e.g., anticonvulsants, antimalarials, alcohol, aminopterin, and methotrexate) are folic acid antagonists and interfere with nucleic acid synthesis.

Elevated levels of folic acid may be seen in patients with pernicious anemia. The folic acid test may be done in conjunction with tests for vitamin B_{12} levels (see Schilling test). This test for folate is often done in the workup for alcoholic patients to assess the patient's nutritional status.

Interfering factors

- Drugs that may cause decreased folic acid levels include alcohol, aminopterin, aminosalicylic acid (PAS), ampicillin, antimalarials, chloramphenicol, erythromycin, estrogens, methotrexate, oral contraceptives, penicillin, phenobarbital, phenytoin, and tetracyclines.

Procedure and patient care
Before
- Explain the procedure to the patient.
- Tell the patient that no fasting is usually required. (However, some laboratories prefer an 8-hour fast.)
- Instruct the patient not to consume alcoholic beverages before the test.
- Draw the specimen before starting folate therapy.

During
- Collect approximately 7 to 10 ml of venous blood in a red-top tube.
- Avoid hemolysis.
- Indicate on the laboratory slip any medications that can affect test results.

After
- Apply pressure or a pressure dressing to the venipuncture site.
- Assess the venipuncture site for bleeding.
- Transport the blood immediately to the laboratory after collection.

Abnormal findings
Increased levels
- Pernicious anemia

Decreased levels
- Folic acid deficiency anemia
- Hemolytic anemia
- Malnutrition
- Malabsorption syndrome (e.g., sprue, celiac disease)
- Malignancy
- Liver disease
- Pregnancy

Notes

galactose-1-phosphate uridyl transferase
(Gal-1-PUT, Galactosemia screening)

Type of test Blood

Normal findings 18.5-28.5 U/g hemoglobin

Test explanation and related physiology

Galactosemia is an inborn error of metabolism that causes a disorder of carbohydrate metabolism. This inherited disorder is characterized by lack of the enzyme Gal-1-PUT, which prevents the infant from converting galactose to glucose. This impairs normal glucose metabolism. The most common form of galactate is milk, which contains lactose.

Galactosemia is manifested by mental retardation, cataracts, jaundice, hepatomegaly, cirrhosis of the liver, and failure to thrive. Therapy consists of eliminating galactose from the diet. As with phenylketonuria (PKU), detection and treatment should begin in the first several weeks of life. (This test can also be ordered for adults to detect a carrier state of this disorder of carbohydrate metabolism.)

Several screening tests may be used to detect galactosemia. The most popular are the Paigen assay and the Beutler fluorometric test. Because the Paigen assay depends on the presence of an elevated blood galactose level, milk ingestion is necessary. The Beutler assay does not depend on milk ingestion. Both these tests can be performed on filter paper blood spots.

Procedure and patient care

Before

■ Inform the patient or parents about the purpose of this test and the method of obtaining the specimen.

During

■ Collect approximately 1 ml of blood by a heel stick for infants.
■ Note the patient's age on the laboratory slip.
■ Collect approximately 5 ml of venous blood in a green-top or lavender-top tube for adults.

After

- Apply pressure or a pressure dressing to the puncture site. Assess for bleeding.
- If the infant's test results are positive, inform the parents that dietary therapy should begin at once. Foods containing galactose, especially milk, should be removed from the infant's diet.
- Instruct adults who are heterozygous carriers of galactosemia to make certain their infants are screened at birth for galactosemia.

Abnormal finding

Galactosemia

Notes

gallbladder scanning (Hepatobiliary scintigraphy, Hepatobiliary imaging, Biliary tract radionuclide scan, Cholescintigraphy, DISIDA scanning, HIDA scanning, IDA gallbladder scanning)

Type of test Nuclear scan

Normal findings Gallbladder, common bile duct, and duodenum visualize within 60 minutes after radionuclide injection. (This confirms patency of the cystic and common bile ducts.)

Test explanation and related physiology

Through the use of iminodiacetic acid analogues (IDAs) labeled with technetium-99m (^{99m}Tc), the biliary tract can be evaluated in a safe, accurate, and noninvasive manner. These radionuclide compounds are extracted by the liver and excreted into the bile. Cholescintigraphy is valuable in evaluating patients for suspected gallbladder disease. The primary use of this study is to diagnose acute cholecystitis in patients who have acute right upper quadrant abdominal pain. Failure to visualize the gallbladder 60 to 120 minutes after injection of the radionuclide dye is virtually diagnostic of an obstruction of the cystic duct, which occurs in the pathophysiology of acute cholecystitis. Delayed filling of the gallbladder is associated with chronic or acalculus cholecystitis. This procedure is also helpful in diagnosing biliary duct obstructions.

This procedure is superior to oral cholecystography, IV cholangiography, ultrasonography, and computed tomography of the gallbladder in the detection of cholecystitis. Also, with cholescintigraphy, gallbladder function can be numerically determined by calculating the capability of the gallbladder to eject its contents. It is believed that an ejection fraction below 35% indicates primary gallbladder disease.

Contraindication

- Pregnancy, because of the risk of fetal damage

Interfering factor

- If the patient has not eaten for more than 24 hours, the radionuclide may not fill the gallbladder. This would give a false positive test result.

Procedure and patient care
Before

- Explain the procedure to the patient.
- Assure the patient that he or she will not be exposed to large amounts of radioactivity.
- Instruct the patient to fast for at least 2 hours before the test. This fasting is preferable, but not mandatory.

During

- Note the following procedural steps:

  1. After IV administration of a ^{99m}Tc-labeled IDA analogue (e.g., DISIDA, PIPIDA, HIDA), the right upper quandrant of the abdomen is scanned.
  2. Serial images are obtained over 1 hour.
  3. Subsequent images can be obtained at 15- to 30-minute intervals.
  4. If the gallbladder, common bile duct, or duodenum are not visualized within 60 minutes after injection, delayed images are obtained up to 4 hours later.
  5. Images are recorded on Polaroid or x-ray film.
  6. When an ejection fraction is to be determined, the patient is given a fatty meal or cholecystokinin to evaluate emptying of the gallbladder. The gallbladder is continually scanned to measure the percentage of isotope ejected.

- Note that a radiologist performs this study in 1 to 4 hours in the nuclear medicine department.
- Tell the patient that the only discomfort associated with this procedure is the IV injection of radionuclide.

After

- Obtain a meal for the patient if indicated.

Abnormal findings

Acute cholecystitis
Chronic cholecystitis
Common bile duct obstruction
  secondary to gallstones,
  tumor, or stricture
Acalculus cholecystitis

Notes

gallium scan

Type of test Nuclear scan

Normal findings

Diffuse low level of gallium uptake, especially in the liver and spleen

No increased gallium uptake within the body

Test explanation and related physiology

A gallium scan of the total body is usually performed 24, 48, and 72 hours after an IV injection of radioactive gallium. Gallium is a radionuclide that is concentrated by areas of inflammation and infection, by abscesses, and by benign and malignant tumors. Not all types of tumors, however, will concentrate gallium. Lymphomas are particularly susceptible for concentrating gallium. Other tumors that can be detected by gallium scan include sarcomas, hepatomas, and carcinomas of the gastrointestinal tract, kidney, uterus, stomach, and testicle.

This test is useful in detecting metastatic tumor, especially lymphoma, even when other diagnostic imaging tests are normal. The gallium scan also is useful in demonstrating a source of infection in patients who have a fever of unknown origin. Unfortunately, this test is not specific enough to differentiate among tumor, infection, inflammation, or abscess.

Some organs (liver, spleen, bone, colon) normally retain gallium. Therefore a normal total-body gallium scan study would demonstrate some uptake in these organs. However, this uptake is much less concentrated than in pathologic areas (e.g., tumor, inflammation).

Contraindication

- Pregnancy, because of the risk of fetal damage

Procedure and patient care

Before

- Explain the procedure to the patient.
- Usually, administer a cathartic or enema to the patient to minimize increased gallium uptake within the bowel.

During

- Note the following procedural steps:

  1. The unsedated patient is injected with gallium.
  2. A total-body scan may be performed 4 to 6 hours later by slowly passing a radionuclide detector over the body.
  3. The images provided by the detector are recorded on x-ray or Polaroid film.
  4. Additional scans are usually taken 24, 48, and 72 hours later.
  5. During the scanning process the patient is positioned in the supine, prone, and lateral positions.

- Note that a nuclear medicine technologist performs each scan is approximately 30 to 60 minutes. Repeated scanning, however, is required. Repeated injections are not necessary.
- Inform the patient that test results are interpreted by a physician trained in nuclear medicine and are usually available 72 hours after the injection.
- Tell the patient that no pain or discomfort is associated with this procedure other than the IV injection. However, it occasionally can be uncomfortable to lay still on a hard table for the duration required.
- Tell the patient that no pain or discomfort is associated with this procedure other than the IV injection. However, it occasionally can be uncomfortable to lay still on a hard table for the duration required.

After

- Assure the patient that only tracer doses of radioisotopes have been used and that no precautions against radioactive exposure to others are necessary.

Abnormal findings

Tumor	Noninfectious inflammation
Infection	Abscess

Notes

gamma-glutamyl transpeptidase (GGTP, γ-GTP, Gamma-glutamyl transferase, [GGT])

Type of test Blood

Normal findings

Male and female, over age 45: 8-38 U/L
Female, under age 45: 5-27 U/L
Elderly: slightly higher than adult
Child: similar to adult
Newborn: five times higher than adult

Test explanation and related physiology

The enzyme GGTP participates in the transfer of amino acids and peptides across the cellular membrane and also possibly participates in glutathione metabolism. Highest concentrations of this enzyme are found in the liver, kidney, spleen, and prostate gland. This test is used to detect liver cell dysfunction. It very accurately reveals evidence of cholestasis. As with leucine aminopeptidase and 5'-nucleotidase, the elevation of GGTP generally parallels that of alkaline phosphatase. However, GGTP is more sensitive. Also, as with 5'-nucleotidase and leucine aminopeptidase, GGTP is not increased in bone diseases as is alkaline phosphatase. A normal GGTP level with an elevated alkaline phosphatase level would imply skeletal disease. An elevated GGTP and elevated alkaline phosphatase level would imply hepatic disease.

Another important clinical aspect of GGTP is that it can detect alcohol ingestion. This enzyme rises rapidly after even a small intake of alcohol. It is therefore very useful in evaluation of alcoholic patients. GGTP is elevated in approximately 75% of these patients.

Why this enzyme is elevated 4 to 10 days after an acute myocardial infarction is not clear, but it may represent the associated hepatic insult.

Interfering factors

- Values may be decreased in late pregnancy.
- Drugs that may cause increased GGTP levels include alcohol, phenytoin (Dilantin), and phenobarbital.

- Drugs that may cause decreased levels include clofibrate and oral contraceptives.

Procedure and patient care
Before

- Explain the procedure to the patient.
- Tell the patient that no fasting is required.

During

- Collect approximately 7 to 10 ml of venous blood in a red-top tube.
- Indicate on the laboratory slip any medications the patient may be taking that can affect test results.

After

- Apply pressure or a pressure dressing to the venipuncture site.
- Assess the venipuncture site for bleeding. Patients with liver dysfunction often have prolonged clotting times.

Abnormal findings
Increased levels

Hepatitis
Cirrhosis
Hepatic necrosis
Hepatic ischemia
Myocardial infarction
  (4-10 days after)

Congestive heart failure
Hepatic tumor
Hepatotoxic drugs
Cholestasis
Alcohol ingestion

Notes

gastric analysis (Tube gastric analysis, Tubeless gastric analysis/Diagnex Blue test)

Type of test Fluid analysis

Normal findings

Tube gastric analysis: basal acid output, 2-5 mEq/hr
                       maximal acid output, 10-20 mEq/hr
Tubeless gastric analysis: detectable dye in urine

Test explanation and related physiology

With gastric analysis the contents of the stomach are aspirated to determine the amount of acid produced by the parietal cells within the stomach lining during the resting or basal state (basal acid output [BAO]) and during the stimulated state (maximal acid output [MAO]). This information is useful in the following clinical settings:

1. To determine whether a gastric ulcer is benign or malignant. Because a benign peptic ulcer requires the presence of acid, ulcerations that occur in the absence of acid (as determined by gastric analysis) will usually be malignant. However, differentiation between benign and malignant can be better determined by biopsy directed by esophagogastroduodenoscopy (EGD, see p. 321).

2. To determine the presence of the Zollinger-Ellison (ZE) syndrome. In this disease a pancreatic islet cell tumor secretes high levels of gastrin, which constantly and maximally stimulates the stomach to secrete acid. Therefore the stomach is always in the stimulated state and is never found in the resting state. This causes the value of the BAO to approach that of the MAO. The BAO/MAO ratio would then be greater than 0.6 in ZE syndrome. However, because of the development of direct measurement of serum gastrin levels, gastric analysis is no longer used for this purpose.

3. To determine the efficacy of medical or surgical antiulcer therapy. To be therapeutic, medical or surgical treatment of peptic ulcer disease must substantially decrease the acid output of the stomach. Baseline values are determined by a pretreatment gastric analysis.

The study is repeated during treatment. Effective therapy is indicated by a 50% reduction in the quantity of acid produced. This last indication is probably the only present use for gastric analysis.

Contraindications
- Patients with carcinoid syndrome

Potential complications
- Because histamine is the most frequently used drug to stimulate gastric acid, patients with congestive heart failure, carcinoid syndrome, or hypertension may have their conditions exacerbated.

Interfering factors
- Surgical vagotomy can alter test results.
- Smoking stimulates secretion of the gastric cells.
- Food or fluid alters gastric acid secretion.
- Drugs that may affect test results include anticholinergics and H_2-blocking agents (e.g., Tagamet, Zantac, Pepcid).

Procedure and patient care
Before
- Explain the procedure to the patient. Most patients are very apprehensive about this study.
- Instruct the patient to keep NPO after midnight on the day of the test.
- Instruct the patient to abstain from anticholinergic medications, which may inhibit the stimulating action of the histamine.
- Instruct the patient to abstain from smoking, which stimulates gastric acid secretion.

During
- Note the following procedural steps:

Tube gastric analysis
1. To assess the gastric acid secretion reliably, a nasogastric (NG) tube must be inserted into the dependent portion of the stomach.
2. A syringe is attached to the tube while initial gastric acid is aspirated and discarded.
3. Four subsequent samples are aspirated at 15-minute intervals. These are maked as BAO. The BAO is de-

termined by multiplying the number of milliequiva-
lents in the highest basal sample by four. Then, 0.04
mg/kg body weight of histamine is administered subcutaneously to the patient. (Occasionally, betazole hydrochloride is administered.)
4. Eight subsequent specimens are taken at 15-minute
intervals. These are the MAO specimens. The MAO is
determined by multiplying the number of milliequiva-
lents of the highest measurement by four.

Tubeless gastric analysis

1. In this type of test, which uses Diagnex Blue (Diagnex Blue test), the patient is asked to ingest a gastric
stimulant (e.g., a tablet of caffeine).
2. A resin dye such as Diagnex Blue is then ingested. If
the gastric contents contain hydrochloric acid (HCl),
the stomach acid displaces the dye from the Diagnex
resin.
3. The dye is absorbed by the bowel and excreted in the
urine in approximately 2 hours. The urine will be
changed to a blue color. The absence of a blue color
in the urine usually indicates the absence of HCl in
the stomach.

- Note that the gastric analysis is usually performed by a
nurse or physician in approximately 3 hours. It can be
performed in a laboratory or at the patient's bedside.
- Tell the patient that, except for the initial gagging usually
associated with insertion of the NG tube, this test is not
uncomfortable. (No NG tube insertion is needed for the
tubeless test.)

After

- Observe the patient for side effects of the histamine injection. They may include uterine, intestinal, or bronchial
spasm.
- Observe the patient for capillary dilation, which may be
evidenced by increased pulse rate and mildly decreased
blood pressure.
- If the tubeless gastric analysis uses Diagnex, inform the
patient that the urine may stay blue or blue-green for several days.

Abnormal findings

Zollinger-Ellison syndrome
Peptic ulceration
Inadequate therapeutic effect from surgical vagotomy
Inadequate therapeutic antipeptic ulcer medication

Notes

G

gastric cytology

Type of test Microscopic examination

Normal findings No malignant cells present

Test explanation and related physiology

Gastric cells can be collected and examined microscopically to detect malignancy. Tumor cells are often shed into the gastric lumen. These cells can be collected by gastric aspiration and examined. It is important to realize that the value of this test depends totally on the ability of the cytologist to read the slides accurately. By itself, a negative cytology report does not rule out malignancy. It reinforces other clinical data that suggest a benign gastric condition exists. A clearly positive cytology does indicate cancer. However, cells can appear suspicious and be benign, especially when inflammatory conditions exist.

Gastric cytology is rarely performed because gastrointestinal (GI) endoscopy has become such a routine part of diagnosing upper GI complaints. Gastric cytology and other intestinal cytologies are an indirect method to determine malignancy. Endoscopy, on the other hand, provides direct visualization, biopsy, and, occasionally, removal of GI tumors. Sometimes the position or size of the neoplasm prevents endoscopic biopsy. In these situations, under direct endoscopic vision, a small brush is passed over the neoplasm. The specimen on the brush is then examined cytologically. This is explained more completely under esophagogastroduodenoscopy (EGD, see p. 321).

Potential complication

- Tracheal misplacement of the nasogastric (NG) tube for gastric aspiration
  The patient will show signs of gasping, inspiratory stridor, and difficulty breathing. The tube should be removed immediately.

Interfering factor

- Food in the stomach

Procedure and patient care

Before

- Explain the procedure to the patient.
- Instruct the patient to keep NPO after midnight on the day of the test.
- Explain to the patient that some discomfort will be associated with the passage of the NG tube. Assure the patient that this is not a painful test.

During

- Note the following procedural steps:
  1. Gastric aspiration for cytology can be obtained during gastroscopy or with the insertion of an NG tube.
  2. When using an NG tube, approximately 100 ml of saline solution is instilled into the stomach.
  3. The patient is asked to turn 360 degrees several times. This ensures that saline has come into contact with all walls of the stomach.
  4. The fluid is aspirated and sent to the cytology laboratory in covered containers.
  5. Brush cytology may also be performed endoscopically.
  6. The NG tube or gastroscope is removed.
  7. Once at the laboratory, the fluid is centrifuged, and the precipitate containing cells from the gastric lining is examined microscopically.

- Note that this procedure is usually performed by a nurse in approximately 30 minutes. If endoscopy is required, a physician trained in endoscopy performs the procedure.
- Remind the patient that the only discomfort associated with this test is placement of the NG tube.

After

- Inform patients they may have a mild sore throat as a result of the tube placement.

Abnormal findings

Gastric cancer
Gastritis

Notes

gastric emptying scan

Type of test Nuclear scan

Normal findings

No delay in gastric emptying
Gastric emptying complete in 90 minutes

Test explanation and related physiology

This study involves having the patient ingest a solid or liquid "test meal" containing a radionuclide such as technetium (Tc). The stomach is then scanned until gastric emptying is complete. This study is used to assess the stomach's ability to empty solids or liquids and to evaluate disorders that may cause delay in gastric emptying, such as obstruction (caused by peptic ulcers or gastric malignancies) and gastroparesis. This scan also is useful in determining the patency of a gastrointestinal anastomosis.

Contraindications

- Patients who are pregnant or lactating

Before

- Explain the procedure to the patient.
- Assure the patient that no pain is associated with this study.
- Inform the patient that only a small dose of nuclear material is ingested. Reassure the patient that this is a safe dose.
- Instruct the patient to keep NPO after midnight on the day of the test.

During

- Note the following procedural steps:
  1. In the nuclear medicine department the patient is asked to ingest a test meal. In the *solid-emptying* study the patient eats a cooked egg white containing Tc. In the *liquid-emptying* study the patient drinks orange juice containing Tc.
  2. After ingestion of the test meal, the patient lies supine

under a gamma ray detector camera, which records images until gastric emptying has been complete. This may take several hours.

- Note that this procedure lasts approximately 90 minutes, depending on gastric emptying time.
- Inform the patient that the test is interpreted by a nuclear medicine physician and that results are available the same day.
- Remind the patient that no discomfort is associated with the test.

After

- Assure the patient that he or she has ingested only a small amount of nuclear material. No radiation precautions need to be taken against the patient or his or her bodily secretions.

Abnormal findings

Gastric obstruction caused by gastric ulcer or cancer
Nonfunctioning gastrointestinal anastomosis
Gastroparesis caused by diabetes or neuropathy

Notes

gastrin

Type of test Blood

Normal findings <200 pg/ml or <200 ng/L (SI units)

Test explanation and related physiology

Gastrin is a hormone produced by the G cells located in the distal part of the stomach (antrum). Gastrin is a potent stimulator of gastric acid. In normal gastric physiology an alkaline environment (created by food) stimulates the release of gastrin. Gastrin then stimulates the parietal cells of the stomach to secrete gastric acid. The pH environment in the stomach is thereby reduced. By negative feedback, this low pH environment suppresses further gastrin secretion.

Zollinger-Ellison (ZE) syndrome (gastrin-producing pancreatic tumor) and G-cell hyperplasia (overfunctioning of G cells in the distal stomach) are associated with high serum gastrin levels. Patients with these tumors have aggressive peptic ulcer disease. Unlike the patient with routine peptic ulcers, the patient with ZE syndrome or with G-cell hyperplasia has a high incidence of complicated and recurrent peptic ulcers. It is important to identify this latter group of patients to institute more appropriate aggressive medical and surgical therapy. The serum gastrin level will be normal in the patient with routine peptic ulcer and will be greatly elevated in patients with ZE syndrome or G-cell hyperplasia.

It is important to note, however, that patients who are taking antacid peptic ulcer medicines or who have had peptic ulcer surgery will have a high serum gastrin level. However, levels are not usually as high as in patients with ZE syndrome or G-cell hyperplasia.

Not all patients with ZE syndrome exhibit increased levels of serum gastrin. Some may have "top" normal gastrin levels, which makes these patients difficult to differentiate from patients who have routine peptic ulcer disease. These "top" normal patients can be identified, however, with gastrin stimulation tests using calcium or secretin. Patients with ZE syndrome or G-cell hyperplasia will have greatly increased serum gastrin levels associated with the infusion of these drugs.

Interfering factors

- Peptic ulcer surgery
  This creates a persistent alkaline environment, which is the strongest stimulant to gastrin.
- Diabetic patients taking insulin may have falsely elevated levels.
- Drugs that may increase serum gastrin levels include antacids, H_2-blocking agents (e.g., Tagamet, Zantac), and hydrogen pump inhibitors (e.g., Losec).

Procedure and patient care

Before

- Explain the procedure to the patient.
- Usually, instruct the patient to fast for 12 hours. Water is permitted.
- Tell the patient to avoid alcohol for at least 24 hours.

During

- Collect approximately 5 to 7 ml of venous blood in a red-top tube.
- For the *calcium infusion test,* administer calcium gluconate intravenously for 3 hours. A preinfusion serum gastrin level is then compared to specimens taken every 30 minutes for 4 hours.
- For the *secretin test,* administer secretin intravenously. Preinjection and postinjection serum gastrin levels are taken at 15-minute intervals for 1 hour after injection.
- Indicate on the laboratory slip any drugs that can affect test results.

After

- Apply pressure or a pressure dressing to the venipuncture site.
- Observe the venipuncture site for bleeding.

Abnormal findings

Increased levels

Zollinger-Ellison syndrome
G-cell hyperplasia
Pernicious anemia

Notes

gastroesophageal reflux scan (GE reflux scan, Aspiration scan)

Type of test Nuclear scan

Normal findings No evidence of gastroesophageal reflux

Test explanation and related physiology

GE reflux scans are used to evaluate patients with symptoms of heartburn, regurgitation, vomiting, and dysphagia. Also, these scans are used to evaluate the medical or surgical treatment of patients with GE reflux. Finally, *aspiration scans* may be used to detect aspiration of gastric contents into the lungs.

Contraindications

- Patients who cannot tolerate abdominal compression
- Patients who are pregnant or lactating

Procedure and patient care

Before

- Explain the procedure to the patient.
- Assure the patient that no pain is associated with this test.
- Instruct the patient to eat a full meal just before the study.

During

- Note the following procedural steps:

  1. The patient is placed in the supine position and asked to swallow a tracer cocktail (e.g., orange juice, diluted hydrochloric acid, and technetium-99-labeled colloid).
  2. Images are taken of the patient over the esophageal area.
  3. The patient is asked to assume other positions to determine whether GE reflux occurs and, if so, in what position.
  4. A large abdominal binder that contains an air-inflatable cuff is placed on the patient's abdomen. This is insufflated to increase abdominal pressure.
  5. Images are again taken over the esophageal area to determine if any GE reflux occurs.

Aspiration scans

1. These scans may be performed by adding a radionuclide to the patient's evening meal and keeping the patient in the supine position until the next morning.
2. Images are made over the lung fields to detect esophagotracheal aspiration of the tracer.

- In infants being evaluated for chalasia, note that the tracer is added to the feeding or formula. Nuclear tracer films are then taken over the next hour, with delayed films as needed.
- Note that this procedure is performed in the nuclear medicine department in approximately 30 minutes.
- Remind the patient that no discomfort is associated with this test.

After

- Assure the patient that he or she has ingested only a small dose of nuclear material. No radiation precautions need to be taken against the patient or his or her bodily secretions.

Abnormal findings

Gastroesophageal reflux
Pulmonary aspiration

Notes

gastrointestinal bleeding scan (Abdominal scintigraphy, GI scintigraphy)

Type of test Nuclear scan

Normal findings No collection of radionuclide in GI tract

Test explanation and related physiology

The GI bleeding scan is a test used to localize the site of bleeding in patients who are having GI hemorrhage. The scan also can be used in patients who have intraabdominal hemorrhage from an unknown source. Localization of the source of GI bleeding can be quite difficult. When surgery is required under these circumstances, it is difficult, cumbersome, and prolonged. The surgeon may have extreme difficulty finding the source of bleeding.

Endoscopy has proved to be extremely useful in determining the source of intestinal bleeding. However, endoscopy is not helpful if the source of bleeding is within the small intestine or in the colon. Although colonoscopy allows excellent visualization of the colon when it is cleared out, it is extremely difficult to see when acute active intestinal bleeding is occurring. Arteriography can determine the site of bleeding. However, the rate of bleeding must exceed 0.5 ml per minute for detection by arteriography. Also, GI bleeding can be intermittent and the arteriogram could be falsely negative.

A GI scintigram is much more sensitive in locating the site of GI bleeding. However, it is not very specific in pinpointing the site of bleeding. Usually, when positive, the exact source of bleeding cannot be localized any more accurately than indicating the affected quadrant of the abdomen (e.g., right upper, left lower). This test is usually performed by injecting sulfur colloid labeled with technetium-99m (^{99m}Tc) or ^{99m}Tc-labeled red blood cells (RBCs) into the patient. If the patient is bleeding at a rate in excess of 0.05 ml per minute, pooling of the radionuclide will ultimately be detected in the abnormal segment of the intestine. Few false positive results occur. The test will only localize the bleeding; it will not indicate the exact pathologic condition causing the bleeding. With this test result, if surgery is required, the surgeon is directed to the abnormal area and, it is hoped, can detect and resect the pathologic bleeding source.

Contraindications

- Patients who are pregnant or lactating
- Medically unstable patients whose stay in the nuclear medicine department may be risky

Interfering factor

- Barium within the GI tract can mask a small source of bleeding

Procedure and patient care

Before

- Explain the procedure to the patient.
- Assess the patient's vital signs to ensure that they are stable for the patient's transfer to and from the nuclear medicine department.
- Accompany the patient to the nuclear medicine department if vital signs are questionably stable.
- Assure the patient that only a small amount of nuclear material will be administered.
- Instruct the patient to notify the nuclear medicine technologist if the patient has a bowel movement during the test. Blood in the GI tract can act as a cathartic.
- Inform the patient that no pretest preparation is required.
- Inform the nuclear medicine technologist to notify the nurse of all bloody bowel movements that occur while the patient is in the nuclear medicine department.

During

- Note the following procedural steps:

  1. Ten millicuries of freshly prepared ^{99m}Tc-labeled sulfur colloid is administered intravenously to the patient. If ^{99m}Tc-labeled RBCs are to be used, 3 to 5 ml of the patient's own blood is combined with the ^{99m}Tc and reinjected into the patient.
  2. Immediately after administration of the radionuclide, the patient is placed under a scintillation camera.
  3. Multiple images of the abdomen are obtained at short intervals (5 to 15 minutes). Scintigrams are recorded on Polaroid or x-ray film.

4. Detection of radionuclide in the abdomen indicates the site of bleeding. If no bleeding sites are noted in the first hour, the scan is repeated at hourly intervals for as long as 24 hours.

- Note that areas of the bowel hidden by the liver or spleen may not be adequately evaluated by this procedure. Also, the rectum cannot be easily evaluated because of other pelvic structures (e.g., the bladder) obstruct the view. If the initial study is negative and subsequent films give evidence of active bleeding, a repeat scan may be performed.
- Note that this test is usually performed in approximately 20 to 30 minutes by a technologist in the nuclear medicine department.
- Tell the patient that the only discomfort associated with this study is the injection of the radioisotope.

After

- Reevaluate the patient's vital signs on return to the nursing unit.
- Assure the patient that only tracer doses of radioisotopes have been used and that no precautions against radioactive exposure to others are necessary.

Abnormal findings

Ulcers
Angiodysplasia
Diverticulosis

Tumors
Polyps
Inflammatory bowel disease

Notes

glucose, blood (Blood sugar, Fasting blood sugar [FBS])

Type of test Blood

Normal findings

Cord: 45-96 mg/dl or 2.5-5.3 mmol/L (SI units)
Premature infant: 20-60 mg/dl or 1.1-3.3 mmol/L
Neonate: 30-60 mg/dl or 1.7-3.3 mmol/L
Infant: 40-90 mg/dl or 2.2-5.0 mmol/L
Child less than age 2 years: 60-100 mg/dl or 3.3-5.5
   mmol/L
Child over age 2 years to adult: 70-105 mg/dl or 3.9-5.8
   mmol/L
Elderly: increase in normal range after age 50

Possible critical values

Adult male: <50 and >400 mg/dl
Adult female: <40 and >400 mg/dl
Infant: <40
Newborn: <30 and >300 mg/dl

Test explanation and related physiology

The serum glucose test is helpful in diagnosing many metabolic diseases. Serum glucose levels must be evaluated according to the time of the day they are performed. For example, a glucose level of 135 mg/dl may be abnormal if the patient is in the fasting state. However, this level would be within normal limits if the patient had eaten a meal within the last hour.

In general, true glucose elevations indicate diabetes mellitus. However, one must be aware of many other possible causes of hyperglycemia. Similarly, hypoglycemia has many causes. The most common cause, however, is inadvertent insulin overdose in patients with brittle diabetes. Glucose determinations must be performed frequently in new diabetic patients to monitor closely the insulin dosage to be administered.

Interfering factors

- Many forms of stress (e.g., trauma, general anesthesia, cerebrovascular accident, myocardial infarction) can cause increased serum glucose levels.

- Caffeine may cause increased levels.
- Drugs that may cause increased levels include antidepressants (tricyclics), beta-adrenergic blocking agents, corticosteroids, dextrose IV infusion, dextrothyroxine, diazoxide, diuretics, epinephrine, estrogens, glucagon, isoniazid (INH), lithium, phenothiazines, phenytoin, salicylates (acute toxicity), and triamerene.
- Drugs that may cause decreased levels include acetaminophen, alcohol, anabolic steroids, clofibrate, disopyramide, gemfibrozil, insulin, monoamine oxidase inhibitors, pentamidine, propranolol, tolazamide, and tolbutamide.

Procedure and patient care

Before

- Explain the procedure to the patient.
- For an FBS, keep the patient fasting at least 8 hours. Water is permitted.
- The patient should not fast longer than 16 hours in order to prevent starvation, which may artificially raise the glucose levels.
- Withhold insulin or oral hypoglycemics until after blood is obtained.

During

- Collect approximately 7 ml of venous blood in a red-top or gray-top tube.

After

- Apply pressure or a pressure dressing to the venipuncture site.
- Observe the venipuncture site for bleeding.
- Be certain that the patient receives a meal after fasting blood work.

Abnormal findings

Increased levels (hyperglycemia)	Decreased levels (hypoglycemia)
Diabetes mellitus	Insulinoma
Acute stress response	Hypothyroidism
Cushing's disease	Hypopituitarism
Pheochromocytoma	Addison's disease
Hyperparathyroidism	Extensive liver disease

Adenoma of the pancreas
Pancreatitis
Diuretic therapy
Corticosteroid therapy
Acromegaly

Notes

glucose, postprandial (2-Hour postprandial glucose [2-hour PPG], 2-Hour postprandial blood sugar)

Type of test Blood

Normal findings
0-50 years: 70-140 mg/dl or <7.8 mmol/L (SI Units)
50-60 years: 70-150 mg/dl
60 years and older: 70-160 mg/dl

Test explanation and related physiology
The 2-hour PPG test is a measurement of the amount of glucose in the patient's blood 2 hours after a meal (postprandial) is ingested. For this study a meal acts as a glucose challenge to the body's metabolism. In normal patients, insulin is secreted immediately after a meal in response to the elevated blood glucose level, thus causing the level to return to the premeal range within 2 hours. In diabetic patients the glucose level is usually still elevated 2 hours after the meal.

The PPG is an easily performed screening test for diabetes mellitus. If the results are abnormal, a glucose tolerance test (see p. 388) may be performed to confirm the diagnosis.

Interfering factors
- Smoking during the testing period may increase the blood glucose level.
- Stress can increase glucose levels.

Procedure and patient care
Before
- Explain the procedure to the patient.
- Instruct the patient to eat the entire meal (of at least 75 g of carbohydrates) and then not to eat anything else until the blood is drawn.
- Instruct the patient not to smoke during the testing.
- Inform the patient that he or she should rest during the 2-hour interval.

During
- Collect approximately 7 ml of blood in a red-top or gray-top tube at exactly 2 hours after eating.

After

- Apply pressure or a pressure dressing to the venipuncture site.
- Observe the venipuncture site for bleeding.

Abnormal findings
Increased levels

Diabetes mellitus
Cushing's syndrome
Acromegaly
Malnutrition
Hyperthyroidism
Pheochromocytoma

Decreased levels

Addison's disease
Steatorrhea
Islet cell adenoma
Anterior pituitary insufficiency

Notes

glucose, urine (Urine sugar, Urine glucose)

Type of test Urine

Normal findings

Random specimen: Negative
24-hour specimen: <0.5 g/day or <2.78 mmol/day (SI units)

Test explanation and related physiology

A qualitative glucose test is usually part of a routine urinalysis. This screening test for the presence of glucose within the urine may indicate the likelihood of diabetes mellitus. This diagnosis must be confirmed by other tests (e.g., glucose tolerance test, glycosylated hemoglobin test). Urine glucose tests are also used to monitor the effectiveness of diabetes therapy. However, this is largely supplanted today by finger stick determinations of blood glucose levels.

In diabetic patients whose conditions are not well controlled with hypoglycemic agents, blood glucose levels can become very high. High glucose levels can also be produced artificially by IV administration of dextrose-containing fluids. When the blood glucose level exceeds 180 mg/dl (the renal threshold), glucose begins to spill over into the urine (glycosuria). As the blood glucose level increases further, the amount of glucose spilling into the urine also increases.

Interfering factors

- Drugs that may cause increased urine glucose levels include aminosalicylic acid (PAS), cephalosporins, chloral hydrate, chloramphenicol, dextrothyroxine, diazoxide, diuretics (loop and thiazide), estrogens, glucose infusions, isoniazid (INH), levodopa, lithium, nafcillin, nalidixic acid, and nicotinic acid (large doses).
- Drugs that may cause false positive tests with Clinitest but not with Clinistix or Tes-Tape include acetylsalicylic acid, aminosalicylic acid (PAS), ascorbic acid, cephalothin, chloral hydrate, nitrofurantoin, streptomycin, and sulfonamides.
- Drugs that may cause false negative tests include ascorbic acid (Clinistix, Tes-Tape), levodopa (Clinistix), and phenazopyridine (Clinistix, Tes-Tape)

Procedure and patient care
Before
- Explain the procedure to the patient.
- Read the directions on the bottle or container of the reagent strips.
- Check the expiration date on the bottle before use.
- Inform the patient that urine tests for glucose may be performed at specified times during the day, generally before meals and at bedtime, and that test results may be used to determine insulin requirements.

During
- Because accuracy is necessary, collect a "fresh" urine specimen. The stagnant urine that has been in the bladder for several hours will not accurately reflect the serum glucose level at testing.
- Preferably, obtain a *double-voided specimen:*
  1. Collect a urine specimen 30 to 40 minutes before the time the urine specimen is actually needed.
  2. Discard this first specimen.
  3. Give the patient a glass of water to drink.
  4. At the required time obtain a second specimen, which is tested for glucose.
- Inform the patient that testing for glucose can be easily performed using enzyme tests such as Clinistix, Diastix, or Tes-Tape.
- Remember that urine glucose can also be determined using the Clinitest method (a copper-reducing approach).
- If a 24-hour specimen (see p. 325) is required, refrigerate the urine during the collection period.

After
- Record the urine glucose results on the patient's chart.

Abnormal findings
Increased levels

Diabetes mellitus	Infection
Cushing's syndrome	Drug therapy
Severe stress (e.g., trauma, surgery)	Pregnancy
	Low renal threshold

glucose-6-phosphate dehydrogenase (G-6-PD screen)

Type of test Blood

Normal findings Negative (screening test) or 8-8.6 U/g hemoglobin

Test explanation and related physiology

G-6-PD is an enzyme used in glucose metabolism. In the red blood cell a G-6-PD deficiency causes precipitation of hemoglobin and cellular membrane changes. This may result in hemolysis of variable severity. This disease is a sex-linked, recessive trait carried on the X chromosome. Affected males inherit this abnormal gene from their mothers, who are usually asymptomatic. Hemolytic episodes in these individuals may be triggered by drugs (e.g., sulfonamides, nitrofurantoin, phenacetin, antipyretics, primaquine), infections, acidosis, stress, or certain foods (e.g., fava beans). The two common types of G-6-PD deficiency are Mediterranean, affecting Sephardic Jews, and type A, affecting the black population. This test is used to diagnose G-6-PD deficiency in suspected individuals.

Interfering factors

- Drugs that may cause increased G-6-PD levels include antipyretics, ascorbic acid, aspirin, nitrofurantoin (Furadantin), phenacetin, primaquine, quinidine, sulfonamides, thiazide diuretics, tolbutamide (Orinase), and vitamin K.

Procedure and patient care

Before

- Explain the procedure to the patient.
- Tell the patient that no fasting is required.

During

- Collect approximately 5 ml of venous blood in a lavender-top or green-top tube.
- Avoid hemolysis.

After

- Apply pressure or a pressure dressing to the venipuncture site.
- Assess the venipuncture site for bleeding.
- If the test indicates that a G-6-PD deficiency, give the patient a list of drugs that can precipitate hemolysis. Instruct patients with the Mediterranean variant of this disease not to eat fava beans. Teach patients to read labels on any over-the-counter drugs for the presence of agents (e.g., aspirin, phenacetin) that may cause hemolytic anemia.

G

Abnormal findings

Increased levels

Pernicious anemia
Myocardial infarction
Hepatic coma
Hyperthyroidism
Chronic blood loss
Megaloblastic anemia

Decreased levels

G-6-PD deficiency
Hemolytic anemia
Infections
Septicemia
Diabetic acidosis

Notes

glucose tolerance test (GTT, Oral glucose tolerance test [OGTT])

Type of test Blood; urine

Normal findings

Serum test
Fasting: 70-115 mg/dl or <6.4 mmol/L (SI units)
30 minutes: <200 mg/dl or <11.1 mmol/L
1 hour: <200 mg/dl or <11.1 mmol/L
2 hours: <140 mg/dl or <7.8 mmol/L
3 hours: 70-115 mg/dl or <6.4 mmol/L
4 hours: 70-115 mg/dl or <6.4 mmol/L
Urine test: negative

Test explanation and related physiology

In the GTT the patient's ability to tolerate a standard oral glucose load is evaluated by obtaining serum and urine specimens for glucose level determinations before glucose administration and then at 30 minutes, 1 hour, 2 hours, 3 hours, and sometimes 4 hours after the glucose administration. Patients with an appropriate insulin response are able to tolerate the dose quite easily, with only a minimal and transient rise in serum glucose levels within 1 hour after ingestion. In normal patients, glucose will not spill over into the urine.

Diabetic patients, who have a deficiency of active insulin, will not be able to tolerate this load. As a result, their serum glucose levels will be greatly elevated from 1 to 5 hours. Also, glucose can be detected in their urine.

Gestational diabetes can also be diagnosed by the GTT. Generally the diagnosis of diabetes can be made if two or more of the results exceed the following:

Fasting: 105 mg/dl
1 hour: 190 mg/dl
2 hours: 165 mg/dl
3 hours: 145 mg/dl

Occasionally a patient is unable to tolerate the oral glucose load (e.g., patients with prior gastrectomy, short bowel syndrome, or malabsorption). In these instances an *intravenous glucose tolerance test* (IV-GTT) can be performed by administering the glucose load intravenously. The values for the IV-GTT differ slightly from those of the oral GTT because the IV glucose is absorbed faster.

Contraindications

- Patients with serious concurrent infections, endocrine disorders, or infections, because glucose intolerance will be observed even though these patients may not be diabetic.

Potential complications

- Dizziness, tremors, anxiety, sweating, euphoria, or fainting during testing
  If these symptoms occur, a blood specimen is obtained. If the glucose level is too high, the test may need to be stopped and insulin administered.

Interfering factors

- Smoking during the testing period stimulates glucose because of the nicotine.
- Stress (e.g., from surgery, infection) can increase glucose levels.
- Exercise during the testing can affect glucose levels.
- Drugs that may cause glucose intolerance include antihypertensives, antiinflammatory drugs, aspirin, beta blockers, furosemide, nicotine, oral contraceptives, psychiatric drugs, steroids, and thiazide diuretics.

Procedure and patient care

Before

- Explain the procedure to the patient.
- Educate the patient about the importance of having adequate food intake with adequate carbohydrates for at least 3 days before the test.
- Instruct the patient to fast 12 hours before the test.
- Instruct the patient to discontinue drugs that could interfere with the test results.
- Give the patient written instructions explaining the pretest dietary requirement.
- Obtain the patient's weight to determine the appropriate glucose loading dose.

During

- Obtain fasting blood and urine specimens.
- Administer the oral glucose solution, usually a 75 to 100 g carbohydrate load.
- Give pediatric patients a carbohydrate load of 1.75 g/kg body weight up to a maximum of 75 g.
- Instruct the patient to ingest the entire glucose load.
- Tell the patient that he or she cannot eat anything until the test is completed. However, encourage the patient to drink water. No other liquids should be taken.
- Inform the patient that tobacco, coffee, and tea are not allowed because they cause physiologic stimulation.
- Collect approximately 5 ml of venous blood in a gray-top tube at 30 minutes and at hourly periods. Apply pressure or a pressure dressing to the sites.
- Collect urine specimens at hourly periods.
- Mark on the tubes the time that the specimens are collected.
- Assess the patient for reactions such as dizziness, sweating, weakness, and giddiness. (These are usually transient.)
- For the IV-GTT, administer the glucose load intravenously over 3 to 4 minutes.
- Indicate on the laboratory any drugs that can affect test results.

After

- Send all specimens promptly to the laboratory.
- Allow the patient to eat and drink normally.
- Administer insulin or oral hypoglycemics if ordered.
- Assess the venipuncture sites for bleeding.

Abnormal findings

Diabetes mellitus
Gestational diabetes
Hypoglycemia

Cushing's syndrome
Pancreatic cancer

Notes

glycosylated hemoglobin (GHb, GHB, Glycohemoglobin [Hb A$_{1c}$], Diabetic control index)

Type of test   Blood

Normal findings   Vary with laboratory method employed

Adult/elderly: 2.2%-4.8%
Child: 1.8%-4.0%
Good diabetic control: 2.5%-6%
Fair diabetic control: 6.1%-8%
Poor diabetic control: >8%

G

Test explanation and related physiology

The GHb test provides an accurate long-term index of the patient's average blood glucose level by measuring the patient's glycohemoglobin or GHb. Glycohemoglobin is a minor hemoglobin (A$_1$ components). These A$_1$ components (hemoglobin A$_{1a}$, A$_{1b}$, and A$_{1c}$), which make up about 4% to 8% of the total hemoglobin, are glycosylated, that is, they have glucose attached to them. Hb A$_{1c}$ is usually measured. (If Hb A$_1$ is measured, its value is always 2.4% higher than that of the A$_{1c}$ component.)

As the red blood cell (RBC) circulates, it combines some of its hemoglobin with some of the glucose in the bloodstream to form glycohemoglobin. This glycosylation is irreversible. The amount of GHb depends on the amount of glucose available in the bloodstream over the RBC's 120-day life span. Since old RBCs are constantly being destroyed and new ones are being formed, determination of the GHb value reflects the average blood sugar level for the 100- to 120-day period *before* the test. The more glucose the RBC was exposed to, the greater the GHb percentage. One important advantage of this test is that the sample can be drawn at any time because it is not affected by short-term variations (e.g., food intake, exercise, stress, hypoglycemic agents, patient cooperation).

The GHb test is particularly beneficial for:

1. Evaluating the success of diabetic treatment
2. Comparing and contrasting the success of past and new forms of diabetic therapy

3. Determining the duration of hyperglycemia in newly diagnosed diabetic patients
4. Providing a sensitive estimate of glucose imbalance in patients with mild diabetes
5. Individualizing diabetic control regimens
6. Providing a feeling of reward for many patients when the test shows achievement of good diabetic control

Interfering factors

- Low values may occur with sickle cell anemia, with chronic renal failure, and in pregnancy.
- Falsely elevated values occur when the RBC life span is lengthened (as in thalassemia).

Procedure and patient care

Before

- Explain the procedure to the patient.
- Tell the patient that fasting is not indicated.

During

- Collect approximately 5 ml of venous blood in a gray-top or lavender-top tube.

After

- Apply pressure or a pressure dressing to the venipuncture site.
- Assess the venipuncture site for bleeding.

Abnormal findings

Newly diagnosed diabetic patient
Poorly controlled diabetic patient
Hemolytic anemia in nondiabetic persons
Chronic renal failure
Pregnancy

Notes

gonorrhea culture

Type of test Microscopic examination

Normal findings No evidence of *Neisseria gonorrhoeae*

Test explanation and related physiology

Cultures for gonococcal infections are performed on men and women with suspected gonorrhea. If the culture is positive, sexual partners should be evaluated and treated. Cervical cultures are usually done for women; urethral cultures are done for men. Rectal and throat cultures are performed in persons who have engaged in anal and oral intercourse. Because rectal gonorrhea accompanies genital gonorrhea in a high percentage of women, rectal cultures may be recommended in all women with suspected gonorrhea. Performing a culture for gonorrhea is also part of the prenatal workup. If the culture is positive, treatment during pregnancy can prevent possible fetal complications (e.g., ophthalmia neonatorum) and maternal complications. Rectal and orogastric cultures should be done on neonates of infected mothers.

Gram stains of smears or bacterial cultures should be taken before a patient begins antibiotic therapy. Bacterial cultures use a special medium such as Thayer-Martin, designed for the cultivation of *N. gonorrhoeae.*

Interfering factors

- *N. gonorrhoeae* is very sensitive to lubricants and disinfectants.
- Menses can alter test results.
- Female douching within 24 hours of a cervical culture makes fewer organisms available for culture.
- Male voiding within 1 hour of a urethral culture washes secretions out of the urethra.
- Fecal material may contaminate an anal culture.

Procedure and patient care

Before

- Explain the purpose and procedure to the patient. Use a matter-of-fact, nonjudgmental approach.
- Tell the patient that no fasting or sedation is required.

During

- Obtain cultures as follows:

Cervical culture

1. The female patient is told to refrain from douching and tub bathing before the cervical culture.
2. The patient is placed in the lithotomy position, and a nonlubricated vaginal speculum is inserted to expose the cervix.
3. Cervical mucus is removed with a cotton ball held in a ring forceps.
4. A sterile cotton-tipped swab is inserted into the endocervical canal and moved from side to side to obtain the culture.

Anal canal culture

1. An anal culture of the female or male is taken by inserting a sterile, cotton-tipped swab about 1 inch into the anal canal.
2. If stool contaminates the swab, a repeat swab is taken.

Urethral culture

1. The urethral specimen should be obtained from the man before voiding. Voiding within 1 hour of collection washes secretions out of the urethra, making fewer organisms available for culture.
2. A culture is taken by inserting a sterile swab gently into the anterior urethra.
3. It is advisable to place the male patient in the supine position to prevent falling if vasovagal syncope occurs during introduction of the cotton swab or wire loop into the urethra.
4. The patient is observed for hypotension, bradycardia, pallor, sweating, nausea, and weakness.

Oropharyngeal culture

1. This culture should be obtained in men and women who have engaged in oral intercourse.
2. A throat culture is best obtained by depressing the patient's tongue with a wooden tongue blade and touching the posterior wall of the throat with a sterile cotton-tipped swab.

- Note that gonorrheal cultures are obtained by a physician or nurse in several minutes.
- Tell the person that little discomfort is associated with these procedures.

After

- Place the swabs in a Thayer-Martin medium and roll them from side to side.
- Label and send the culture bottle to the microbiology laboratory.
- Transport the specimen to the laboratory as soon as possible. Handle all specimens as though they were capable of transmitting disease.
- Do not refrigerate the specimen.
- Mark the laboratory slip with the collection time, date, source of specimen, patient's age, current antibiotic therapy, and clinical diagnosis.
- Advise the patient to avoid intercourse and all sexual contact until test results are available.
- If the culture results are positive, tell the patient to receive treatment and to have sexual partners evaluated.
- Note that repeat cultures should be taken after completion of treatment to evaluate therapy.

Abnormal finding

Gonorrhea

Notes

granular casts

Type of test Urine

Normal findings Occasional casts present

Test explanation and related physiology

Casts are clumps of materials or cells. They are formed in the renal collecting tubule and have the shape of the tubule, thus the term *cast*. Granular casts result from the disintegration of cellular material in white and epithelial blood cells into granular particles. Granular casts are found after exercise and in patients with various renal diseases.

Procedure and patient care
Before
- Explain the procedure to the patient.

During
- Collect a fresh urine specimen in a urine container.
- Note that if the specimen is contaminated by vaginal discharge or bleeding, a "clean-catch" or "midstream" specimen will be needed. This requires meticulous cleansing of the urinary meatus with an iodine preparation to reduce contamination of the specimen by external organisms. Then the cleansing agent must be completely removed, or it will contaminate the specimen. The midstream collection is obtained by:
  1. Having the patient begin to urinate in a bedpan, urinal, or toilet and then stop urinating (This washes the urine out of the distal urethra.)
  2. Correctly positioning a sterile urine container, into which the patient voids 3 to 4 ounces of urine
  3. Capping the container
  4. Allowing patient to finish voiding

After
- Send the specimen immediately to the laboratory.
- Do *not* allow the specimen to sit, since the casts will break up. Urine should be checked for casts when it is fresh.

Abnormal findings
Increased levels

Acute tubular necrosis
Urinary tract infection
Glomerulonephritis
Pyelonephritis
Nephrosclerosis

Chronic lead poisoning
Reaction after exercise
Stress
Renal transplant rejection

Notes

haptoglobin

Type of test Blood

Normal findings

Adult: 100-150 mg/dl or 16-31 μmol/L (SI units)
Newborn: 0-10 mg/dl

Possible critical values <40 mg/dl

Test explanation and related physiology

The serum haptoglobin test is used to detect intravascular destruction (hemolysis) of red blood cells (RBCs). Haptoglobins are glycoproteins produced by the liver. These haptoglobins are powerful, free hemoglobin–binding proteins. In hemolytic anemias associated with hemolysis of RBCs, the released hemoglobin is quickly bound to haptoglobin, and the new complex is quickly catabolized. This causes a greatly decreased amount of free haptoglobin in the serum, and this decrease cannot be quickly compensated for by normal liver production. As a result, the patient demonstrates a transient reduced level of haptoglobin in the serum.

Haptoglobins are also decreased in patients with primary liver disease not associated with hemolytic anemias. This occurs because the diseased liver is unable to produce these glycoproteins.

Elevated haptoglobin concentrations are found in many inflammatory diseases and can therefore be used as a nonspecific test of disease in much the same way as a sedimentation rate test (see p. 314).

Interfering factors

- Ongoing infection can cause falsely elevated test results.
- Drugs that may cause increased haptoglobin levels include androgens and steroids.
- Drugs that may cause decreased levels include chlorpromazine, diphenhydramine, indomethacin, isonazid (INH), nitrofurantoin, oral contraceptives, quinidine, and streptomycin.

Procedure and patient care

Before

- Explain the procedure to the patient.
- Tell the patient that no fasting is required.

During

- Collect at least 2 ml of venous blood in a red-top tube.
- Avoid hemolysis, which could alter test results.

After

- Apply pressure or a pressure dressing to the venipuncture site.
- Assess the venipuncture site for bleeding.

Abnormal findings

Increased levels

Collagen diseases
Infections
Tissue destruction
Biliary obstruction
Nephritis
Pyelonephritis
Ulcerative colitis
Peptic ulcer
Myocardial infarction
Acute rheumatic disease
Neoplasia

Decreased levels

Hemolytic anemias
Transfusion reactions
Prostatic heart valves
Systemic lupus erythematosus
Primary liver disease not associated with hemolytic anemia
Erythroblastosis fetalis
Hematoma
Tissue hemorrhage
Chronic liver disease

Notes

hematocrit (Hct, Packed red cell volume, Packed cell volume [PCV])

Type of test Blood

Normal findings

Male: 42%-52%
Female: 37%-47% (pregnancy, >33%)
Elderly: values may be slightly decreased.
Child: 31%-43%
Infant: 30%-40%
Newborn: 44%-64%

Possible critical values <15%

Test explanation and related physiology

The Hct is a measure of the percentage of red blood cells (RBCs) in the total blood volume. It is routinely performed as part of a complete blood count (CBC). Therefore the Hct closely reflects the hemoglobin (Hgb) and RBC values. The Hct in percentage points is usually about three times the Hgb concentration in grams per deciliter when the RBCs are of normal size and contain normal amounts of Hgb. Normal values also vary according to sex and age. Abnormal values indicate the same pathologic states as abnormal RBC counts and Hgb concentrations (see pp. 617 and 402).

Interfering factors

- Abnormalities in RBC size may alter Hct values.
- Extremely elevated white blood cell (WBC) counts can affect values.
- Hemodilution and dehydration can affect the Hct level.
- Pregnancy usually causes slightly decreased values because of hemodilution.
- Living in high altitudes causes increased values.
- Values may not be reliable immediately after hemorrhage.
- Drugs that may cause decreased levels include chloramphenicol and penicillin.

Procedure and patient care

Before

- Explain the procedure to the patient.
- Tell the patient that no fasting is required.

During

- Collect approximately 5 to 7 ml of venous blood in a lavender-top tube. However, only 0.5 ml is required when using capillary tubes.
- Avoid hemolysis.

After

- Apply pressure or a pressure dressing to the venipuncture site.
- Assess the venipuncture site for bleeding.

Abnormal findings

Increased levels

Congenital heart disease
Polycythemia vera
Severe dehydration
Shock
Erythrocytosis
Severe diarrhea
Eclampsia
Trauma
Surgery
Burns
Dehydration

Decreased levels

Anemia
Hyperthyroidism
Cirrhosis
Hemolytic reaction
Hemorrhage
Dietary deficiency
Bone marrow failure
Hodgkin's disease
Organ failure
Normal pregnancy
Rheumatoid arthritis
Multiple myeloma
Malnutrition
Leukemias

Notes

hemoglobin (Hb, Hgb)

Type of test Blood

Normal findings
Male: 14-18 g/dl or 8.7-11.2 mmol/L (SI units)
Female: 12-16 g/dl or 7.4-9.9 mmol/L (pregnancy, >11 g/dl)
Elderly: values are slightly decreased.
Child: 11-16 g/dl
Infant: 10-15 g/dl
Newborn: 14-24 g/dl

Possible critical values <5.0 g/dl

Test explanation and related physiology

The Hgb concentration is a measure of the total amount of Hgb in the peripheral blood. The test is normally performed as part of a complete blood count (CBC). Hgb serves as a vehicle for oxygen and carbon dioxide transport. As with the red blood cell (RBC) count, normal values vary according to sex and age. The clinical implications of this test closely parallel those of the RBC count (see p. 617). In addition, however, changes in plasma volume are more accurately reflected by the Hgb concentration. Dilutional overhydration decreases the concentration, whereas dehydration tends to cause an artificially high value. Slight decreases in the values of Hgb and the hematocrit during pregnancy reflect the expanded blood volume. The number of cells is actually increased during pregnancy.

Interfering factors

- Slight Hgb decreases normally occur during pregnancy because of the expanded blood volume.
- Living in high-altitude areas causes high Hgb values.
- Drugs that may cause increased levels include gentamicin and methyldopa (Aldomet).
- Drugs that may cause decreased levels include antibiotics, antineoplastic drugs, aspirin, indomethacin (Indocin), rifampin, and sulfonamides.

Procedure and patient care

Before

- Explain the procedure to the patient.
- Tell the patient that no fasting is required.

During

- Collect approximately 5 to 7 ml of venous blood in a lavender-top tube.
- Avoid hemolysis.
- List on the laboratory slip any drugs that can affect test results.

After

- Apply pressure or a pressure dressing to the venipuncture site.
- Observe the venipuncture site for bleeding.

Abnormal findings

Increased levels	Decreased levels
Congenital heart disease	Anemia
Polycythemia vera	Severe hemorrhage
Hemoconcentration of the blood	Hemolysis
	Hodgkin's disease
Chronic obstructive pulmonary disease	Hemoglobinopathies
	Cancer
Congestive heart failure	Nutritional deficiency
High altitudes	Lymphoma
Severe burns	Systemic lupus erythematosus
Dehydration	Sarcoidosis
	Kidney diseases
	Chronic hemorrhage
	Splenomegaly
	Sickle cell anemia

Notes

hemoglobin electrophoresis

Type of test   Blood

Normal findings

Adult/elderly
Hgb A_1: 95%-98%
Hgb A_2: 2%-3%
Hgb F: 0.8%-2%
Hgb S: 0%
Hgb C: 0%
Children: Hgb F
Newborn: 50%-80%
6 months: 8%
Over 6 months: 1%-2%

Test explanation and related physiology

The hemoglobin (Hgb) electrophoresis is a test that enables abnormal forms of Hgb (hemoglobinopathies) to be detected. Although many different Hgb variations have been described, the more common types are A_1, A_2, F, S, and C. Each major Hgb type is charged to varying degrees. When placed in an electromagnetic field, the Hgb variants migrate at different rates and therefore spread apart from each other. One is able to quantitate each band as a percentage of the total Hgb.

Hgb A_1 constitutes the major component of Hgb in the normal red blood cell (RBC). Hgb A_2 is only a minor component (2% to 3%) of the normal Hgb total. Hgb F is the major Hgb in the fetus but exists in only minimal quantities in the normal adult. Levels of Hgb F greater than 2% in patients over age 3 years are considered abnormal. Hgb F is able to transport oxygen when only small amounts of oxygen are available (as in fetal life). In patients requiring compensation for prolonged chronic hypoxia (as in congenital cardiac abnormalities), Hgb F may be found in increased levels to assist in the transport of the available oxygen.

Hgb S is an abnormal form of Hgb associated with sickle cell anemia, which occurs predominantly in American blacks. Hgb S is a relatively insoluble variant. When little oxygen is available, it assumes a crescent (sickle) shape that greatly distorts the RBC morphology. Vascular sludging is a consequence of the localized sickling and may lead to organ infarction.

Hgb C is another Hgb variant that exists in American blacks. RBCs containing Hgb C have a decreased life span and are more readily lysed than normal RBCs. Mild to severe hemolytic anemia may result.

The Hgb contents of the common hemoglobinopaties, as determined by electrophoresis, are as follows:

Sickle cell disease (homozygous SS)
  Hgb S: 80%-100%
  Hgb A_1: 0%
  Hgb A_2: 2%-3%
  Hgb F: <2%
Sickle cell trait (heterozygous SA)
  Hgb S: 20%-40%
  Hgb A_1: 60%-80%
  Hgb A_2: 2%-3%
  Hgb F: 2%
Hemoglobin C disease (homozygous)
  Hgb C: 90%-100%
  Hgb A_1: 0%
  Hgb A_2: 2%-3%
  Hgb F: 2%
Hemoglobin H disease
  Hgb A_1: 65%-90%
  Hgb A_2: 2%-3%
  Hgb H: 5%-30%
Thalassemia major (homozygous)
  Hgb A_1: 5%-20%
  Hgb A_2: 2%-3%
  Hgb F: 65%-100%
Thalassemia minor (heterozygous)
  Hgb A_1: 50%-85%
  Hgb A_2: 4%-6%
  Hgb F: 1%-3%

Interfering factors

- Blood transfusions within the previous 12 weeks can alter test results.

Procedure and patient care
Before

- Explain the procedure to the patient.
- Tell the patient that no fasting is required.

During

- Collect approximately 7 ml of venous blood in a lavender-top tube.

After

- Apply pressure or a pressure dressing to the venipuncture site.
- Assess the venipuncture site for bleeding.

Abnormal findings

Sickle cell disease
Sickle cell trait
Hemoglobin C disease

Hemoglobin H disease
Thalassemia major
Thalassemia minor

Notes

hepatitis virus studies (Hepatitis-associated antigen [HAA], Australian antigen)

Type of test Blood

Normal findings Negative

Test explanation and related physiology

Hepatitis is an inflammation of the liver caused by a virus. Three common viruses are now recognized to cause this disease: hepatitis A virus, hepatitis B virus, and hepatitis non-A, non-B virus (also called hepatitis C virus).

Hepatitis A virus (HAV) was originally called "infectious hepatitis." It has a short incubation period of 2 to 6 weeks. HAV is excreted in the stool and transmitted via the oral-fecal route. Although tests are not yet available to detect HAV, two types of antibodies to HAV can be detected.

The first type of antibody to HAV is immunoglobulin M (IgM) antibody (HAV-Ab/IgM), which appears approximately 3 to 4 weeks after exposure or just before hepatocellular enzyme elevations occur. These IgM levels usually return to normal in about 8 weeks.

The second type of antibody is IgG (HAV-Ab/IgG), which appears approximately 2 weeks after the beginning of the IgM increase and slowly returns to normal levels. The IgG enzyme can remain detectable for more than 10 years after the infection. If the IgM antibody is elevated in the absence of the IgG antibody, acute hepatitis is suspected. If, on the other hand, IgG is elevated in the absence of IgM elevation, this indicates the convalescent or chronic stage of HAV viral infection.

Hepatitis B virus (HBV) is commonly known as "serum hepatitis." It has a long incubation period of 5 weeks to 6 months. HBV is most frequently transmitted by blood transfusion; however, it can also be contracted via other body fluids. HBV may cause a severe and unrelenting form of hepatitis ending in liver failure and death. Its incidence is increased among blood transfusion recipients, male homosexuals, dialysis patients, transplant patients, IV drug abusers, and patients with leukemia or lymphoma.

The HBV, also called the Dane particle, is made up of an inner core surrounded by an outer capsule. The outer capsule contains the hepatitis B surface antigen (HBsAg), formerly called Australian antigen. The inner core contains HBV core antigen (HBcAg). The hepatitis B e-antigen (HBeAg) is also found within the core. Antibodies to these antigens are called HBsAb, HBcAb, and HBeAb. The tests used to detect these antigens and antibodies are as follows:

1. *Hepatitis B surface antigen* (HBsAg). This is the most frequently and easily performed test for hepatitis B. This is the first test to become abnormal. HBsAg rises before the onset of clinical symptoms, peaks during the first week of symptoms, and returns to normal by the time jaundice subsides. HBsAg generally indicates active infection by HBV. If the level of this antigen persists in the blood, the patient is considered to be a carrier.

2. *Hepatitis B surface antibody* (HBsAb). This antibody appears approximately 4 weeks after the disappearance of the surface antigen and signifies the end of the acute infection phase. HBsAb also signifies immunity to subsequent infection. Concentrated forms of this agent constitute the hyperimmunoglobulin given to patients who have come in contact with HBV-infected patients (e.g., contact by an inadvertent needle prick from a needle previously used on a patient with HBV infection). HBsAb is the antibody that denotes immunity after administration of hepatitis B vaccine.

3. *Hepatitis B core antigen* (HBcAg). No tests are currently available to detect this antigen.

4. *Hepatitis B core antibody* (HBcAb). This antibody appears approximately 1 month after HBsAg and declines (although remains elevated) over several years. HBcAb is also present in patients who have chronic hepatitis. The HBcAb level is elevated during the time lag between the disappearance of HBsAg and the appearance of HBsAb. This interval is called the *core window*. During the core window, HBcAb is the only detectable marker of a recent hepatitis infection.

5. *Hepatitis B e-antigen* (HBeAg). This antigen is generally not used for diagnostic purposes but rather is an index of infectivity. The presence of HBeAg correlates with early and active disease as well as with high infectivity in acute HBV infection. The persistent presence

of HBeAg in the blood predicts the development of chronic HBV infection.

6. *Hepatitis B e-antibody (HBeAb)*. This antibody indicates that an acute phase of HBV infection is over or almost over and that the chance of infectivity is greatly reduced.

Non-A, non-B hepatitis, also called hepatitis C, is transmitted in a manner similar to HBV. The incubation period is 2 to 12 weeks after exposure. The clinical manifestations of the illness parallel HBV. Most patients with hepatitis caused by blood transfusion have the non-A, non-B type. A hepatitis non-A, non-B viral titer is now available to detect these infections. However, no vaccine protection exists against this form of hepatitis.

Procedure and patient care
Before

- Explain the procedure to the patient.
- Tell the patient that no fasting is required.

During

- Collect approximately 5 to 7 ml of venous blood in a red-top tube.
- Note that most of the testing for hepatitis is done by radioimmunoassay. Usually, a hepatitis profile that includes several HBV antigens and antibodies is performed.

After

- Apply pressure or a pressure dressing to the venipuncture site.
- Assess the venipuncture site for bleeding.
- Handle the specimen as if it were capable of transmitting hepatitis.
- Immediately discard the needle in the appropriate receptacle.
- Send the specimen promptly to the laboratory.

Abnormal findings
Increased levels

Hepatitis A
Hepatitis B
Non-A, non-B hepatitis

Chronic carrier state, hepatitis B
Chronic hepatitis B

herpes genitalis (Herpesvirus type 2, Herpes simplex virus type 2 [HSV 2])

Type of test Microscopic examination

Normal findings No virus present

Test explanation and related physiology

The herpes simplex virus (HSV) can be classified as either type 1 or type 2. Type 1 is primarily responsible for oral lesions. HSV 2 is a sexually transmitted viral infection of the urogenital tract. Vesicular lesions may occur on the penis, scrotum, vulva, perineum, perianal region, vagina, or cervix. Because most infants become infected if they pass through a birth canal containing HSV, determining its presence at delivery is necessary. Congenital infections may result in problems such as microcephaly, chorioretinitis, and mental retardation in the newborn. Disseminated neonatal herpesvirus infections carry a high incidence of infant mortality. A vaginal delivery is possible if no virus is present, and cesarean birth is needed if HSV is present. Viral testing can be performed on males or females to determine risk of sexual transmission.

Procedure and patient care

Before

- Explain the procedure to the patient.
- Tell the the female patient to refrain from douching and tub bathing before the cervical culture is performed.
- Obtain the urethral specimen from the male patient before voiding.

During

- Obtain cultures as follows:

Urethral culture

1. A culture is taken by inserting a sterile swab gently into the anterior urethra of the male patient.
2. It is advisable to place the male patient in the supine position to prevent falling if vasovagal syncope occurs during introduction of the cotton swab or wire loop into the urethra.
3. The patient is observed for hypotension, bradycardia, pallor, sweating, nausea, and weakness.

Cervical culture

1. The female patient is placed in the lithotomy position, and a vaginal speculum is inserted.
2. Cervical mucus is removed with a cotton ball.
3. A sterile cotton-tipped swab is inserted into the endocervical canal and moved from side to side to obtain the culture.

- For pregnant women with herpes genitalis, note that the cervix is cultured weekly for the herpesvirus beginning 4 to 6 weeks before the due date. Vaginal delivery is possible if the following criteria are met:

1. The two most recent cultures are negative.
2. The woman is not experiencing any symptoms.
3. No lesions are visible on inspection of the vagina and vulva.
4. Throughout her pregnancy, the woman has not had more than one positive culture during which she was symptom free.

After

- Inform the patient how to obtain the test results.

Abnormal finding

Herpesvirus infection

Notes

HLA-B27 antigen (Human lymphocyte antigen B27)

Type of test Blood

Normal findings Negative

Test explanation and related physiology

The HLA antigens are the major histocompatibility (tissue compatibility) antigens important in tissue recognition. These antigens are under direct genetic control and share a locus on the chromosome. Many HLA antigens exist, but the one with the most clinical relevance is HLA-B27. This antigen is often found in patients with ankylosing spondylitis and Reiter's syndrome. HLA-B27 is used to detect and confirm these diagnoses. HLA-B27 is found in 5% to 7% of normal patients, but approximately 80% to 90% of patients with ankylosing spondylitis or Reiter's syndrome have HLA-B27.

For this test, lymphocytes from the patient are extracted and incubated with anti-HLA-B27 cytotoxic antibody. If the patient has HLA-B27 antigen, a complex will be formed on the cell surface. Serum complement is then added to the mixture, thereby killing the lymphocyte and recognizing the titer of HLA-B27.

Procedure and patient care

Before

- Explain the procedure to the patient.
- Tell the patient that no fasting or special preparation is required.

During

- Collect at least 10 ml of venous blood in a heparinized solution.

After

- Apply pressure or a pressure dressing to the venipuncture site.
- Assess the venipuncture site for bleeding.

Abnormal findings
Increased levels

Ankylosing spondylitis
Reiter's syndrome

Notes

Holter monitoring (Ambulatory monitoring,
Ambulatory electrocardiography)

Type of test Electrodiagnostic

Normal findings Normal sinus rhythm

Test explanation and related physiology

Holter monitoring is a continuous recording of the electrical activity of the heart. This can be performed for periods up to 48 hours. With this technique, an electrocardiogram (EKG) is recorded continuously on magnetic tape during unrestricted activity, rest, and sleep. The Holter monitor is equipped with a clock that permits accurate time monitoring on the EKG tape. The patient is asked to carry a diary and record daily activities and any cardiac symptoms that may develop during the period of monitoring. Most units in present use are equipped with an "Event marker." This is a button the patient can push when symptoms such as chest pain, syncope, or palpitations are experienced.

The Holter monitor is used primarily to identify suspected cardiac rhythm disturbances and to correlate these disturbances with symptoms such as dizziness, syncope, palpitations, or chest pain. The monitor also is used to assess pacemaker function and the effectiveness of antiarrhythmic medications.

After completion of the determined time period, the Holter monitor is removed from the patient, and the record tape is played back at high speeds. The EKG tracing is usually interpreted by computer, which can detect any significant abnormality that occurred during the testing. A report can then be generated as to the frequency and severity of abnormal cardiac events, especially in relation to the patient's symptoms.

Contraindications

- Patients who are unable to cooperate with maintaining the lead placement from the monitor to the body
- Patients who are unable to maintain an accurate diary of significant activities or events

Interfering factor

- Interruption in the electrode placement

Procedure and patient care

Before

- Explain the procedure to the patient.
- Instruct the patient about care of the Holter monitor.
- Inform the patient about the necessity of ensuring good contact of the electrodes to skin.
- Teach the patient how to maintain an accurate diary. Stress the need to record significant symptoms.
- Instruct the patient to note in the diary if any interruption in Holter monitoring occurs.
- Assure the patient that the electrical flow is coming *from* the patient and that he or she will not experience any electrical stimulation from the machine.
- Instruct the patient not to bathe during the period of cardiac monitoring.
- Tell the patient to minimize the use of electrical devices (e.g., electric toothbrushes, shavers), which may cause artificial changes in the EKG tracing.

During

- Prepare the sites for electrode placement with alcohol. (This is usually done in the cardiology department by a technologist.)
- Securely place the gel and electrodes at the appropriate sites. Usually the chest and abdomen are the most appropriate locations for limb lead electrode placement. The precordial leads may also be placed.
- Usually, do not use the extremities for electrode placement in order to minimize alterations in tracing that occur with normal physical activity.
- Encourage the patient to call if he or she has any difficulties.

After

- Gently remove the tape and other paraphenalia securing the electrodes.
- Wipe the patient clean of electrode gel.
- Inform the patient that the Holter monitoring interpretation will be available in a few days.

Abnormal findings

Cardiac arrhythmias (dysrhythmias)

human placental lactogen (HPL, Human chorionic somatomammotropin [HCS])

Type of test Blood

Normal findings Value should rise progressively during pregnancy.

Test explanation and related physiology

HPL is a hormone produced by the placenta and is used to evaluate placental functioning. HPL can be detected in the maternal serum as early as the fifth week of gestation. Levels gradually rise until week 36 of pregnancy and then tend to stabilize. Values less than 4 mg/dl are rarely found in the last 10 weeks of pregnancy. Low HPL levels may indicate fetal distress, threatened abortion, toxemia, intrauterine growth retardation, and postmaturity. HPL levels may be high with maternal sickle cell disease, maternal liver disease, maternal diabetes, Rh sensitization, or multiple pregnancies.

Interfering factors

- Recent radioactive scans

Procedure and patient care

Before

- Explain the procedure to the patient.
- Collect approximately 7 to 10 ml of blood in a red-top tube.

After

- Apply pressure or a pressure dressing to the venipuncture site.
- Assess the venipuncture site for bleeding.

Abnormal findings

Increased levels	Decreased levels
Maternal sickle cell disease	Fetal distress
Maternal liver disease	Threatened abortion
Maternal diabetes	Toxemia
Rh sensitization	Intrauterine growth retardation
Multiple pregnancies	Postmaturity

hyaline casts

Type of test Urine

Normal findings Occasional casts present

Test explanation and related physiology

Casts are clumps of materials or cells. They are formed in the renal collecting tubule and have the shape of the tubule, thus the term *cast*. Hyaline casts are conglomerations of protein and indicate proteinuria. A few hyaline casts can normally be found, especially after strenuous exercise.

Procedure and patient care

Before

- Explain the procedure to the patient.

During

- Collect a fresh urine specimen in a urine container.
- If the specimen is contaminated by vaginal discharge or bleeding, a "clean-catch" or "midstream" specimen will be needed. This requires meticulous cleansing of the urinary meatus with an iodine preparation to reduce contamination of the specimen by external organisms. Then the cleansing agent must be completely removed, or it will contaminate the specimen. The midstream collection is obtained by:

  1. Having the patient begin to urinate in a bedpan, urinal, or toilet and then stop urinating (This washes the urine out of the distal urethra.)
  2. Correctly positioning a sterile urine container, into which the patient voids 3 to 4 ounces of urine
  3. Capping the container
  4. Allowing the patient to finish voiding

After

- Send the specimen immediately the laboratory.
- Do *not* allow the specimen to sit, since the casts will break up. Urine should be checked for casts when it is fresh.

Abnormal findings
Increased levels

Proteinuria

Fever

Strenuous exercise

Stress

Glomerulonephritis

Pyelonephritis

Congestive heart failure

Chronic renal failure

Notes

17-hydroxycorticosteroids (17-OCHS)

Type of test Urine (24 hour)

Normal findings

Male
Under age 8 years: <1.5 mg/24 hr
Under age 12 years: <4.5 mg/24 hr
Adult: 4.5-10 mg/24 hr
Elderly: values lower than for adult
Female
Under age 8 years: <1.5 mg/24 hr
Under age 12 years: <4.5 mg/24 hr
Adult: 2.5-10 mg/24 hr
Elderly: values lower than for adult

Test explanation and related physiology

This urine study is used to assess adrenocortical function by measuring the cortisol (17-OCHS) metabolites in a 24-hour urine collection. Since the excretion of cortisol metabolites follows a diurnal variation, a 24-hour collection is necessary. Elevated levels of 17-OCHS are seen in patients with hyperfunctioning of the adrenal gland (Cushing's syndrome), whether this condition is caused by pituitary or adrenal tumor, bilateral adrenal hyperplasia, or ectopic tumors producing adrenocorticotropic hormone (ACTH). Low levels of 17-OCHS are seen in patients who have a hypofunctioning adrenal gland (Addison's disease) as a result of destruction of the adrenals (by hemorrhage, infarction, metastatic tumor, or autoimmunity), surgical removal of adrenals without appropriate steroid replacement, congenital enzyme deficiency, hypopituitarism, or adrenal suppression after prolonged exogenous steroid ingestion.

Testing the urine for this hormone metabolite is only an indirect measure of adrenal function. Urine and plasma levels of cortisol (see pp. 239 and 237) provide a much more accurate measurement of adrenal function.

Interfering factors

- Emotional and physical stress (e.g., infection) and licorice ingestion can cause increased adrenal activity.

- Drugs that may cause increased 17-OCHS levels include acetazolamide, chloral hydrate, chlorpromazine, colchicine, erythromycin, meprobamate, paraldehyde, quinidine, quinine, and spironolactone.
- Drugs that may cause decreased levels include estrogens, oral contraceptives, phenothiazines, and reserpine.

Procedure and patient care

Before

- Explain the procedure to the patient.
- Note that drugs are usually withheld several days before the urine collection. Check with the physician and laboratory for specific guidelines.
- Assess the patient for signs of stress and report these to the physician.

During

- Do not administer the patient any drugs that may interfere with test results.
- Begin the 24-hour urine collection after the patient urinates. Discard this urine and note this as the start time of the test.
- Collect all urine passed by the patient during the next 24 hours.
- Post the hours for the urine collection in a prominent spot.
- Note that it is not necessary to measure each urine specimen.
- Tell the patient to void before defecating so that the urine is not contaminated by feces.
- Inform the patient that toilet paper should not be placed in the collection container.
- Encourage the patient to drink fluids during the 24 hours unless this is contraindicated for medical purposes.
- Collect the last specimen as close as possible to the end of the 24-hour collection. Add this to the container.
- Keep the urine specimen refrigerated or on ice during the entire collection.

After

- Send the urine to the chemistry laboratory as soon as the test is completed.

- List on the laboratory slip any medications the patient may be taking that can affect test results.

Abnormal findings
Increased levels

Cushing's syndrome
Pituitary tumor
Adrenal tumor
Bilateral adrenal hyperplasia
Ectopic ACTH-producing tumor
Acromegaly
Thyrotoxicosis
Severe hypertension
Stress

Decreased levels

Addison's disease
Adrenal infarction
Adrenal hemorrhage
Surgical removal of the adrenals
Congenital enzyme deficiency
Adrenal suppression from steroid therapy
Hypopituitarism
Hypothyroidism
Adrenogenital syndrome

H

Notes

5-hydroxyindoleacetic acid (5-HIAA)

Type of test   Urine (24 hour)

Normal findings   2-9 mg/24 hr (female levels lower than male levels)

Test explanation and related physiology

Quantitative analysis of urine levels of 5-HIAA is used to detect and follow the clinical course of patients with carcinoid tumors. Carcinoid tumors are serotonin-secreting tumors that may grow in the appendix, intestine, lung, or any tissue derived from the neuroectoderm. These tumors contain *argentaffin (enteroendocrine) cells,* which produce serotonin and other powerful neurohormones that are metabolized by the liver to 5-HIAA and are excreted in the urine. These powerful neurohormones are responsible for the clinical presentation of carcinoid syndrome (bronchospasm, flushing, diarrhea). This test is used not only to identify patients with carcinoid tumor, but also to reevaluate those with known tumor by using serial levels of urinary 5-HIAA. Rising levels of 5-HIAA indicate progression of tumor; falling levels of 5-HIAA indicate a therapeutic response of the tumor to antineoplastic therapy.

Interfering factors

- Drugs that may cause increased 5-HIAA levels include acetanilid, acetophenetidin (phenacetin), glyceryl guaiacolate (guaifenesin [Robitussin]), methocarbamol, and reserpine.
- Drugs that may cause decreased levels include chlorpromazine, ethyl alcohol, heparin, imipramine (Tofranil), isoniazid (INH), levodopa, MAO inhibitors, methenamine, methyldopa (Aldomet), phenothiazines, promethazine (Phenergan), and tricyclic antidepressants.

Procedure and patient care

Before

- Explain the procedure to the patient.
- Instruct the patient to refrain from eating foods containing serotonin (e.g., plums, pineapples, bananas, eggplant,

tomatoes, avocados, walnuts) for several days (usually 3) before and during testing.

During

- To begin the 24-hour urine collection, discard the patient's initial specimen and start the timing at that point.
- Collect all urine passed during the next 24 hours.
- Show the patient where to store the urine specimen.
- Keep the specimen on ice or in a refrigerator during the 24-hour collection. A preservative is needed to keep the specimen at an appropriate pH.
- Post the hours for urine collection in a noticeable place to prevent accidental discarding of the specimen.
- Instruct the patient to void before defecating so that urine is not contaminated by stool.
- Tell the patient not to put toilet paper in the urine container.
- Collect the last specimen as close as possible to the end of the 24-hour collection. Add this urine to the container.

After

- Send the urine specimen to the laboratory promptly.
- List on the laboratory slip any medications that can affect test results.

Abnormal findings
Increased levels

Carcinoid tumors

Notes

hysterosalpingography (Uterotubography, Uterosalpingography, Hysterogram)

Type of test X-ray with contrast dye

Normal findings
Patent fallopian tubes
No defects in uterine cavity

Test explanation and related physiology
In hysterosalpingography the uterine cavity and fallopian tubes are radiographically visualized after the injection of contrast material through the cervix. Uterine tumors, intrauterine adhesions, and developmental anomalies can be seen. Tubal obstruction caused by internal scarring, tumor, or kinking can also be detected. A possible therapeutic effect of this test is that the passage of dye through the tubes may clear mucous plugs, straighten kinked tubes, or break up adhesions. This test may also be used to document adequacy of surgical tubal ligation.

Contraindications
- Patients with infections of the vagina, cervix, or fallopian tubes, since there is risk of extending the infection.
- Patients with uterine bleeding, since contrast material may enter the open blood vessels
- Patients with suspected pregnancy, since contrast material might induce abortion

Potential complications
- Infection of the endometrium (endometritis)
- Infection of the fallopian tubes (salpingitis)
- Uterine perforation
- Allergic reaction to iodinated dye or shellfish
  This rarely occurs, since the dye is not administered intravenously.

Interfering factors
- Fecal material or gas in the bowel could obscure visualization.
- Tubal spasm or excessive traction may cause the appearance of a stricture in normal fallopian tubes.

- Excessive traction can displace adhesions, making tubes appear normal.

Procedure and patient care

Before

- Explain the procedure to the patient. Ask the patient when she had her last menstrual period. If pregnancy is suspected, the test is not done at that time.
- Obtain informed consent if required by the institution.
- Assess the patient for allergy to iodine dye or shellfish. Report positive findings to the radiologist. (Allergic reactions in this study are rare, since the dye is not administered intravenously.)
- Instruct the patient to take laxatives the night before the test, if ordered.
- Administer enemas or suppositories on the morning of the test, if ordered.
- Administer sedatives (e.g., diazepam [Valium]) or antispasmodics, if ordered, before the test.
- Tell the patient that no food or fluid restrictions are needed.

During

- Note the following procedural steps:

  1. A plain x-ray film of the abdomen is often taken before the test to ensure that the preparation adequately eliminated gastrointestinal gas or feces.
  2. After voiding, the patient is placed on the fluoroscopy table in the lithotomy position.
  3. A speculum is inserted into the vagina, and the cervix is visualized and cleansed.
  4. Contrast material is injected during fluoroscopy, and x-ray films are taken.
  5. More dye is injected so that the entire upper genital tract (uterus and tubes) can be filled.
  6. This test can be considered satisfactorily performed only if the uterus and the tubes are distended to their maximal capacity or if fluid flows through the fallopian tubes.

- Note that this procedure is performed by a physician in approximately 15 to 30 minutes.
- Tell the patient that she may feel occasional transient

menstrual-type cramping and that she may have shoulder pain caused by subphrenic irritation from the dye as it leaks into the peritoneal cavity.

After

- Inform the patient that a vaginal discharge (sometimes bloody) may be present for 1 to 2 days after the test. A perineal pad should be worn.
- Evaluate the patient for delayed reaction to dye (dyspnea, rash, tachycardia, hives). If this occurs, treat with antihistamines or steroids.
- Inform the patient that cramping and dizziness may occur following this study.
- Evaluate the patient for signs and symptoms of infection (e.g., fever, increased pulse rate, pain). Instruct the patient to call her physician and report these symptoms if they occur.

Abnormal findings

Uterine tumors (e.g., leiomyomas)
Internal scarring
Kinking secondary to adhesions
Extrauterine pregnancy
Uterine fistulas
Developmental anomalies (e.g., uterus bicornis)
Intrauterine adhesions
Tumor
Fallopian tube occlusion
Uterine masses

Notes

immunoglobulin electrophoresis
(Gammaglobulin electrophoresis)

Type of test Blood

Normal findings

IgG: 565-1765 mg/dl
IgA: 85-385 mg/dl
IgM: 55-375 mg/dl
IgD and IgE: minimal

Test explanation and related physiology

The protein within the blood is made up of albumin and globulin. Several types of globulin exist, one of which is gammaglobulin. Antibodies are made of gammaglobulin protein and are called immunoglobulins. There are many classes of immunoglobulins (antibodies). Immunoglobulin G (IgG) comprises approximately 75% of the serum immunoglobulins; therefore it constitutes the majority of circulating blood antibodies. IgA constitutes about 15% of the immunoglobulins within the body and is present primarily in the secretions of the gastrointestinal tract, saliva, and tears. IgM is an immunoglobulin primarily responsible for ABO blood grouping and rheumatoid factor. IgE often mediates an allergic response and is measured to detect allergic diseases. IgD, which constitutes the smallest portion of the immunoglobulins, is rarely evaluated or detected.

Serum electrophoresis is used to detect diseases of hypersensitivity, immune deficiencies, autoimmune diseases, chronic infections, multiple myeloma, chronic viral infections, and intrauterine fetal infections. For this test the serum is placed on a slide containing agar gel, and an electric current is passed through this gel. Immunoglobulins are separated out and electrophoresed according to the quantity and difference in electrical charge. Specific antisera are placed alongside the slide to identify the specific type of immunoglobulin present.

Interfering factors

- Drugs that may cause increased immunoglobulin levels include gamma globulin, hydralazine, isoniazid (INH), phenytoin (Dilantin), procainamide, and tetanus toxoid and antitoxin.

Procedure and patient care

Before

- Explain the procedure to the patient.
- Tell the patient that no fasting or special preparation is required.

During

- Collect 7 to 10 ml of venous blood in a red-top tube.
- Indicate on the laboratory slip if the patient has received any vaccinations or immunizations within the past 6 months. Also, list any drugs that can affect test results.

After

- Apply pressure or a pressure dressing to the venipuncture site.
- Observe the venipuncture site for bleeding.

Abnormal findings

Increased IgG

Chronic infection
Hyperimmunization
Severe malnutrition
Sarcoidosis
Rheumatic fever
Liver disease
IgG multiple myeloma
Rheumatoid arthritis

Decreased IgG

Agammaglobulinemia
Lymphoid hyperplasia
Amyloidosis
Congenital IgG deficiencies
Preeclampsia
Leukemia

Increased IgE

Allergy (e.g., hay fever, asthma, anaphylaxis)

Decreased IgE

Agammaglobulinemia

Increased IgA

Cirrhosis
Rheumatic fever
Inflammatory bowel disease
Alcoholism
Chronic infections
Carcinoma, especially involving the gastrointestinal or hepatobiliary tracts

Increased IgM

Macroglobulinemia
Rheumatoid arthritis
Brucellosis
Lymphosarcoma
Other autoimmune diseases
Viral infections (e.g., infectious mononucleosis)
Malaria
Fungal infections

Decreased IgA

Agammaglobulinemia
Malignancies
Use of lymphopenic drugs (e.g., chemotherapy, steroids)
Protein-losing gastroenteropathies (e.g., inflammatory bowel disease)

Decreased IgM

Agammaglobulinemia
Lymphoid hyperplasia
Leukemia
Amyloidosis

Notes

insulin assay

Type of test Blood

Normal findings

5-24 µU/ml or 36-179 pmol/L (SI units)
Newborn: 3-20 µU/ml

Possible critical values >30 µU/ml

Test explanation and related physiology

The hormone insulin can be measured successfully by radioimmunoassay in most larger laboratories. Insulin regulates blood glucose levels by facilitating the movement of glucose out of the bloodstream. Insulin secretion is primarily determined by the blood glucose level. Normally, as the blood glucose level increases, the insulin level also increases; as the glucose level decreases, insulin release stops. This test is used to diagnose insulinoma and to evaluate abnormal lipid and carbohydrate metabolism.

Some investigators believe that measuring the ratio of the blood sugar and the insulin levels together on the same specimen during the oral glucose tolerance test (GTT, see p. 388) is more reliable than measuring the insulin levels alone. The insulin assay, when compared with the oral GTT, can show characteristic curves in certain situations. For example, patients with juvenile diabetes have low fasting insulin levels and display flat GTT curves because of little or no increase in insulin levels. Patients who are mildly diabetic have normal fasting insulin levels and display GTT curves with a delayed rise. After the patient fasts 12 to 14 hours, the insulin/glucose ratio should be less than 0.3. Patients with insulinoma have ratios greater than this.

Interfering factors

- Food intake and obesity can cause increased insulin levels.
- Recent administration of radioisotopes can affect test results.
- Drugs that may cause increased insulin levels include corticosteroids, levodopa, and oral contraceptives.

Procedure and patient care
Before
- Explain the procedure to the patient.
- Keep the patient NPO for 8 hours.

During
- Collect approximately 5 ml of venous blood in a red-top tube and pack it in ice.
- Avoid hemolysis.
- If the serum insulin level will be measured during the GTT, collect the blood sample before the oral ingestion of the glucose load and often at designated intervals after glucose ingestion.

After
- Apply pressure or a pressure dressing to the venipuncture site.
- Observe the venipuncture site for bleeding.
- Transport the specimen immediately to the laboratory.

Abnormal findings

Increased levels	Decreased levels
Insulinoma	Diabetes
Cushing's syndrome	
Acromegaly	
Obesity	

Notes

intravenous pyelography (IVP, Excretory urography [EUG], Intravenous urography [IUG, IVU])

Type of test X-ray with contrast dye

Normal findings

Normal size, shape, and position of the kidneys, renal pelvis, ureters, and bladder

Normal kidney excretory function, as evidenced by length of time for passage of contrast material through the kidneys

Test explanation and related physiology

IVP is an x-ray study that uses radiopaque contrast material to visualize the kidneys, renal pelvis, ureters, and bladder. The dye is injected intravenously, filtered out at the kidney by the glomeruli, and then passed through the renal tubules. X-ray films taken at set intervals over the next half hour will show passage of the dye material through the kidneys and ureters and into the bladder.

If the artery leading to one of the kidneys is blocked, the dye cannot enter that part of the renal system and that kidney will not be visualized. If the artery is partially blocked, the length of time required for the appearance of the contrast material will be prolonged.

With primary glomerular disease (e.g., glomerulonephritis), the glomerular filtrate is reduced, which causes a reduction in the quantity of dye filtered. Therefore it requires more time for enough dye to enter the kidney filtrate and allow for renal opacification. As a result, kidney visualization is delayed. This provides an estimate of renal function.

Defects in the dye filling of the kidney can indicate renal tumors or cysts. Often, intrinsic tumors, stones, extrinsic tumors, and scarring can partially or completely obstruct the flow of dye through the collecting system (pelvis, ureters, bladder). If the obstruction has been of sufficient duration, the collecting systems proximal to the obstruction will be dilated (hydronephrosis). Retroperitoneal and pelvic tumors, aneurysms, and enlarged lymph nodes can also produce extrinsic compression and distortions of the opacified collecting system.

IVP is also used to assess the effect of trauma on the urinary system. Renal hematomas distort the renal contour. Renal artery laceration is suggested by nonopacification of one kidney. Laceration of the kidneys, pelvis, ureters, or bladder often causes urine leaks, which are identified by dye extravasation from the urinary system.

IVP is also used to assess a patient for congenital absence or malposition of kidneys. Horseshoe kidneys (connection of the two kidneys), double ureters, and pelvic kidneys are typical congenital abnormalities.

Nephrotomography provides radiographic visualization of the kidney using tomographic technique following the IV injection of a radiopaque dye. Tomography is a radiographic technique by which a sequence of x-ray films, each representing a visual "slice" through the organ, is taken. Tomography permits examination of a single layer or plane of the organ that would otherwise be obscured by the surrounding structures. Nephrotomography permits visualization of different planes of the kidney for the purpose of differentiating solid renal and adrenal tumors from benign renal cysts.

Contraindications

- Patients who are allergic to shellfish or iodinated dyes and who have not received premedication with prednisone and diphenhydramine (Benadryl)
- Patients who are severely dehydrated, since this can cause renal shutdown and failure
  Geriatric patients are particularly vulnerable.
- Patients with renal insufficiency, as evidenced by a blood urea nitrogen (BUN) greater than 40 mg/dl, since the iodinated nephrotoxic dye can worsen kidney function
- Patients with multiple myeloma, since the iodinated nephrotoxic dye can worsen renal function

Potential complications

- Allergic reaction to iodinated dye
  Allergic reactions vary from mild flushing, itching, and urticaria to severe, life-threatening anaphylaxis (evidenced by respiratory distress, drop in blood pressure, shock). In the unusual event of anaphylaxis the patient may be treated with diphenhydramine (Benadryl), steroids, and epinephrine. Oxygen and endotracheal equipment should be on hand for immediate use.
- Infiltration of contrast dye

This is avoided by ensuring the patency of the IV line. In the event of infiltration, a local injection of hyaluronidase may be given to hasten the absorption of iodine and the resolution of the reaction.

- Renal failure
  This occurs most often in elderly patients who are chronically dehydrated before the dye injection.

Interfering factors

- Fecal material, gas, or barium in the bowel can obscure visualization of the renal system.
- Abnormal renal function studies may prevent adequate visualization of the urinary tract.
- Retained barium from previous studies can obscure visualization. Studies using barium (e.g., barium enema) should be scheduled *after* an IVP.

Procedure and patient care

Before

- Explain the procedure to the patient. Inform the patient that several x-ray films will be taken over ½ hour.
- Obtain informed consent if required by the institution.
- Check for allergies to iodinated dye and shellfish.
- Inform the radiologist if an allergy to iodine is suspected. The radiologist may prescribe a Benadryl and steroid preparation to be administered before the test. Usually a hypoallergenic, non-ionic contrast will be used during the test.
- Give the patient a laxative (e.g., castor oil) or a cathartic, as ordered, the evening before the test.
- Inform the patient of the required food and fluid restrictions. Some institutions prefer abstinence from solid foods for 8 hours before testing. Some allow a clear-liquid breakfast on the test day.
- Ensure adequate hydration for the patient (IV or oral) before and after the test to avoid dye-induced renal failure.
- Note that pediatric patients will have decreased fasting times, as ordered on an individual basis.
- Note that elderly and debilitated patients should have fasting times indicated specifically for them.
- Note that patients receiving high rates of IV fluids may have infusion rates decreased for several hours before the

study to increase the concentration of the dye within the urinary system.

- Assess the patient's BUN and creatinine levels. Abnormal renal function could deteriorate as a result of the dye injection.
- Schedule any barium studies *after* completion of the IVP.
- Give the patient an enema or suppository on the morning of the study, if ordered.

During

- Note the following procedural steps:
  1. The patient is taken to the radiology department and placed in the supine position.
  2. A plain film of the abdomen (KUB) is taken to ensure that no residual stool obscures visualization of the renal system. This also screens for calculi in the renal collecting system.
  3. Skin testing for iodine allergy is often done.
  4. A peripheral IV line is started (if not in place), and a contrast dye (e.g., Hypaque, Renografin) is given.
  5. X-ray films are taken at specific times, usually at 1, 5, 10, 15, 20, and 30 minutes and sometimes longer, to follow the course of the dye from the cortex of the kidney to the bladder.
  6. Tomography may be performed to identify a mass.
  7. The patient is taken to the bathroom and asked to void.
  8. A postvoiding film is taken to visualize the empty bladder.

- Note that occasionally it is necessary to occlude the ureters temporarily to obtain a better film of the collecting system in the upper part of the ureters. This is done by compressing the abdomen with an inflatable rubber tube, which is wrapped tightly around the abdomen slightly below the umbilicus.
- For *nephrotomography,* note that the x-ray tube and the film cassette are rapidly moved in opposite directions while the x-ray film is taken. This technique effectively blurs all tissue planes except that plane or "slice" being studied.
- Note that this test is performed by a radiologist in approximately 45 minutes.

- Inform the patient that the dye injection often causes a transitory flushing of the face, a feeling of warmth, a salty taste in the mouth, or even transient nausea. Initial IV needle placement and lying on a hard x-ray table are the only other discomforts associated with IVP.

After

- Assess the patient's urinary output. A decreased output may be an indication of renal failure.
- Evaluate the patient for delayed reaction to dye (dyspnea, rashes, tachycardia, hives). This usually occurs within the first 2 to 6 hours after the test. Treat with antihistamines or steroids.
- Encourage the patient to drink fluids to counteract fluid depletion caused by test preparation.
- Evaluate elderly and debilitated patients for weakness because of the combination of fasting and catharsis necessary for test preparation. Instruct these patients to ambulate only with assistance.
- Maintain the patient on adequate oral or IV hydration for several hours after the IVP.

Abnormal findings

Pyelonephritis
Glomerulonephritis
Kidney tumors (benign and malignant)
Renal hematomas
Tumors of the collecting system
Bladder tumors
Absence of a kidney
Renal or ureteral calculi
Hydronephrosis
Prostate enlargement (male)
Congenital abnormalities
Extrinsic compression of the collecting system (e.g., caused by tumor, aneurysm)

Notes

iron level and total iron-binding capacity
(Fe and TIBC, Transferrin saturation)

Type of test Blood

Normal findings

Iron: 60-190 µg/dl or 13-31 µmol/L (SI units)
TIBC: 25-420 µg/dl or 45-73 µmol/L (SI units)
Transferrin saturation: 30%-40%

Test explanation and related physiology

Abnormal levels of iron and TIBC are characteristic of many diseases, including iron deficiency anemia. Most of the iron in the body is found in the hemoglobin of the red blood cells (RBCs). Iron, supplied by the diet, is absorbed in the small intestine and transported to the plasma. There the iron is bound to a globulin protein called *transferrin* and carried to the bone marrow for incorporation into hemoglobin. The serum iron determination is a measurement of the quantity of iron bound to transferrin. The TIBC is a direct, quantitative measurement of transferrin. The percentage of saturation is calculated by dividing the serum iron level by the TIBC:

$$\text{Transferrin saturation (\%)} = \frac{\text{Serum iron level}}{\text{TIBC}} \times 100\%$$

The normal value for transferrin saturation is 30% to 40%. Calculation of transferrin saturation is helpful in determining the cause of abnormal iron and TIBC levels.

Iron deficiency anemia has many causes, including:

1. Insufficient iron intake
2. Inadequate gut absorption
3. Increased requirements (as in growing children and late pregnancy)
4. Loss of blood (as in menstruation, bleeding peptic ulcer, and colon neoplasm)

Iron deficiency results in a decreased production of hemoglobin, which in turn results in a small, pale (microcytic, hypochromic) RBC. A decreased serum iron level, an elevated TIBC, and a low transferrin saturation value are characteristic of iron deficiency anemia. A decrease in the mean corpuscular volume and mean corpuscular hemoglobin concentration (MCV, MCHC; see p. 620) is also found.

Chronic illness (e.g., infections, neoplasia, cirrhosis) is characterized by a low serum iron level, a decreased TIBC, and a normal transferrin saturation. Pregnancy is marked by high levels of protein, including transferrin. Because iron requirements are high, it is not unusual to find low serum iron levels, high TIBC, and a low percentage of transferrin saturation in late pregnancy.

Increased intake or absorption of iron (as in hemochromatosis) leads to elevated iron levels. In such cases the TIBC is unchanged, and as a result the percentage of transferrin saturation is very high. Excess iron is usually deposited in the brain, liver, and heart and causes severe dysfunction of these organs. Massive blood transfusions may also cause elevated serum iron levels.

Because serum iron levels may vary significantly during the day, the specimen for them should be drawn in the morning, especially when the results are used to monitor iron replacement therapy. The patient should refrain from eating for about 12 hours to avoid artificially high iron measurements caused by eating food with a high iron content. Blood transfusions will also greatly increase the iron level, although only transiently, and should be avoided before serum iron level determinations.

TIBC, on the other hand, varies minimally according to intake. The TIBC is more of a reflection of liver function (transferrin is produced by the liver) and nutrition than of iron metabolism. TIBC values often are used to monitor the course of patients receiving hyperalimentation.

Contraindications

- Patients with hemolytic diseases, since they may have an artificially high iron content

Interfering factors

- Recent blood transfusions can affect test results.
- Recent ingestion of a meal containing high iron content can affect test results.
- Hemolytic diseases may be associated with an artificially high iron content.
- Drugs that may cause increased iron levels include chlor-

amphenicol, dextran, estrogens, ethanol, iron preparations, methyldopa, and oral contraceptives.
- Drugs that may cause decreased iron levels include adrenocorticotropic hormone (ACTH), cholestyramine, chloramphenicol, colchicine, deferoxamine, methicillin, and testosterone.
- Drugs that may cause increased TIBC levels include fluorides and oral contraceptives.
- Drugs that may cause decreased TIBC levels include ACTH and chloramphenicol.

Procedure and patient care
Before
- Explain the procedure to the patient.
- Keep the patient fasting except for water for 12 hours before the blood test.
- Assess the patient for a history of recent blood transfusion and recent meals high in iron content. Both can affect test results.

During
- Collect approximately 5 to 7 ml of venous blood in a red-top tube. The specimen should always be obtained using a 20-gauge or larger needle.
- Avoid hemolysis because the iron contained in the RBC will pour out into the serum and cause artificially high iron levels.
- Indicate on the laboratory slip any drugs that can affect test results.

After
- Apply pressure or a pressure dressing to the venipuncture site.
- Assess the venipuncture site for bleeding.

Abnormal findings

Increased serum iron levels

Hemosiderosis
Hemochromatosis
Hemolytic anemias
Hepatitis
Hepatic necrosis
Lead toxicity
Iron poisoning

Decreased serum iron levels

Insufficient dietary iron
Chronic blood loss
Inadequate absorption of
  iron
Pregnancy (late)
Iron deficiency anemia
Neoplasia
Chronic gastrointestinal
  blood loss
Chronic hematuria
Chronic heavy physiologic
  or pathologic menstrua-
  tion

Increased TIBC levels

Oral contraceptives
Pregnancy (late)
Polycythemia vera
Iron deficiency anemia

Decreased TIBC levels

Hypoproteinemia
Inflammatory diseases
Cirrhosis
Hemolytic anemia
Pernicious anemia
Sickle cell anemia

Notes

ketones (Urine ketones, Urine acetones)

Type of test Urine

Normal findings Negative

Test explanation and related physiology

As part of the routine urinalysis, the urine is tested for the presence of ketones. Normally, no ketones are present in the urine. However, a poorly controlled diabetic patient who is hyperglycemic has massive fatty acid catabolism. The purpose of this catabolism is to provide an energy source when glucose cannot be transferred into the cell because of an insufficiency of insulin. Ketones (beta-hydroxybutyric acid, acetoacetic acid, and acetone) are the end product of this fatty acid breakdown. As with glucose, ketones spill over into the urine when the blood levels of diabetic patients are elevated. The excess production of ketones in the urine is usually associated with poorly controlled diabetes. This test for ketonuria is also important for evaluating ketoacidosis associated with the following: alcoholism, fasting, starvation, high-protein diets, and isopropanol ingestion. Infants and children may have ketonuria with febrile illnesses.

Interfering factors

- Special diets (e.g., carbohydrate free, high protein, high fat) may cause ketonuria.
- Drugs that may cause false positive test results include bromosulfophthalein (BSP, Bromsulphalein), isoniazid (INH, high doses), isopropanol (isopropyl alcohol), levodopa, paraldehyde, phenazopyridine (Pyridium), and PSP dye.

Procedure and patient care

Before

- Explain the procedure to the patient.
- Tell the patient that no fasting is required.

During

- Collect the patient's urine in a plastic urine container.
- Note that the test can be done immediately after collecting by placing a drop of urine on an Acetest tablet. If

K

acetone is present, varying shades of lavender will appear in the designated time.

- For Ketostix, dip the reagent strip into the urine specimen and remove it. Read the strip in 15 seconds by comparing it to a color chart.

After

- Refrigerate the sample if it cannot be tested immediately.
- If indicated, transport the specimen to the laboratory promptly following collection.

Abnormal findings

Uncontrolled diabetes
  mellitus
Starvation
Excessive aspirin ingestion
Ketoacidosis of alcoholism
Febrile illnesses in infants
  and children
Weight reduction diets

Following anesthesia
Prolonged vomiting
Anorexia
Fasting
High-protein diets
Isopropanol ingestion
Dehydration

Notes

17-ketosteroids (17-KS)

Type of test Urine (24 hour)

Normal findings
Male: 8-15 mg/24 hr
Female: 6-12 mg/24 hr
Elderly: values decrease with age.
Child: under 12 years, <5 mg/24 hr
      12-15 years, 5-12 mg/24 hr

Test explanation and related physiology
This urine test is used to measure adrenocortical functioning by measuring 17-KS in the urine. 17-KS are metabolites of the sex hormones that are secreted from the adrenal cortex and the testes. In men, approximately one third of the hormone metabolites come from the testes and two thirds from the adrenal cortex. In women and children, almost all the excreted hormones (androgens) are derived from the adrenal cortex. Therefore this test is very useful in diagnosing adrenocortical dysfunction. Elevated 17-KS levels are frequently seen in patients with congenital adrenal hyperplasia and testosterone- or estrogen-secreting tumors of the adrenal glands, ovaries, or testes. Low levels of 17-KS occur in patients with Addison's disease (chronic adrenocortical insufficiency) and in those who have had their ovaries or testes removed.

Interfering factors
- Stress can increase adrenal activity.
- Drugs that may cause increased 17-KS levels include antibiotics, chloramphenicol, chlorpromazine, dexamethasone, meprobamate, phenothiazines, quinidine, secobarbital, and spironolactone (Aldactone).
- Drugs that may cause decreased levels include estrogen, oral contraceptives, probenecid, promazine, reserpine, salicylates (prolonged use), and thiazide diuretics.

Procedure and patient care
Before
- Explain the procedure to the patient.

- Withhold all drugs (with physician approval) for several days beforehand.
- Assess the patient for signs of stress and report these to the physician.

During

- Begin the 24-hour urine collection after the patient urinates; discard this specimen.
- Collect all urine passed by the patient during the next 24 hours.
- Post the hours for the urine collection in a prominent spot.
- Remember that it is not necessary to measure each urine specimen.
- Tell the patient to void before defecating so that the urine is not contaminated by feces.
- Inform the patient that toilet paper should not be placed in the collection container.
- Encourage the patient to drink fluids during the 24 hours unless this is contraindicated for medical purposes.
- Remember that the urine collection needs a preservative.
- Refrigerate the urine throughout the collection.
- Collect the last specimen as close as possible to the end of the 24-hour period. Add this to the urine collection.

After

- Indicate on the laboratory slip the start and end times of the specimen collection.
- List on the laboratory slip any medications that can affect test results.
- Send the specimen to the laboratory as soon as the test is completed.

Abnormal findings
Increased levels

Congenital adrenal
  hyperplasia
Pregnancy
Adrenocorticotropic
  hormone (ACTH)
  administration
Cushing's syndrome
Testosterone- or estrogen-
  secreting tumors of the
  adrenals, ovaries, or
  testes
Severe stress or infection
Hyperpituitarism
Ovarian neoplasia

Decreased levels

Addison's disease
Hypogonadism
Hypopituitarism
Myxedema
Severe debilitating disease
Nephrosis
Gout
Castration
Thyrotoxicosis

Notes

K

kidney sonogram (Renal ultrasonography)

Type of test   Ultrasound

Normal findings   Normal size, shape, and position of the kidneys

Test explanation and related physiology

Through the use of reflected sound waves, ultrasonography provides accurate visualization of the kidney structures for many diagnostic purposes. The technique of ultrasonography requires the emission of high-frequency sound waves from the transducer to penetrate the organ being studied. The sound waves are bounced back to the transducer and electronically converted into a pictorial image. A realistic Polaroid picture or x-ray film of the organ studied is then obtained.

Ultrasonography of the kidney is used to diagnose and locate renal cysts, to differentiate renal cysts from solid renal tumors, to demonstrate renal or pelvic calculi, to document hydronephrosis, and to guide a percutaneously inserted needle for cyst aspiration or biopsy. One advantage of a kidney sonogram over intravenous pyelography (IVP, see p. 432) is that it can be performed on patients who have impaired renal function or an iodine allergy.

Interfering factors

- Barium or gas can reflect the sound waves and alter the test results. This test should be performed before x-ray studies with barium.

Procedure and patient care

Before

- Explain the procedure to the patient.
- Tell the patient that no fasting is required.

During

- Note the following procedural steps:
  1. The patient is placed on the ultrasonography table in a prone position.
  2. A greasy, conductive paste is applied to the patient's

back. This paste is used to enhance sound wave transmission and reception.

3. A transducer is passed over the skin, and pictures are taken of the reflections.
4. The patient is told to inspire deeply so that the upper poles of the kidneys can be visualized.

- Note that this test is completed in approximately 20 minutes, usually by an ultrasound technologist, and interpreted by a radiologist.
- Tell the patient that no discomfort is associated with this safe procedure.

After

- Remove the coupling agent (grease) from the patient's back.
- Note: if a biopsy was done, refer to p. 631.

Abnormal findings

Renal cysts
Renal tumors
Renal calculi
Hydronephrosis
Ureteral obstruction

Perirenal abscess
Glomerulonephritis
Pyelonephritis
Perirenal hematoma

K

Notes

kidney, ureter, and bladder x-ray study
(KUB)

Type of test   X-ray

Normal finding
No evidence of calculi
Normal gastrointestinal (GI) gas pattern

Test explanation and related physiology
The KUB is a *flat plate,* or simple x-ray film of the lower abdomen. It is often referred to as a *plain film,* or *scout film,* of the abdomen. The KUB is similar to an *obstruction series* (see p. 527) and can be done to demonstrate the size, shape, location, and malformations of the kidneys and bladder. The KUB can also be used to identify calculi in these organs and in the ureters. This is often one of the first studies done to diagnose other intraabdominal diseases, such as intestinal obstruction, soft tissue masses, and a ruptured viscus. The KUB is useful in detecting abnormal accumulations of gas within the GI tract and finding ascites. This study involves no contrast medium and poses no risk to the patient.

Contraindications
- Patients who are pregnant

Interfering factors
- Retained barium from previous studies can obscure visualization.

Procedure and patient care
Before
- Explain the procedure to the patient.
- Tell the patient that no fasting or sedation is required.
- Schedule this study before any barium studies.
- Ensure that the male patient has a lead sheet over his testicles to prevent their irradiation.
- Note that the female ovaries cannot be shielded because of their proximity to the kidneys, ureters, and bladder.

During

- Note that in the radiology department, the patient is placed in the supine position with the arms extended overhead. X-ray films are taken of the patient's abdomen.
- Note that the KUB is performed by a radiologic technologist in a few minutes and is interpreted by a radiologist.
- Inform the patient that results are available in about 1 hour.
- Tell the patient that no discomfort is associated with this study.

After

- Schedule intravenous pyelography (IVP) or GI studies after completion of the KUB.

Abnormal findings

Malformations
Calculi
Abnormal accumulation of
  gas

Ascites
Intestinal obstruction
Soft tissue masses
Ruptured viscus

Notes

K

lactic dehydrogenase (LDH)

Type of test Blood

Normal findings

Adult/elderly: 45-90 U/L (30° C), 115-225 IU/L, or
   0.4-1.7 μmol/L (SI units)
Isoenzymes in adult/elderly values
   LDH-1: 17%-27%
   LDH-2: 27%-37%
   LDH-3: 18%-25%
   LDH-4: 3%-8%
   LDH-5: 0%-5%
Child: 60-170 U/L (30° C)
Infant: 100-250 U/L
Newborn: 160-450 U/L

Test explanation and related physiology

The enzyme LDH is found in many body tissues, especially the heart, liver, kidneys, skeletal muscle, brain, red blood cells, and lungs. The serum LDH level rises within 24 to 72 hours after a myocardial infarction (MI), peaks in 3 to 4 days, and returns to normal in approximately 14 days. This makes the serum LDH level especially useful for a delayed diagnosis of patients with MI (e.g., where the patient reports having had severe chest pain 4 days ago). Because LDH is widely distributed through the body, the total LDH level is not a specific indicator of myocardial disease. LDH, as with creatinine phosphokinase (CPK, see p. 248), is more useful diagnostically when fractionated into isoenzymes. Five LDH isoenzymes, called LDH-1 through LDH-5, may be separated by electrophoresis. Isoenzyme LDH-1 comes mainly from the heart and red blood vessels; LDH-2 primarily from the reticuloendothelial system; LDH-3 from the lungs and other tissues; LDH-4 from the kidney, placenta, and pancreas; and LDH-5 mainly from the liver and striated muscle. Normally, serum levels of LDH-2 are higher than those of the other four isoenzymes.

In patients with MI, the LDH-1 level is a more sensitive and specific indicator of MI than the total LDH level. Its sensitivity is greater than 95%. When LDH-1 activity is greater than LDH-2 activity, this strongly supports the diagnosis of MI. This is referred to as a *flipped* LDH because the normal LDH-1/LDH-2 ratio of less than 1 is reversed. In an acute MI the flipped LDH ratio usually appears in 12 to 24 hours and is present within 48 hours in approximately 80% of patients. When LDH-2 is greater than LDH-1 (a normal LDH-1/LDH-2 ratio), it is considered reliable evidence against MI. The patient may have had a severe ischemic episode or only minimal heart damage. Other diseases (e.g., pulmonary infarction, hemolysis, congestive heart failure) that cause an increase in LDH levels may obscure the enzyme diagnosis of MI unless isoenzyme levels are determined.

Some laboratories measure only the LDH-1 level. An elevated LDH level with greater than 40% LDH-1 is considered diagnostic of myocardial damage.

Interfering factors

- Hemolysis of blood will cause false positive LDH levels.
- Drugs that may cause increased LDH levels include alcohol, anesthetics, aspirin, clofibrate, fluorides, mithramycin, narcotics, and procainamide.
- Drugs that may cause decreased levels include ascorbic acid.

Procedure and patient care

Before

- Explain the procedure to the patient.
- Tell the patient that no fasting is required.
- Inform the patient if he or she will be receiving frequent venipuncture for the evaluation of an MI.

During

- Collect approximately 7 to 10 ml of venous blood in a red-top tube.
- Since many diseases cause an increased LDH level, identify disease conditions on the laboratory slip.
- Record the data and time when blood was drawn on the laboratory slip for an accurate evaluation of the temporal pattern of enzyme elevations.

After

- Apply pressure or a pressure dressing to the venipuncture site.
- Assess the venipuncture site for bleeding.

Abnormal findings
Increased values

Myocardial infarction
Pulmonary diseases (e.g., infarction)
Hepatic diseases (e.g., hepatitis)
Red blood cell diseases (e.g., hemolytic anemias)
Skeletal muscle disease and injury
Renal parenchymal diseases (e.g., infarction)
Intestinal ischemia and infarction

Cerebrovascular accident (CVA)
Neoplastic states
Infectious mononucleosis
Heat stroke
Pancreatitis
Collagen diseases
Fracture
Muscular dystrophy
Shock
Hypotension

Notes

lactose tolerance test

Type of test Blood

Normal findings Adult/elderly: rise in plasma glucose levels >20 mg/dl

Test explanation and related physiology

This test is performed to detect lactose intolerance. Lactose is a disaccharide typically found in dairy products. During digestion, lactose is broken down into glucose and galactose by the intestinal enzyme lactase. Because lactose-intolerant patients have an absence of lactase, lactose digestion will not occur. Thus the small bowel is flooded with a high lactose load. Bacterial metabolism of the lactose occurs within the intestine. This creates a strong cathartic effect. Symptoms of lactose intolerance include abdominal cramping, flatus, abdominal bloating, and diarrhea.

In this test the patient is provided a lactose load. If lactose is not present in sufficient quantities, lactose is not metabolized to glucose and galactose. Plasma levels of glucose do not rise as expected. Therefore lower-than-expected serum glucose levels suggest intestinal lactase deficiency.

Interfering factors

- Enterogenous steatorrhea
- Strenuous exercise
- Smoking, which may increase blood glucose levels

Procedure and patient care
Before

- Explain the procedure to the patient. Inform the patient that four blood samples will be needed.
- Instruct the patient to fast 8 hours before testing.
- Instruct the patient to avoid strenuous exercise for 8 hours before testing. This may fictitiously affect the blood glucose level.
- Inform the patient that smoking is prohibited before testing. This may falsely increase the blood sugar level.

During

- Obtain 5 to 7 ml of venous blood in a gray-top tube from the fasting patient.
- Provide a specified dose of lactose for the patient. Usually, dilute 100 g of lactose into 200 ml of water for ingestion in adults.
- Note that pediatric doses of lactose are based on weight.
- Collect three more blood samples at 30, 60, and 120 minutes after the ingestion of lactose.
- Tell the patient that the only discomfort is the venipuncture. However, patients with lactase deficiency will have the symptoms previously described.

After

- Apply pressure or a pressure dressing to the venipuncture site.
- Observe the venipuncture site for bleeding.
- Note that patients with abnormal test results may receive a monosaccharide tolerance test (e.g., a glucose or galactose tolerance test).

Abnormal findings
Decreased levels

Lactase insufficiency
Enterogenous diarrhea

Notes

laparoscopy (Pelvic endoscopy, Gynecologic laparoscopy)

Type of test Endoscopy

Normal findings Normal-appearing female reproductive organs

Test explanation and related physiology

During a laparoscopy the female abdominal organs can be visualized by inserting a fiberoptic scope through the abdominal wall and into the peritoneum. This is particularly helpful in diagnosing pelvic adhesions, ovarian tumors and cysts, and other tubal and uterine causes of infertility. Also, endometriosis, ectopic pregnancy, ruptured ovarian cyst, and salpingitis can be detected during an evaluation for pelvic pain. This procedure is also used to stage carcinomas. Surgical procedures (e.g., biopsy specimen removal from abdominal organs, lysis of adhesions, removal of intraabdominal intrauterine devices [IUDs], tubal ligation) can easily be performed with the laparoscope. General surgical procedures (e.g., cholecystectomy, appendectomy) are now being performed with laparoscopy.

Contraindications

- Patients with local peritonitis, since laparoscopy may spread the infection throughout the abdominal cavity
- Patients who have had multiple surgical procedures, since adhesions may have formed between the viscera and the abdominal wall
- Patients with suspected intraabdominal hemorrhage, since visualization through the scope will be obscured by the blood

Potential complications

- Perforation of the bowel, with spilling of intestinal contents into the peritoneum
- Hemorrhage
- Acidosis, from carbon dioxide inflation of the abdominal cavity

L

Interfering factors

- Adhesions or extreme obesity may obstruct the field of vision.

Procedure and patient care

Before

- Explain the procedure to the patient.
- Ensure that an informed consent for this procedure is obtained.
- If enemas are ordered to clear the bowel, assist the patient as needed and record the results.
- Since the procedure is usually performed with the patient under general anesthesia, follow the routine general anesthesia precautions.
- Shave and prepare the patient's abdomen, as ordered.
- Keep the patient NPO after midnight on the day of the test. Fluids may be given intravenously.
- Instruct the patient to void before going to the operating room, since a distended bladder can be easily penetrated.

During

- Note the following procedural steps:

  1. Pelvic endoscopy is usually performed in the operating room. The patient is placed in a modified lithotomy or Trendelenburg position so that the intestines move away from the pelvis, thus permitting better visualization of the pelvic organs.
  2. After the abdominal skin is cleansed, a blunt-tipped needle is inserted through a small incision in the sub-umbilical area into the peritoneal cavity.
  3. The peritoneal cavity is filled with approximately 3 to 4 L of carbon dioxide to separate the abdominal wall from the intraabdominal viscera, thus enhancing visualization of pelvic and abdominal structures.
  4. A laparoscope is inserted to examine the pelvic organs in the upper abdomen.
  5. After the desired procedure (inspection, tubal ligation, biopsy removal) is completed, the laparoscope is removed and the carbon dioxide is allowed to escape.
  6. The incision is closed with a few skin stitches and covered with an adhesive bandage.

- Note that laparoscopy is usually performed by a surgeon in approximately 20 to 40 minutes.
- Inform the patient who will be under general anesthesia that she will feel no discomfort. However, most patients will have mild incisional pain later and may also complain of shoulder or subcostal discomfort from pneumoperitoneum.

After

- Instruct the patient not to walk or stand immediately after the legs have been removed from the stirrups. The orthostasis that may result from standing erect may cause dizziness and fainting.
- Assess the patient frequently for signs of bleeding (increased pulse rate, decreased blood pressure), perforated viscus (abdominal tenderness, guarding, decreased bowel sounds), and acidosis (increased respiratory rate). Report any significant findings to the physician.
- If the patient has shoulder or subcostal discomfort from pneumoperitoneum, assure her that this usually lasts only 24 hours. Minor analgesics usually relieve this discomfort.

Abnormal findings

Pelvic adhesions
Ovarian tumors
Ovarian cysts
Endometriosis
Ectopic pregnancy
Ruptured ovarian cyst
Salpingitis
Pelvic inflammatory disease
  (PID)

Cancer
Uterine fibroids
Abscess
Infection
Ascites
Liver nodules
Portal hypertension
Other abdominal organ
  pathology

Notes

leucine aminopeptidase (LAP)

Type of test Blood; urine (24 hour)

Normal findings

Blood: male, 80-200 U/ml
            female, 75-185 U/ml
Urine: 2-18 U/24 hr

Test explanation and related physiology

LAP, produced exclusively by the liver, is used in diagnosing liver disorders and in the differential diagnosis of increased levels of alkaline phosphatase (ALP, see p. 26). LAP levels tend to parallel ALP levels in hepatic disease. LAP is a sensitive indicator of cholestasis. However, unlike ALP, LAP remains normal in bone disease. LAP can be detected in both the blood and the urine. Patients with elevated serum LAP levels will always show urine elevations. However, when the urine LAP level is elevated, the blood level may have already returned to normal.

Interfering factors

- Pregnancy may cause increased values.
- Drugs that may cause increased LAP levels include estrogens and progesterones.

Procedure and patient care

Before

- Explain the procedure to the patient.
- Tell the patient that no fasting is required.

During

- Collect approximately 7 to 10 ml of venous blood in a red-top tube.
- If a urine sample is needed, follow the procedure for a 24-hour urine collection (see p. 325).
- Indicate on the laboratory slip any medications the patient may be taking that can affect test results.

After

- Apply pressure or a pressure dressing to the venipuncture site.
- Assess the venipuncture site for bleeding. Patients with liver dysfunction often have prolonged clotting times.

Abnormal findings
Increased levels

Hepatitis
Cirrhosis
Hepatic necrosis
Hepatic ischemia

Hepatic tumor
Hepatotoxic drugs
Cholestasis

Notes

L

leukocyte esterase (WBC esterase)

Type of test Urine

Normal findings Negative

Test explanation and related physiology

Leukocyte (white blood cell [WBC]) esterase is a screening test used to detect leukocytes in the urine. This test, which indicates a possible urinary tract infection, is frequently part of the urinalysis. This macroscopic examination employs chemical testing with a leukocyte esterase dipstick. Any shade of purple is considered positive. Some laboratories have established a screening protocol in which a microscopic examination is only performed if a leukocyte esterase test is positive.

Interfering factors

- False positive results may occur in specimens contaminated with vaginal secretions (e.g., heavy mucous discharge, *Trichomonas* infection, parasites).
- False negative results may occur in specimens containing high levels of protein and ascorbic acid.

Procedure and patient care

Before

- Explain the procedure to the patient.

During

- Collect a fresh, random urine specimen in a urine container.
- Note that a "clean-catch" urine or "midstream" collection is preferable in women to avoid vaginal contamination. This requires meticulous cleansing of the urinary meatus with an iodine preparation to reduce contamination of the specimen by external organisms. Then the cleansing agent must be completely removed, or it will contaminate the specimen. The midstream collection is obtained by:

  1. Having the patient begin to urinate in a bedpan, urinal, or toilet and then stop urinating (This washes the urine out of the distal urethra.)

2. Correctly positioning a sterile urine container, into which the patient voids 3 to 4 ounces of urine
3. Capping the container
4. Allowing the patient to finish voiding

After

- Follow the manufacturer's directions exactly for the leukocyte esterase test.
- If the specimen cannot be processed immediately, refrigerate it.

Abnormal findings

Possible urinary tract infections

Notes

L

lipase

Type of test Blood

Normal findings 0-110 units/L or 0-417 U/L (SI units) (values are method dependent)

Test explanation and related physiology

The most common cause of an elevated serum lipase level is acute pancreatitis. Lipase is an enzyme secreted by the pancreas into the duodenum to break down triglycerides into fatty acids. As with amylase (see p. 43), lipase appears in the bloodstream following damage to the pancreatic acinar cells. Since lipase is produced only in the pancreas, elevated serum levels are specific to pathologic pancreatic conditions.

In acute pancreatitis, elevated lipase levels usually parallel serum amylase levels. However, the lipase levels usually rise 24 to 48 hours after the onset of pancreatitis and remain elevated for 5 to 7 days. Thus they peak later and remain elevated longer than the serum amylase levels. Therefore serum lipase levels are more useful in the late diagnosis of acute pancreatitis. Lipase levels are less useful in more chronic pancreatic diseases (e.g., chronic pancreatitis, pancreatic carcinoma).

Interfering factors

- Drugs that may cause increased lipase levels include bethanechol, cholinergics, codeine, indomethacin, meperidine, methacholine, and morphine.
- Drugs that may cause decreased levels include calcium ions.

Procedure and patient care

Before

- Explain the procedure to the patient.
- Instruct the patient to remain NPO except for water for 8 to 12 hours before the test.

During

- Collect 5 to 7 ml of venous blood in a red-top tube.
- Indicate on the laboratory slip drugs that can affect test results.

After

- Apply pressure or a pressure dressing the venipuncture site.
- Observe the venipuncture site for bleeding.

Abnormal findings

Acute pancreatitis
Chronic relapsing pancreatitis
Acute cholecystitis

Notes

lipoproteins (High-density lipoprotein [HDL], Low-density lipoprotein [LDL], Very low-density lipoprotein [VLDL])

Type of test Blood

Normal findings

HDL: male, >45 mg/dl
       female, >55 mg/dl
LDL: 60-180 mg/dl
VLDL: 25%-50%

Test explanation and related physiology

Lipoproteins are proteins in the blood whose main purpose is to transport cholesterol, triglycerides, and other fats. With the use of electrophoresis, these lipoproteins can be grouped into chylomicrons, which are primarily triglycerides; low-density lipoproteins (LDLs), composed primarily of cholesterol; very low-density lipoproteins (VLDLs), which are mainly triglycerides; and high-density lipoproteins (HDLs), predominantly composed of protein.

HDL is a carrier of cholesterol. It is suspected that the purpose of HDL is to remove the cholesterol from the peripheral tissues and transport this to the liver for excretion. Also, HDLs may have a protective effect by preventing cellular uptake of cholesterol and lipids. These potential actions may be the source of the protective cardiovascular characteristics associated with HDLs within the blood. The HDL/total cholesterol ratio should be at least 1:5, with 1:3 as an ideal ratio.

LDLs are also cholesterol rich. Cholesterol carried by LDLs can be deposited into the peripheral tissues and is associated with an increased risk of arteriosclerotic heart and peripheral vascular disease. Therefore high levels of LDL are atherogenic. The LDL level should be less than 160 mg/dl in persons with coronary artery disease and less than 180 mg/dl in those without disease.

VLDLs, although carrying a small amount of cholesterol, are the predominant carriers of blood triglycerides. To a lesser degree, VLDLs are also associated with an increased risk of arteriosclerotic occlusive disease.

The HDL, LDL, and VLDL levels are a part of a lipid

profile test that also evaluates cholesterol (see p. 190) and triglycerides (see p. 736). The lipoproteins test is used to assess the risk of coronary artery disease. High levels of the "protective" HDL are associated with a decreased risk of coronary disease, whereas high levels of LDL and VLDL are associated with an increased risk of coronary occlusive disease.

Levels of HDL are increased in patients who engage in frequent physical activity or who use moderate doses of alcohol. On the other hand, LDL and VLDL are known to be increased in patients who have poor dietary habits associated with an increased intake of animal fats and snack foods. Genetic makeup, however, is probably the most important determinant of lipoprotein level.

The VLDL is usually expressed as a percentage of total cholesterol. Levels in excess of 25% to 50% are associated with increased risk of coronary disease. The LDL is derived by subtracting the HDL minus one fifth of the triglycerides from the total cholesterol:

$$\text{LDL} = \text{Total cholesterol} - (\text{HDL} - \text{Triglycerides}/5)$$

There are other formulas to derive LDL, which may account for different sets of normal values.

Interfering factors

- Smoking and alcohol ingestion decrease HDL levels.
- Binge eating can alter lipoprotein values.
- Exercise can raise HDL levels.
- Drugs that may cause increased lipoprotein levels include aspirin, oral contraceptives, phenothiazines, steroids, and sulfonamides.

Procedure and patient care

Before

- Instruct the patient to fast for 12 to 14 hours before testing. Only water is permitted.
- Inform the patient that dietary indiscretion within the previous few weeks may influence lipoprotein levels.

During

- Collect 5 to 10 ml of venous blood in a red-top tube.
- Indicate on the laboratory slip any drugs that can affect test results.

After

- Apply pressure or a pressure dressing to the venipuncture site.
- Observe the venipuncture site for bleeding.
- Instruct patients with high lipoprotein levels regarding diet, exercise, and appropriate body weight.

Abnormal findings
Increased HDL levels

Liver disease

Decreased HDL levels

Increased risk of arteriosclerotic heart disease

Increased LDL and VLDL levels

Hyperlipidemia
Increased ingestion of fatty foods and animal fats

Decreased LDL and VLDL levels

Malnutrition
Malabsorption

Notes

liver biopsy

Type of test Microscopic examination of tissue

Normal findings Normal liver histology

Test explanation and related physiology

Liver biopsy is a safe, simple, and valuable method of diagnosing pathologic liver conditions. For this study a specially designed needle is inserted through the abdominal wall and into the liver. A piece of liver tissue is removed for microscopic examination. Percutaneous liver biopsy is used in the diagnosis of various liver disorders, such as cirrhosis, hepatitis, drug reaction, granuloma, and tumor. Biopsy is indicated for:

1. Patients with unexplained hepatomegaly
2. Patients with persistently elevated liver enzymes
3. Patients with suspected primary or metastatic tumor, as determined by other studies
4. Patients with unexplained jaundice
5. Patients with suspected hepatitis
6. Patients with suspected infiltrative diseases (e.g., sarcoidosis, amyloidosis)

Contraindications

- Uncooperative patients who cannot remain still and hold their breath during sustained exhalation
- Patients with impaired hemostasis
- Anemic patients who could not tolerate major blood loss associated with inadvertent puncture of a intrahepatic blood vessel
- Patients with infections in the right pleural space or right upper quadrant, since the biopsy may spread the infection
- Patients with obstructive jaundice
  In these patients, bile within the ducts is under pressure and may subsequently leak into the abdominal cavity after needle penetration.
- Patients with a hemangioma
  This is a very vascular tumor, and bleeding after a biopsy may be severe.

Potential complications

- Hemorrhage caused by inadvertent puncture of a blood vessel within the liver
- Chemical peritonitis caused by inadvertent puncture of a bile duct, with subsequent leakage of bile into the abdominal cavity
- Pneumothorax (collapsed lung) caused by improper placement of the biopsy needle into the adjacent chest cavity

Procedure and patient care

Before

- Explain the procedure to the patient. Many patients are apprehensive about this procedure.
- Obtain an informed consent.
- Ensure that all coagulation tests are normal.
- Instruct the patient to keep NPO after midnight on the day of the test.
- Administer any sedative medications as ordered.

During

- Note the following procedural steps:
  1. The patient is placed in the supine or left lateral position.
  2. The skin area used for puncture is anesthetized locally.
  3. The patient is asked to exhale and hold the exhalation. This causes the liver to descend and reduces the possibility of a pneumothorax. Frequently, the patient practices exhalation two or three times before insertion of the needle.
  4. During the patient's sustained exhalation, the physician rapidly introduces the biopsy needle into the liver and obtains liver tissue.
     a. Several types of needles are available.
     b. Occasionally, the biopsy needle is inserted under computed tomography (CT) guidance. This is especially useful when tissue from a specific area of the liver is needed.
  5. The needle is withdrawn from the liver.
- Note that this test is performed by a physician in approximately 15 minutes.

- Inform the patient that he or she may have minor discomfort during injection of the local anesthetic and during needle insertion.

After

- Place the tissue sample into a specimen bottle containing formalin and send it to the pathology department.
- Apply a small dressing over the needle insertion site.
- Place the patient on his or her right side for about 1 to 2 hours. In this position the liver capsule is compressed against the chest wall, thereby decreasing the risk of hemorrhage or bile leak.
- Assess the patient's vital signs frequently for evidence of hemorrhage (increased pulse, decreased blood pressure) and peritonitis (increased temperature).

Abnormal findings

Benign tumor
Malignant tumor (primary or metastatic)
Abscess
Cyst

Hepatitis
Infiltrative diseases (e.g., amyloidosis, hemochromatosis, cirrhosis)

L

Notes

liver and pancreatobiliary system ultrasonography (Echogram of the liver, biliary tree, gallbladder, and pancreas)

Type of test Ultrasound

Normal findings Normal pancreas, gallbladder, and biliary ducts without dilation or filling defects

Test explanation and related physiology

Through the use of reflected sound waves, ultrasonography provides accurate visualization of the gallbladder, liver, biliary tree, and pancreas. The technique of ultrasonography requires the emission of high-frequency sound waves from the transducer to penetrate the organ being studied. The sound waves are bounced back to the transducer and electronically converted into a pictorial image. A realistic Polaroid picture or x-ray film of the organ studied is obtained.

Ultrasound is used in detecting cystic structures of the liver (e.g., benign cysts, hepatic abscesses, dilated intrahepatic ducts) and solid intrahepatic tumors (primary and metastatic). The gallbladder and extrahepatic ducts can be visualized and are examined for evidence of gallstones or dilation secondary to obstructive strictures or tumors. The pancreas is examined for evidence of tumor, pseudocyst, pancreatitis, or pancreatic abscess. Ultrasound of the pancreas is frequently performed serially to document and demonstrate resolution of an acute pancreatic process.

Because this study requires no contrast material and has no associated radiation, it is especially useful in patients who are allergic to contrast and in pregnant patients. Also, fasting is not mandatory to obtain accurate results.

Interfering factors

- Barium or gas will distort the sound waves and alter test results. This test should be performed before any x-ray testing with barium.

Procedure and patient care

Before

- Explain the procedure to the patient.
- Tell the patient that no fasting is required. However, the gallbladder is more easily visualized after an 8-hour fast.

During

- Note the following procedural steps:

  1. The patient is placed on an ultrasonography table in the supine position.
  2. A greasy conductive paste is applied to the desired area. This paste is used to enhance sound wave transmission and reception.
  3. A transducer is placed over the skin.
  4. Pictures are taken of the reflections from the organs being studied.

- This test is completed in approximately 20 minutes, usually by an ultrasound technologist, and interpreted by a radiologist.
- Tell the patient that no discomfort is associated with this procedure.

After

- Remove the coupling agent (grease) from the patient's abdomen.

Abnormal findings

Tumor, gallstone, or polyp of the gallbladder
Tumor, abscess, or dilated hepatic ducts within the liver
Tumor, cyst, pseudocyst, abscess, or inflammation of the pancreas
Dilation of the bile ducts
Gallstone, stricture, tumor, and dilation of the bile ducts

Notes

liver scanning (Radioisotope liver scanning)

Type of test Nuclear scan

Normal findings Normal size, shape, and position of the liver

Test explanation and related physiology

This radionuclide procedure is used to outline and detect structural changes of the liver. A radionuclide, usually technetium (Tc) sulfur–labeled albumin colloid, is administered intravenously. Later, a gamma ray detector is placed over the right upper quadrant of the patient's abdomen. This records the distribution of the radioactive particles in the liver. The spleen can also be visualized by this detector when Tc sulfur–labeled colloid is administered. Images are obtained and recorded on Polaroid or x-ray film.

Because the scan can only demonstrate filling defects greater than 2 cm in diameter, false negative results can occur in patients who have space-occupying lesions (e.g., tumors, cysts, granulomas) smaller than 2 cm. The scan may be incorrectly interpreted as positive for filling defects in patients who have cirrhosis because of the distortion of the patient's liver parenchyma. The liver scan can also detect diffuse infiltrative processes affecting the liver (e.g., amyloidosis, sarcoidosis).

Contraindications

- Patients who are pregnant or lactating, because of the risk of damage to the fetus or infant

Interfering factor

- Barium in the GI tract overlying the liver or spleen will produce defects on the scan that can be mistaken for masses.

Procedure and patient care

Before

- Explain the procedure to the patient.
- Tell the patient that no fasting or premedication is required.
- Assure the patient that he or she will not be exposed to

large amounts of radiation because only a tracer dose of isotope is used.

During

- Note the following procedural steps:
  1. The patient is taken to the nuclear medicine department, where the radionuclide is administered intravenously. (For inpatients, a nuclear medicine technologist may administer the radionuclide at the bedside.)
  2. Thirty minutes after injection, a gamma ray detector is placed over the right upper quadrant of the patient's abdomen.
  3. The patient is placed in supine, lateral, and prone positions so that all surfaces of the liver can be visualized.
  4. The radionuclide image is recorded on either x-ray or Polaroid film.

- Note that the procedure is performed by a trained technologist in approximately 1 hour. A physician trained in nuclear medicine interprets the reports.
- Tell the patient that the only discomfort associated with this procedure is the IV injection of the radionuclide.

After

- Because only tracer doses of radioisotopes are used, inform the patient that no precautions need to be taken by others against radiation exposure.

Abnormal findings

Tumors
Abscesses
Hematomas
Infiltrative diseases (e.g., sarcoidosis, amyloidosis)

Hepatic cysts
Tuberculosis

Notes

long-acting thyroid stimulator (LATS, Thyroid-stimulating immunoglobulin [TSIG])

Type of test Blood

Normal findings Negative

Test explanation and related physiology

The LATS antibody is an immunoglobulin directed against the thyroid cell plasma membrane. LATS mimics the action of thyroid-stimulating hormone (TSH). LATS stimulates the thyroid gland to produce and secrete excessive amounts of thyroid hormones. This factor inhibits TSH secretion through the normal negative feedback mechanism. LATS is found in the blood of some hyperthyroid patients. Assessment for LATS is important in the evaluation of some patients with thyroid disease, especially those with malignant exophthalmos. Elevated levels support the diagnosis of Graves' disease. Because LATS crosses the placenta, it may be found in neonates whose mothers have Graves' disease.

Interfering factor

- Recent administration of radioactive iodine may affect test results.

Procedure and patient care

Before

- Explain the procedure to the patient.
- Tell the patient that no fasting or special preparation is required.

During

- Collect approximately 5 ml of venous blood in a red-top tube.
- Notify the laboratory if the patient has received radioactive iodine in the preceding 2 days.
- Handle the blood sample gently. Hemolysis may interfere with interpretation of test results.

After

- Apply pressure or a pressure dressing to the venipuncture site.
- Observe the venipuncture site for bleeding.

Abnormal findings
Increased levels

Hyperthyroidism
Malignant exophthalmos
Graves' disease

Notes

long bones x-ray

Type of test X-ray

Normal findings No evidence of fracture, tumor, infection, or congenital abnormalities

Test explanation and related physiology

X-ray films of the long bones are usually taken when the patient has complaints about a particular body area. Fractures or tumors are readily detected by x-ray studies. In patients who have a severe or chronic infection overlying a bone, an x-ray film may detect the infection involving that bone (osteomyelitis). X-ray studies of the long bones also can detect joint destruction and bone spurring as a result of persistent arthritis. Growth patterns can be followed by serial x-ray studies of a long bone, usually the wrist. Healing of a fracture can also be documented and followed. X-ray films of the joints also reveal the presence of fluid.

Procedure and patient care
Before

- Explain the procedure to the patient.
- Carefully handle any injured parts of the patient's body.
- Instruct the patient that he or she will need to keep the extremity still while the x-ray film is being taken. This can sometimes be difficult, especially when the patient has severe pain associated with a recent injury.
- Shield the patient's testes, ovaries, or pregnant abdomen to avoid exposure from scattered radiation.
- Tell the patient that no fasting or sedation is required.

During

- Note that in the x-ray department, the patient is asked to place the involved extremity in several positions. An x-ray film is taken of each position.
- Note that this test is routinely performed by a radiologic technologist within several minutes.
- Tell the patient that no discomfort is associated with this test, except possibly moving the extremity.

After

- Administer an analgesic for relief of pain (if indicated).

Abnormal findings

Fractures

Tumors

Infection

Osteomyelitis

Joint destruction

Bone spurring

Abnormal growth pattern

Joint fluid

Notes

lumbar puncture and cerebrospinal fluid examination (LP and CSF examination, Spinal tap, Spinal puncture, Cerebrospinal fluid analysis)

Type of test Fluid analysis

Normal findings

Pressure: less than 200 cm H_2O
Color: clear and colorless
Blood: none
Cells: no red blood cells; less than five lymphocytes/mm^3
Culture and sensitivity: no organisms present
Protein: 15-45 mg/dl CSF (up to 70 mg/dl in elderly adults and children)
Glucose: 50-75 mg/dl CSF or 60%-70% of blood glucose level
Chloride: 700-750 mg/dl
Lactic dehydrogenase (LDH): less than 2.0-7.2 U/ml
Cytology: no malignant cells
Serology for syphilis: negative
Glutamine: 6-15 mg/dl

Test explanation and related physiology

By placing a needle in the subarachnoid space of the spinal column, one can measure the pressure of that space and obtain cerebrospinal fluid (CSF) for examination. The examination may assist in the diagnosis of primary or metastatic brain or spinal cord neoplasm, cerebral hemorrhage, meningitis, encephalitis, degenerative brain disease, autoimmune diseases involving the central nervous system, neurosyphilis, and demyelinating disorders (e.g., multiple sclerosis, acute demyelinating polyneuropathy).

LP may be used therapeutically to relieve intracranial pressure, to inject therapeutic or diagnostic agents, and to administer spinal anesthetics. Examination of the CSF includes evaluation for the presence of blood, bacteria, and malignant cells, along with quantitation of the amount of glucose and protein present. Color is noted, and various other tests, such as serologic test for syphilis (STS, see p. 695), are performed.

Pressure. By attaching a sterile manometer to the needle used in LP, the pressure within the subarachnoid space can be measured. A pressure above 200 cm H_2O is considered abnormal. Because the subarachnoid space surrounding the brain is freely connected to the subarachnoid space of the spinal cord, any increase in intracranial pressure will be directly reflected as an increase at the lumbar site. When this normal connection is suspected to be obstructed, a *Queckenstedt-Stookey test* is performed (see "Procedure and patient care").

Color. Normal CSF is clear and colorless. A cloudy appearance may indicate an increase in the white blood cell (WBC) count. Normally, CSF contains no blood. A red tinge to the CSF indicates the presence of blood. This blood may be present because of subarachnoid bleeding or because the needle used in the LP has inadvertently penetrated a blood vessel. These causes of the bleeding must be differentiated. With a traumatic puncture the blood within the CSF will clot. No clotting occurs in a patient with subarachnoid hemorrhage. Also, with a traumatic tap the fluid clears toward the end of the procedure as successive samples are obtained. This clearing does not occur with a subarachnoid hemorrhage.

Blood. Blood within the CSF indicates cerebral hemorrhage into the subarachnoid space or a traumatic tap, as just described.

Cells. The number of red blood cells (RBCs) is merely an indication of the amount of blood present within the CSF. Except for a few lymphocytes, the presence of WBCs in the CSF is abnormal. The presence of polymorphonuclear leukocytes (neutrophils) is indicative of bacterial meningitis or cerebral abscess. When mononuclear leukocytes are present, viral or tubercular meningitis or encephalitis is suspected.

Culture and sensitivity. The organisms that cause meningitis or brain abscess can be cultured from the CSF. Organisms found may also include atypical bacteria, fungi, or *Mycobacterium tuberculosis*. A Gram stain of the CSF may give the clinician preliminary information about the causative infectious agent. This may allow appropriate antibiotic therapy to be initiated before the 24 hours necessary for completion of the culture and sensitivity report.

Protein. Normally, very little protein is found in CSF from the subarachnoid space. The amount of protein is usually lower in CSF obtained from the cisterna magna and even lower in the ventricle. Only small amounts of protein are found in CSF because protein is a large molecule that does not cross the blood-brain barrier. However, disease processes can alter the permeability of this protective membrane, thereby allowing protein to leak into the CSF.

The protein content within CSF is increased in patients who have infectious or inflammatory processes such as meningitis, encephalitis, or myelitis. Tumors may also cause an increase in protein content. Normally, less than 12% to 20% of the total protein consists of gammaglobulin. The proportion of albumin to globulin is higher in CSF than in blood plasma (see p. 592) because albumin is smaller in size than globulin, and therefore albumin can pass more easily through the blood-brain barrier. Patients with multiple sclerosis, neurosyphilis, or degenerative cord or brain disease have an elevation of the globulin fraction of total protein. An increase in the CSF level of immunoglobulin G (IgG), an increase in the ratio of IgG to other proteins (e.g., albumin), and the detection of *oligoclonal gammaglobulin bands* are highly suggestive of inflammatory and autoimmune diseases of the central nervous system, especially multiple sclerosis.

Glucose. The glucose level is decreased when an increase occurs in the number of cells within the CSF using the glucose. These cells may be inflammatory cells in response to infection, shedded tumors, or bacterial cells. A blood sample for glucose (see p. 379) is usually drawn before the spinal tap is performed. A CSF glucose level less than 60% of the blood glucose may indicate meningitis or neoplasm.

Chloride. The chloride concentration in CSF may be decreased in patients with meningeal infections, tubercular meningitis, and conditions of low blood chloride levels. An increase in the chloride level is CSF is not neurologically significant; it correlates with the blood levels of chloride (see p. 179). CSF is not routinely evaluated for chloride; this test is done only if specifically requested.

Lactic dehydrogenase (LDH). Quantitation of LDH (specifically fractions 4 and 5, see p. 450) is helpful in diagnosing bacterial meningitis. The source of LDH is the neutrophils that fight the invading bacteria. When the LDH level is elevated, infection or inflammation is suspected.

Cytology. Examination of the cells in the CSF can determine if they are malignant or benign. Tumors in the central nervous system may shed cells from their surface. These cells can float freely in CSF. Their presence suggests neoplasm as the cause of any neurologic symptoms.

Serology for syphilis. Latent syphilis is diagnosed by performing one of many presently available serologic tests on CSF. These include (1) the Wasserman test, (2) the Venereal Disease Research Laboratory (VDRL) test (see p. 695), and (3) the flourescent treponemal antibody (FTA) test (see p. 695). The FTA test is presently considered to be the most sensitive and specific. When test results are positive, the diagnosis of neurosyphilis is made and appropriate antibiotic therapy initiated.

Glutamine. The CSF can be evaluated for the presence of glutamine. This test is useful in the detection and evaluation of hepatic encephalopathy and coma. Levels of glutamine often are increased in patients with Reye's syndrome.

Contraindications

- Patients with increased intracranial pressure
  The LP may induce cerebral or cerebellar herniation through the foramen magna.
- Patients who have severe degenerative vertebral joint disease
  It is very difficult to pass the needle through the degenerated arthritic interspinal space.
- Patients with infection near the LP site
  Meningitis can result from contamination of CSF with infected material.

Potential complications

- Persistent CSF leak, causing severe headache
- Introduction of bacteria into CSF, causing suppurative meningitis
- Herniation of the brain through the tentorium cerebelli or herniation of the cerebellum through the foramen magnum
  In patients who have increased intracranial pressure, the quick reduction of pressure in the spinal column by the LP may induce hernation of the brain, causing compression of the brainstem. This results in deterioration of the patient's neurologic status and death.
- Inadvertent puncture of the spinal cord, caused by inappropriately high puncture of the spinal cord

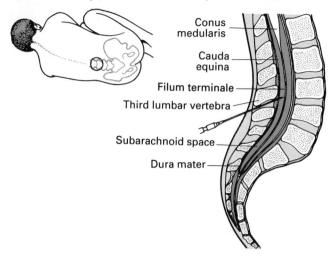

Figure 7 Patient position for lumbar puncture (LP).

- Puncture of the aorta or vena cava, causing serious retro-peritoneal hemorrhage
- Transient back pain and pain or paresthesia in the legs

Procedure and patient care
Before
- Explain the procedure to the patient. Many patients have misconceptions regarding LP. Allay the patients fears and allow time to verbalize concerns.
- Obtain informed consent if required by the institution.
- Perform a baseline neurologic assessment of the legs by assessing the patient's strengths, sensation, and movement.
- Tell the patient that no fasting or sedation is required.
- Instruct the patient to empty the bladder and bowels before the procedure.
- Explain to the patient that he or she must lie very still throughout this procedure. Movement may cause traumatic injury. Encourage the patient to relax and take deep, slow breaths with the mouth open.

During

- Note the following procedural steps:

    1. This study is a sterile procedure that can be easily performed at the bedside. The patient is usually placed in the lateral decubitus (fetal) position (see Figure 7).
    2. The patient is instructed to clasp the hands on the knees to maintain this position. Someone usually helps the patient maintain this position. (A sitting position may also be used.)
    3. A local anesthetic is injected into the skin and subcutaneous tissues after the site has been aseptically cleaned.
    4. A spinal needle containing an inner obturator is placed through the skin and into the spinal canal.
    5. The subarachnoid space is entered.
    6. The insert (obturator) is removed, and CSF can be seen slowly dripping from the needle.
    7. The needle is attached to a sterile manometer, and the pressure (opening pressure) is recorded.
    8. Before the pressure reading is taken, the patient is asked to relax and straighten the legs to reduce the intraabdominal pressure, which causes an increase in CSF pressure.
    9. Three sterile test tubes are filled with 5 to 10 ml of CSF.
    10. The pressure (closing pressure) is measured.

- Note that if blockage in CSF circulation in the spinal subarachnoid space is suspected, a *Queckenstedt-Stookey* test may be performed. For this test the jugular vein is occluded either manually by digital pressure or by a medium-sized blood pressure cuff inflated to approximately 20 mm Hg. Within 10 seconds after jugular occlusion, CSF pressure should increase from 15 to 40 cm H_2O and then promptly return to normal within 10 seconds after release of the pressure. A sluggish rise or fall of CSF pressure suggests partial blockage of CSF circulation. No rise after 10 seconds suggests a complete obstruction within the spinal canal.
- Note that this procedure is performed by a physician in approximately 20 minutes.
- Inform the patient that this procedure is described as un-

comfortable or painful by most patients. Some patients complain of feeling pressure from the needle. Some patients complain of a shooting pain in their legs.

After

- Apply digital pressure and an adhesive dressing to the puncture site.
- Place the patient in the prone position with a pillow under the abdomen to increase the intraabdominal pressure, which will indirectly increase the pressure in the tissues surrounding the spinal cord. This acts to retard continued CSF flow from the spinal canal.
- Encourage the patient to drink increased amounts of fluid with a straw to replace the CSF removed during the lumbar puncture. Drinking with a straw will enable the patient to keep the head flat.
- Usually, keep the patient in a reclining position for up to 12 hours to avoid the discomfort of potential postpuncture spinal headache. Allow the patient to turn from side to side as long as the head is not raised.
- Label and number the specimen jars appropriately and deliver them immediately to the laboratory after the test. Refrigeration will alter test results. A delay between collection time and testing can invalidate results, especially cell counts.
- Assess the patient for numbness, tingling, and movement of the extremities; pain at the injection site; drainage of blood or CSF at the injection site; and the ability to void. Notify the physician of any unusual findings.

Abnormal findings

Brain neoplasm
Spinal cord neoplasm
Cerebral hemorrhage
Meningitis
Encephalitis
Viral or tubercular
  meningitis
Encephalitis
Myelitis
Tumors
Neurosyphilis
Degenerative brain disease
Autoimmune disorders
Hepatic encephalopathy
Coma
Cerebral abscess
Degenerative cord or
  brain disease
Multiple sclerosis
Acute demyelinating
  polyneuropathy
Subarachnoid bleeding
Reye's syndrome

lung biopsy

Type of test Microscopic examination of tissue

Normal findings No evidence of pathology

Test explanation and related physiology

This invasive procedure is used to obtain a specimen of pulmonary tissue for a histologic examination by using either an open or a closed technique. The *open method* involves a limited thoracotomy. The *closed technique* includes methods such as transbronchial lung biopsy, transbronchial needle aspiration biopsy, transcatheter bronchial brushing, and percutaneous needle aspiration biopsy.

Lung biopsy is indicated to determine the pathology of pulmonary parenchymal disease. Carcinomas, granulomas, and sarcoidosis can be diagnosed with this procedure. This procedure is also useful in detecting environmental risks, infections, or familial disease, which may lead to better prevention and treatment.

Contraindications

- Patients with bullae or cysts
- Patients with suspected vascular anomalies
- Patients with bleeding abnormalities
- Patients with pulmonary hypertension
- Patients with respiratory insufficiency

Potential complications

- Pneumothorax
- Pulmonary hemorrhage
- Empyema

Procedure and patient care

Before

- Explain the procedure to the patient.
- Ensure that informed and signed consent is obtained.
- Instruct the patient that fasting is usually ordered. The patient may be kept NPO after midnight on the day of the test.
- Administer the preprocedural medications 30 to 60 minutes before the test, as ordered. Atropine is usually given

to decrease bronchial secretions. Meperidine (Demerol) may be used to sedate anxious patients.

- Instruct the patient to remain still during the lung biopsy. Any movement or coughing could cause perforation of the lung by the biopsy needle.

During

- Note that the patient's position depends on the method used and that the histologic lung specimen may be obtained by several different methods:

Transbronchial lung biopsy
1. This technique is performed via flexible fiberoptic bronchoscopy using cutting forceps.
2. Fluoroscopy is used to ensure proper opening and positioning of the forceps on the lesion.
3. Fluoroscopy also permits visualization of the "tug" of the lung as the specimen is removed.

Transbronchial needle aspiration
1. The specimen is obtained via a fiberoptic bronchoscope using a needle.
2. The bronchoscope is inserted, and the target site is identified by fluoroscopy.
3. The needle is inserted through the bronchoscope and into the tumor or desired area, where aspiration is performed with the attached syringe.
4. The needle is retracted within its sheath, and the entire catheter is withdrawn from the fiberoptic scope.

Transcatheter bronchial brushing
1. This is also performed via a fiberoptic bronchoscope.
2. During bronchoscopy a small brush is moved back and forth over the suspicious area.
3. The cells adhere to the brush, which is then removed and used to make microscopic slides.

Percutaneous needle biopsy
1. In this method for obtaining a closed specimen, the biopsy is obtained after using x-ray determination of the desired site.
2. The procedure is carried out by using a cutting needle or by aspiration with a spinal-type needle to obtain a specimen.
3. The main problem with this procedure is potential damage to major blood vessels.

Open lung biopsy
1. The patient is taken to the operating room, and general anesthesia is provided.
2. The patient is placed in the supine position, and a small incision is made into the chest wall.
3. After a piece of lung tissue is removed, the lung is closed.
4. Chest tube drainage is used for about 24 hours after an open lung biopsy.

- Note that this procedure is performed by a physician in less than ½ hour.
- During the lung biopsy procedure, assess the patient carefully for signs of respiratory distress (e.g., shortness of breath, rapid pulse, cyanosis).
- Tell the patient that most patients describe this procedure as uncomfortable.

After

- Place biopsy specimens in appropriate jars for histologic and microbiologic examinations.
- Observe the patient's vital signs frequently for signs of bleeding (increased pulse, decreased blood pressure) and for shortness of breath.
- Assess the patient's breath sounds, and report any decrease on the biopsy side.
- If ordered, obtain a chest x-ray film to check for complications (e.g., pneumothorax).
- Observe the patient for signs of pneumothorax (e.g., dyspnea, tachypnea, decrease in breath sounds, anxiety, restlessness).

Abnormal findings

Carcinomas
Granulomas

Sarcoidosis
Infections

Notes

---

lung scan (Ventilation/perfusion scanning [VPS], Pulmonary scintiphotography)

Type of test Nuclear scan

Normal findings Diffuse and homogeneous uptake of nuclear material by the lungs

Test explanation and related physiology

This nuclear medicine procedure is used to identify defects in blood *perfusion* of the lung in patients with suspected pulmonary embolism. Blood flow to the lungs is evaluated using a macroaggregated albumin (MAA) tagged with technetium (Tc), which is injected into the patient's peripheral vein. Because the diameter of the radionuclide aggregates is larger than that of the pulmonary capillaries, the aggregates become temporarily lodged in the pulmonary vasculature. A gamma ray detector passed over the patient records the distribution of particles within the lung vasculature.

A homogeneous uptake of particles that fills the entire pulmonary vasculature conclusively rules out pulmonary embolism. If a defect in an otherwise smooth and diffusely homogeneous pattern is seen, a perfusion abnormality exists. This can indicate pulmonary embolism. Unfortunately, many other serious pulmonary parenchymal lesions (e.g., pneumonia, tuberculosis, emphysema) also cause a defect in pulmonary blood perfusion. Therefore, although the scan may be sensitive, it is not specific because many different pathologic conditions can cause the same abnormal results.

The chest x-ray film aids in assessing the perfusion scan, since a defect on the perfusion scan seen in the same area as an abnormality on the chest x-ray film does not indicate pulmonary embolism. Rather, the defect may represent pneumonia, atelectasis, effusion, and so on. However, when a perfusion defect occurs in an area of the lung that is normal on a chest x-ray study, pulmonary embolus is likely.

Specificity of a perfusion scan can also be enhanced by performance of a *ventilation scan,* which detects abnormalities in ventilation. The ventilation scan reflects the patency of the pulmonary airways using krypton gas or Tc-DTPA (diethylenetriamine pentaacetic acid) as an aerosol. When vascular obstruction (embolism) is present, ventilation scans will demonstrate a normal wash-in and a normal wash-out of radioactivity from the embolized lung area. However, if parenchymal disease (e.g., pneumonia) is responsible for the perfusion abnormality, wash-in or wash-out will be abnormal. Therefore the "mismatch" of perfusion and ventilation is characteristic of embolic disorders, whereas the "match" is indicative of parenchymal disease.

Contraindications

- Patients who are pregnant

Interfering factors

- Patients with pulmonary parenchymal problems (e.g., pneumonia, emphysema, pleural effusion, tumors)
  These problems will give the picture of a perfusion defect and will simulate pulmonary embolism.

Procedure and patient care

Before

- Explain the procedure to the patient.
- Obtain informed consent if required by the institution.
- Assure the patient that he or she will not be exposed to large amounts of radioactivity because only tracer doses of isotopes are used.
- Although rarely done, if iodine-131 will be administered, give the patient 10 drops of Lugol's solution several hours before the test as a blocking agent for the thyroid gland. This will prevent iodine uptake by the thyroid gland.
- Tell the patient that no fasting is required.
- Note that a recent chest x-ray film should be available.
- Instruct the patient to remove jewelry around the chest area.

During

- Note the following procedural steps:

  1. The unsedated, nonfasting patient suspected of having a pulmonary embolism is taken to the nuclear medicine department.

  Perfusion scan
  2. The patient is given a peripheral IV injection of radionuclide-tagged MAA.
  3. While the patient lies in the appropriate position, a

gamma ray detector is passed over the patient and records radionuclide uptake on either x-ray or Polaroid film.

4. The patient is placed in the supine, prone, and various lateral positions, which allows for anterior, posterior, lateral, and oblique views, respectively.

5. The results are interpreted by a physician trained in diagnostic nuclear medicine.

Ventilation scan

6. The patient breathes the tracer through a face mask with a mouthpiece.

7. Less patient cooperation is needed with a krypton tracer. Ventilation scans can even be performed on comatose patients using krypton. Krypton images can be obtained before, during, or after perfusion images.

8. In contrast, Tc-DTPA images are usually done before perfusion images and require patient cooperation with deep breathing and appropriate use of breathing equipment to prevent contamination.

- Note that this test is usually performed by a physician in approximately 30 minutes.
- Tell the patient that no discomfort is associated with this test other than the peripheral venipuncture.

After

- Inform the patient that no radiation precautions are necessary.

Abnormal findings

Pulmonary embolism
Pneumonia
Tuberculosis
Emphysema
Tumors
Asthma

Atelectasis
Bronchitis
Chronic obstructive pulmonary disease (COPD)

Notes

lupus erythematosus test (LE cell prep)

Type of test Blood

Normal findings No LE cells seen

Test explanation and related physiology

The LE cell prep is a serologic test used to diagnose systemic lupus erythematosus (SLE). Of the patients with active SLE, 70% to 80% will have a positive LE prep. Patients with SLE have antibodies against the constituents of the nuclei within their own cells. LE preps are usually performed by traumatizing some white blood cells (WBCs) to expose the nuclear material within them. This material is then incubated with the patient's serum, and neutrophils (other WBCs) in the affected patient's serum will phagocytize the traumatized nuclear material. When stained with Wright's stain, the phagocytized complex appears as a blue-staining, amorphous mass in the cytoplasm of the neutrophil. These neutrophils are then called LE cells. When these are seen, the test is considered positive.

The test is used not only to diagnose SLE, but also to monitor its treatment. Often, no LE cells are seen several weeks after successful treatment. Also, some clinicians believe that the severity of SLE is related to the number of LE cells present. Because no LE cells may appear on a preparation one day and many may appear on the succeeding day, most physicians will order LE preps daily for 3 days.

This test is rather nonspecific because many rheumatic diseases and drugs may cause a positive LE prep. The anti-DNA (deoxyribonucleic acid) antibody test may be more specific in detecting SLE and other connective tissue diseases.

Interfering factors

- Drugs that may cause a false positive LE cell prep include acetazolamide, aminosalicylic acid, chlorprothixene, chlorothiazide, griseofluvin, hydralazine, oral contraceptives, penicillin, phenylbutazone, phenytoin sodium, procainamide, streptomycin, sulfonamides, and tetracyclines.
- Drugs that may cause false negative LE cell preps include steroids.

Procedure and patient care

Before

- Explain the procedure to the patient.
- Tell the patient that no fasting is required.

During

- Collect approximately 7 to 10 ml of venous blood in a red-top tube.
- List on the laboratory slip any drugs that can affect test results.

After

- Apply pressure or a pressure dressing to the venipuncture site.
- Assess the venipuncture site for bleeding.
- Review the signs of potential infection at the venipuncture site with SLE patients because they are frequently immunocompromised. Often, they are taking steroids, which further diminishes their immunologic capabilities.

Abnormal findings

Systemic lupus erythematosus
Rheumatoid arthritis
Scleroderma
Drug sensitivities
Other rheumatic diseases

Notes

luteinizing hormone assay (LH assay)

Type of test Blood

Normal findings
Male: 7-24 ImU/ml
Female: >6-30 ImU/ml
   Midcycle peak: > three times the baseline
   Postmenopause: >30 ImU/ml
Child: up to 12 ImU/ml

Test explanation and related physiology
LH is a gonadotropin secreted by the anterior pituitary gland. LH, along with follicle-stimulating hormone (FSH), is necessary for ovulation. FSH is usually measured along with the LH.

Performing an LH assay is an easy way to determine if ovulation has occurred. An LH surge in blood levels indicates ovulation has taken place. Under the influence of LH, the corpus luteum develops from the ruptured graafian follicle. Daily samples of serum LH around the woman's midcycle can detect the LH surge, which is believed to occur on the day of maximal fertility.

LH assays also determine whether a gonadal insufficiency is primary (problem with the ovary/testicle) or secondary (because of insufficient stimulation by the pituitary hormones, e.g., LH). LH hormones are used to study testicular dysfunction in men and to evaluate endocrine problems related to precocious puberty in children.

Interfering factors
- Recent use of radioisotopes can affect test results.
- Drugs that may decrease LH levels include estrogens, progesterone, and testosterone.

Procedure and patient care
Before
- Explain the procedure to the patient.
- Tell the patient that no food or fluid restrictions are needed.

L

During

- Collect approximately 7 to 10 ml of venous blood in a red-top tube.
- Note that the patient can also perform LH assays at home using a home urine test or a 24-hour urine test.
- Indicate the date of the last menstrual period on the laboratory slip. Note if the woman is postmenopausal.

After

- Apply pressure or a pressure dressing to the venipuncture site.
- Assess the venipuncture site for bleeding.

Abnormal findings

Increased levels

Gonadal failure
Precocious puberty
Complete testicular
  feminization syndrome
Hypogonadism
Anorchia
Menopause

Decreased levels

Pituitary failure
Hypothalamic failure

Notes

Lyme disease test

Type of test Blood

Normal findings Negative (low titers of IgM and IgG antibodies)

Test explanation and related physiology

Lyme disease was first recognized in Lyme, Conn., in 1975. The disease usually begins in the summer with a skin lesion called erythema chronicum migrans (ECM), which occurs at the site of a bite by a tick, usually *Ixodes dammini*. Ticks are the best documented vectors of this spirochete, which is the causative agent for Lyme disease.

Weeks to months after the insect bite, some patients develop fatigue, meningoencephalitis, cranial or peripheral neuropathies, myocarditis, atrioventricular nodal block, or arthritis. The last manifestation is joint involvement, which often occurs intermittently in a few large joints for several years.

Currently the *enzyme-linked immunosorbent assay* (ELISA) is the best diagnostic test for Lyme disease. This test determines titers of specific immunoglobulin M (IgM) and specific IgG antibodies to the *I. dammini* spirochete. Levels of specific IgM antibody peak during the third to sixth week after disease onset and then gradually decline.

Titers of specific IgG antibodies are generally low during the first several weeks of illness, reach maximal levels months later during arthritis, and often remain elevated for years. Early in the illness, the diagnosis can usually be determined from the gross appearance of ECM and known exposure to an endemic area. These patients do not require antibody determination. However, in the absence of ECM lesions, Lyme disease can be confused with various viral infections. In these patients a single titer of specific IgM antibody may suggest the correct diagnosis. Acute and convalescent sera can be tested to be certain. Later in the illness, determination of specific IgG antibodies can separate Lyme disease from aseptic meningitis or unexplained cranial or peripheral nerve palsies.

Procedure and patient care

Before

- Explain the procedure to the patient.
- Tell the patient that no fasting or special preparation is required.

During

- Collect approximately 7 to 10 ml of venous blood in a red-top tube.

After

- Apply pressure or a pressure dressing to the venipuncture site.
- Assess the venipuncture site for bleeding.

Abnormal finding

Lyme disease

Notes

lymphangiography (Lymphangiogram, Lymphography)

Type of test X-ray with contrast dye

Normal findings Normal-sized lymph nodes containing no filling defects

Test explanation and related physiology

Lymphangiography provides an x-ray examination of the lymphatic system after the injection of contrast medium into a lymphatic vessel in the foot or hand. The lymphatic system consists of lymph vessels and lymph nodes. Assessment of this system is important because cancer often spreads via the lymphatic system.

Lymphangiography is especially useful in patients suspected of having lymphatic pathology (lymphoma or metastatic tumor). The test allows one to demonstrate the extent and level of lymphatic metastasis. The lymphangiogram is also useful in staging lymphoma patients and in evaluating the results of chemotherapy or radiation therapy. Because the contrast medium remains in the lymph nodes for 6 months to a year, repeat plain x-ray films may be done for continued follow-up of disease progression or response to treatment.

Contraindications

- Patients with an allergy to iodine dye or shellfish
- Patients with severe chronic lung diseases, cardiac disease, or advanced kidney or liver disease

Potential complications

- Lipoid (lipid) pneumonia
  This occurs if the contrast medium flows into the thoracic duct and causes micropulmonary emboli. These small emboli usually disappear after several weeks or months.
- Allergic reaction or allergy to iodine dye
  Allergic reactions vary from flushing, itching, and urticaria to severe, life-threatening anaphylaxis (evidenced by respiratory distress, drop in blood pressure, shock). In the event of anaphylaxis the patient may be treated with

diphenhydramine (Benadryl), steroids, and epinephrine. Oxygen and endotracheal equipment should be on hand for immediate use.

Procedure and patient care

Before

- Explain the procedure to the patient.
- Obtain informed consent if required by the institution.
- Tell the patient that no fasting or sedation is required.
- Inform the radiologist if an allergy to iodinated contrast is suspected. The radiologist may prescribe a Benadryl and steroid preparation to be administered before testing. Usually a hypoallergenic, non-ionic contrast will be used during the test.
- Inform the patient that if a blue-colored dye is used, he or she may note a bluish tinge in the urine. Excessive infiltration or IV administration of the lymphatic stain may create a transient bluish tint to the entire skin surface.

During

- Note the following procedural steps:
  1. In the radiology department the patient is placed on an x-ray table in the supine position.
  2. A lymphatic stain is injected into the subcutaneous tissue between each of the first three toes in each foot to outline the lymphatic vessels. (The stain can also be injected into the web of the skin between the fingers.)
  3. After the stain is taken up by the lymphatic vessels, they can be easily seen.
  4. A local anesthetic is injected.
  5. A small incision is made on the top of the foot (or hand).
  6. The lymphatic vessel is identified and cannulated to infuse the iodine contrast agent.
  7. The dye is slowly infused into the vessel. Usually a low-rate infusion pump is used. The patient must lie very still during the injection.
  8. The flow of iodine dye is followed by fluoroscopy.
  9. When the dye reaches the upper lumbar level, the flow of dye is discontinued.
  10. X-ray films are taken of the chest, abdomen, and pelvis to demonstrate the filling of the lymph nodes.

Often the patient is asked to return in 24 hours to
have additional x-ray studies done.

11. On completion of the injection, the cannula is removed and the incision is sutured closed.

- Note that this procedure is performed by a radiologist in
approximately 3 hours. Additional x-ray films are usually
taken 24 to 48 hours later.
- Inform the patient that discomfort may be felt when the
blue stain is injected subcutaneously and when the feet
are locally anesthetized.

After

- Observe the injection and incision sites for evidence of
cellulitis. If the patient will be returning home, instruct
him or her to evaluate the site for redness, pain, and
swelling.
- Inform the patient that the sutures should be removed 7
to 10 days after the test.

Abnormal findings

Metastatic tumor involving the lymph glands
Nodal lymphoma

Notes

magnetic resonance imaging (MRI, Nuclear magnetic resonance [NMR])

Type of test Magnetic field study

Normal findings No evidence of pathology

Test explanation and related physiology

MRI is a noninvasive diagnostic scanning technique that provides valuable information about the body's biochemistry by placing the patient in a magnetic field. MRI is based on how hydrogen atoms behave when placed in a magnetic field and then disturbed by radiofrequency signals. The unique feature about MRI is that is does not require exposure to ionizing radiation. MRI has several advantages over computed tomography (CT) scanning, including the following:

1. MRI provides better contrast between normal tissue and pathologic tissue.
2. Obscuring bone artifacts that occur in CT scanning do not occur in MRI scanning.
3. Since rapidly flowing blood appears dark because of its quick motion, many blood vessels appear as dark lumens. This provides a natural contrast to the blood vessels when using MRI.
4. Since spatial information depends only on how the magnetic fields are varied in space, it is possible to image the transverse, sagittal, and coronal planes directly with MRI.

Although the full usefulness of MRI is yet to be determined, this scanning shows promise in the evaluation of the following areas:

1. Head and surrounding structures
2. Spinal cord and surrounding structures
3. Face and surrounding structures
4. Neck
5. Mediastinum
6. Heart and great vessels
7. Liver
8. Kidney
9. Prostate
10. Bone and joints

11. Breast
12. Extremities and soft tissues

An important advantage of MRI imaging is that serial studies can be performed on the patient without any known risk. This is useful in assessing the response of cancer to radiotherapeutic agents and chemotherapy. A major disadvantage of MRI is that patient eligibility is reduced compared to CT scanning. For example, examination of patients requiring cardiac monitoring or having metal implants, pacemakers, or cerebral aneurysm clips will result in MRI image degradation and may endanger the patient.

Contraindications

- Patients who are extremely obese (more than 300 pounds)
- Patients who are pregnant, since the long-term effects of MRI are not known at this time
- Patients who are confused or agitated
- Patients who are claustrophobic
- Patients who are unstable and require continuous life-support equipment, since monitoring equipment cannot be used inside the scanner room
- Patients with implantable metal objects such as pacemakers, infusion pumps, aneurysm clips, inner ear implants, and metal fragments in one or both eyes, since the magnet may move the object within the body and may injure the patient

Interfering factors

- Movement during the scan may cause artifacts on MRI

Procedure and patient care
Before

- Explain the procedure to the patient. Inform the patient that there is no exposure to radiation.
- Obtain informed consent if required by the institution.
- Tell the patient that he or she can drive after the procedure without assistance.
- Tell parents that they may read or talk to a child in the scanning room during the procedure because no risk of radiation from the procedure exists.
- Assess the patient for any contraindications for testing (e.g., aneurysm clips).

M

- If possible, show the patient a picture of the scanning machine and encourage verbalization of anxieties. Some patients may experience claustrophobia. Antianxiety medications may be helpful for those with mild claustrophobia.
- Instruct the patient to remove all metal objects (e.g., dental bridges, jewelry, hair clips, belts, credit cards) because they will create artifacts on the scan. The magnetic field can damage watches and credit cards. Also, movement of metal objects within the magnetic field can be detrimental to anyone within the field.
- Inform the patient that he or she will be required to remain motionless during this study. Any movement can cause artifacts on the scan.
- Tell the patient that during the procedure, he or she may hear a thumping sound. Earplugs are available if the patient wishes to use them.
- Inform the patient that no fluid or food restrictions are necessary before MRI.
- Instruct the patient to empty his or her bladder before the test for comfort.

During

- Note the following:
  1. The patient lies on a platform that slides into a tube containing the doughnut-shaped magnet.
  2. The patient is instructed to lie very still during the procedure.
  3. During the scan the patient can talk to and hear the staff via microphone or earphones placed in the scanner.
  4. A contrast medium called gadolinium (Magnevist) has recently been approved by the Food and Drug Administration (FDA). This is a paramagnetic enhancement agent that crosses the blood-brain barrier. It is especially useful for distinguishing edema from tumors. If this is to be administered, approximately 10 to 15 ml is injected in the vein. Imaging can begin shortly after the injection. No dietary restrictions are necessary before using this new agent.
- Note that this procedure is performed by a qualified radiologic technologist in approximately 30 to 90 minutes.

- Tell the patient that the only discomfort associated with this procedure may be lying still on a hard surface and a possible tingling sensation in teeth containing metal fillings. Also, an injection is needed for administration of Magnevist.

After

- Inform the patient that no special postprocedural care is needed.

Abnormal findings

Cerebral lesions
Cerebral infarction
Degenerative vertebral disks
Aneurysms
Arteriovenous malformation
Hemorrhage
Subdural hematoma
Multiple sclerosis
Atherosclerotic plaques

Tumors (primary and metastic)
Joint disorders
Myocardial infarction
Aortic dissection
Aortic occlusion and stenosis
Abscesses
Edema
Congenital heart disease
Dementia

M

Notes

mammography (Mammogram)

Type of test X-ray

Normal findings Negative (no tumor noted)

Test explanation and related physiology

Mammography is an x-ray examination of the breast. Careful interpretation of these x-ray films can identify cancers. In many cases, these cancers can be detected before they become palpable lesions. It is believed that early detection of breast cancer may improve patient survival. Radiographic signs of breast cancer include fine, stippled clustered calcifications (white specks on the breast x-ray films); a poorly defined spiculated mass; asymmetric density; and skin thickening.

Although mammography is not a substitute for breast biopsy, it is reliable and accurate when interpreted by a skilled radiologist. The accuracy of detection of breast cancer with mammography has been approximately 85%. Usually, cancers that are not detected by mammography are in areas of the breast not well imaged by x-ray films (the high axillary tail of the breast). Almost 35% of breast cancers are not palpable and are detected only by mammography. Therefore the combination of mammography and close physical examination provides the best approach to detect breast cancer at its earliest stage.

Some controversy surrounds the role of a mammogram in screening asymptomatic patients. Several large U.S. studies have encouraged mammography yearly after age 40 years. The American Cancer Society's recommendation for asymptomatic patients is a baseline mammogram at ages 35 and 45. Women over age 50 should have a mammogram yearly. Women who are at great risk for breast cancer (e.g., those who have had a cancer on the opposite side) should have mammograms yearly regardless of age.

Mammography also can detect other diseases of the breast. These include acute suppurative mastitis, abscess, fibrocystic changes, gross cysts, benign tumors (e.g., fibroadenoma), and intraglandular lymph nodes.

In the past, radiation exposure was quite significant with mammography. Today, however, because of fast-speed film, little radiation is required to expose mammogram film. Therefore the patient receives minimal radiation exposure during this test.

A *xeromammogram* provides the same information as routine mammography and has the same risks. Unlike regular x-ray films, which are negative films, xeromammograms are positive prints. The form of mammography used depends on the preference of the radiologist who must interpret the mammogram. However, the use of xeroradiography is decreasing. Newer "dedicated" mammogram units provide more accurate and easily interpretable x-ray films.

Contraindications

- Patients who are pregnant because of the risk of fetal damage

Interfering factors

- Talc powder can give the impression of calcification within the breast.
- Jewelry worn around the neck can preclude total visualization of the breast.
- Breast augmentation implants prevent total visualization of the breast.

M

Procedure and patient care

Before

- Explain the procedure to the patient. Inform the patient that some discomfort may be experienced during breast compression. This compression allows better visualization of the breast tissue. Assure the patient that the breast will not be harmed by the compression.
- Tell the patient that no fasting is required.
- Explain to the patient that a minimal radiation dose will be used during the test.
- Instruct the patient to disrobe above the waist and put on an x-ray gown.

During

- Note the following procedural steps:
  1. The patient is taken to the radiology department and is seated in front of a mammogram machine.
  2. One breast is placed on the x-ray plate.
  3. The x-ray cone is brought down on the top of the

breast to compress it gently between the broadened cone and the x-ray plate.

4. The x-ray film is exposed. This is the craniocaudal view.
5. The x-ray plate is turned perpendicular to the floor and placed laterally on the outer aspect of the breast.
6. The broadened cone is brought in medially and again gently compresses the breast. This creates the lateral or axillary view.
7. Occasionally, oblique views are required.

- Note that mammography is performed by a radiologic technologist in approximately 10 minutes. The x-ray films are interpreted by a radiologist.
- Tell the patient that very little discomfort is associated with mammography. Remind the patient that some pain may be caused by the pressure required to compress the breast tissue while the x-ray films are being taken. If the patient has very tender breasts, this may be painful.

After

- Take this opportunity to instruct the patient in breast self-examination.

Abnormal findings

Breast cancer
Benign tumors (e.g., fibroadenomas)
Breast cysts

Fibrocystic changes
Breast abscesses
Suppurative mastitis

Notes

mediastinoscopy

Type of test Endoscopy

Normal findings No abnormal mediastinal lymph node tissue

Test explanation and related physiology

Mediastinoscopy is a surgical procedure in which a mediastinoscope (a lighted instrument scope) is inserted through a small incision made at the suprasternal notch. The scope is passed into the superior mediastinum to inspect the mediastinal lymph nodes and to remove biopsy specimens. Because these lymph nodes receive lymphatic drainage from the lungs, their assessment can provide information on intrathoracic diseases such as carcinoma, granulomatous infections, and sarcoidosis. Therefore mediastinoscopy is used in establishing the diagnosis of various intrathoracic diseases. This procedure is also employed to "stage" patients with lung cancer and to assess if they are surgical candidates. Evidence of metastasis is usually a contraindication to thoracotomy because the tumor is considered inoperable.

M

Potential complications

- Puncture of the esophagus, trachea, or blood vessels

Procedure and patient care
Before

- Explain the procedure to the patient.
- Ensure that the physician has obtained the informed consent for this procedure.
- Check if the patient's blood needs to be typed and cross-matched.
- Provide preoperative care as for any other surgical procedure.
- Keep the patient NPO after midnight on the day of the test.
- Administer preprocedural medication approximately 1 hour before the test, as ordered.

During

- Note the following procedural steps:
  1. The patient is taken to the operating room for this surgical procedure.
  2. The patient is placed under general anesthesia.
  3. An incision is made in the suprasternal notch.
  4. The mediastinoscope is passed through this neck incision into the superior mediastinum.
  5. The lymph nodes are biopsied.
  6. The scope is withdrawn, and the incision is sutured closed.

- Note that this procedure is performed by a surgeon in approximately 1 hour.
- Inform the patient that he or she is asleep during the procedure.

After

- Provide postoperative care as for any other surgical procedure.

Abnormal findings

Lung cancer

Metastasis

Sarcoidosis

Tuberculosis

Hodgkin's disease

Lymphoma

Notes

metyrapone

Type of test Blood; urine (24 hour)

Normal findings

24-hour urine: baseline excretion of the urinary 17-OCHS
more than doubled

Blood: 11-deoxycortisol increased to > 7 μg/dl;
cortisol < 10 μg/dl

Test explanation and related physiology

This test is useful in differentiating adrenal hyperplasia from a primary adrenal tumor by determining whether the pituitary-adrenal feedback mechanism is intact. Metyrapone (Metopirone) is a potent blocker of an enzyme involved in cortisol production. When this drug is given, the resulting fall in cortisol production should stimulate pituitary secretion of adrenocorticotropic hormone (ACTH) by way of a negative feedback system. However, since cortisol itself cannot be synthesized because of the metyrapone inhibition of the 11-beta-hydroxylation step, an abundance of cortisol precursors (11-deoxycortisol) will be formed; these can be detected in the urine or in the blood. This test is similar to the ACTH stimulation test (see p. 11).

In patients with adrenal hyperplasia the cortisol precursors are greatly increased, even more than in normal patients. No response to metyrapone occurs in patients with Cushing's syndrome that results from adrenal adenoma or carcinoma, since the tumors are autonomous and therefore insensitive to changes in ACTH secretion. This test has no significant advantage over the ACTH stimulation test in the differential diagnosis of Cushing's disease.

Contraindications

- Patients with possible adrenal insufficiency, since metyrapone inhibits cortisol production

Potential complications

- Addison's disease and Addisonian crisis, since metyrapone inhibits cortisol production

Interfering factors

- Recent administration of radioisotopes will interfere with test results.
- Chlorpromazine (Thorazine) interferes with the response to metyrapone and therefore should not be administered during this testing.

Procedure and patient care
Before

- Explain the procedure to the patient.
- Obtain a baseline 24-hour urine specimen for 17-hydroxycorticosteroid (17-OCHS) level (see p. 419) for the urine test.
- Obtain a baseline cortisol level (see p. 237) for the blood test.

During

Blood
- Administer 2 to 3 g of metyrapone at 11 PM the night before the blood specimen is collected. Collect a blood specimen in the morning.

Urine
- Obtain a 24-hour urine specimen for 17-OCHS level as a baseline. Then collect a 24-hour urine specimen for 17-OCHS level during and again 1 day after the oral administration of 500 to 750 mg of metyrapone, which is given every 4 hours for 24 hours.

After

- Assess the patient for impending signs of Addisonian crisis (muscle weakness, mental and emotional changes, anorexia, nausea, vomiting, hypotension, hyperkalemia, vascular collapse).
- Note that Addisonian crisis is a medical emergency that must be treated vigorously. Basically the immediate treatment includes replenishing steroids, reversing shock, and restoring blood circulation.

Abnormal findings

Adrenal hyperplasia
Adrenal tumor
Ectopic ACTH syndrome

mononucleosis spot test (Mononuclear heterophil test, Heterophil antibody test, Monospot test)

Type of test Blood

Normal findings Negative (<1:28 titer)

Test explanation and related physiology

The mononucleosis test is performed to aid in the diagnosis of infectious mononucleosis, a disease caused by the Epstein-Barr virus (EBV). An EBV titer may also be done (see p. 311). Usually young adults are affected by mononucleosis. The clinical presentation is fever, pharyngitis, lymphadenopathy, and splenomegaly. Approximately 2 weeks after the onset of the disease, many patients are found to have immunoglobulin M (IgM) antibodies in their serum that react against warm red blood cells (RBCs). When these antibodies are present in serial dilutions of greater than 1:56, infectious mononucleosis can be strongly considered. However, false positive results occur; occasionally, patients with lymphoma or systemic lupus erythematosus (SLE) may also have this antibody. Patients with Burkitt's lymphoma, leukemia, and some gastrointestinal cancers also have false positive test results. Burkitt's lymphoma is strongly associated with EBV.

Several heterophil agglutination tests are available, but the most frequently performed is the spot test for infectious mononucleosis (mono spot test). Heterophil antibodies produced by humans react with RBCs of another species. The test is performed by placing the serially diluted patient serum on one side of the slide and mixing it with guinea pig kidney antigen (containing only Forssman antigen). On the other side of the slide the patient's serum is mixed with beef RBCs (containing only infectious mononuclear antigen). Horse RBCs (containing Forssman and infectious mononucleosis antigens) are then applied to each slide. Agglutination of the beef RBCs indicates the presence of the infectious mononuclear heterophil antibody-antigen complexes and thus confirms the diagnosis of infectious mononucleosis.

M

Procedure and patient care

Before

- Explain the procedure to the patient.
- Tell the patient that no fasting or special preparation is required.

During

- Collect approximately 7 to 10 ml of venous blood in a red-top tube.

After

- Apply pressure or a pressure dressing to the venipuncture site.
- Observe the venipuncture site for bleeding.

Abnormal findings

Infectious mononucleosis
Chronic Epstein-Barr viral infection
Chronic fatigue syndrome
Burkitt's lymphoma
Some forms of chronic hepatitis

Notes

myelography (Myelogram)

Type of test X-ray with contrast dye

Normal findings Normal spinal canal

Test explanation and related physiology

By placing radiopaque dye (or air) into the subarachnoid space of the spinal canal, the contents of the canal can be fluoroscopically outlined. Cord tumors, meningeal tumors, metastatic spinal tumors, herniated intravertebral disks, and arthritic bone spurs can readily be detected by this study. These lesions appear as canal narrowing or as varying degrees of obstruction to the flow of the dye column within the canal. The entire canal (from lumbar to cervical areas) can be examined. This test is indicated in patients with severe back pain or localized neurologic signs that suggest the canal as the location of these injuries. Because this test is usually performed by lumbar puncture (LP, see p. 478), all the potential complications of that procedure exist.

Different types of contrast material can be used for myelography. Pantopaque is most often used as the *oil-based* medium. An oil-based dye must be aspirated as much as possible after the procedure before removing the spinal needle because the dye persists indefinitely. The patient's head is then kept elevated above the level of the spine to prevent upward dispersion of the dye, which could cause meningeal irritation. Because the oil base is heavier than cerebrospinal fluid (CSF), it stays in the lower canal. The dye is completely removed, and the patient is kept flat for up to 12 hours.

A *water-soluble* contrast material, metrizamide (Amipaque), is now frequently used for myelography. This dye is absorbed by the blood and excreted by the kidneys. Metrizamide has two advantages over the oil-based medium. First, metrizamide does not need to be removed at the end of the procedure, since it is water soluble and will be completely reabsorbed. This feature reduces the length of the procedure and minimizes the discomfort associated with dye removal. Second, metrizamide is less viscous than the iodine, oil-based dye and therefore permits better visualization of small areas (nerves, nerve roots, nerve sheaths). Also, metrizamide can flow freely through narrow canals and afford better differentiation of complete and incomplete spinal blockages. The disadvantage associated with metrizamide is that it may precipitate seizure activity after the procedure. To prevent this, the patient should be well hydrated and should avoid medications (e.g., phenothiazines, tricyclics, antidepressants, central nervous system [CNS] stimulants, amphetamines) that could decrease the seizure threshold. A new water-soluble contrast agent, Omnipaque, has a significantly lower risk of CNS toxicity than does metrizamide.

After the procedure the patient's head and thorax should be elevated 30 to 50 degrees for about 6 to 8 hours to reduce upward dispersion of the dye and to prevent contact of the water-soluble agent with the cerebral meninges, which could precipitate a seizure. Bed rest may be ordered for up to 24 hours.

To avoid some of the side effects associated with radiopaque substances, some neurosurgeons prefer to use *air-contrast myelography*. After air myelography the patient is positioned with the head lower than the trunk to prevent air from gravitating to the cerebral space and causing headaches. This position is usually maintained for approximately 48 hours. Most of the air will be absorbed by this time, and the head can then be elevated.

Contraindications

- Patients with multiple sclerosis, since exacerbation may be precipitated by myelography
- Patients with increased intracranial pressure, since LP may cause herniation of the brain
- Patients with infection near the LP site, since this may precipitate a bacterial meningitis
- Patients who are allergic to shellfish or iodinated dye

Potential complications

- Headache
- Meningitis
- Herniation of the brain
- Seizures
- Allergic reaction to iodinated dye
  Allergic reactions vary from mild flushing, itching, and urticaria to severe, life-threatening anaphylaxis (evidenced by respiratory distress, drop in blood pressure, shock). In

the unusual event of anaphylaxis the patient may be treated with diphenhydramine (Benadryl), steroids, and epinephrine. Oxygen and endotracheal equipment should be on hand for immediate use.

Procedure and patient care

Before

- Explain the procedure to the patient.
- Ensure that the physician has obtained written and informed consent for this procedure.
- Assess the patient for allergies to iodinated contrast dye or shellfish.
- Inform the radiologist if an allergy to iodinated contrast is suspected. The radiologist may prescribe a Benadryl and steroid preparation to be administered before testing. Usually a hypoallergenic, non-ionic contrast will be used during the test.
- Ascertain if the patient has recently taken phenothiazines, tricyclics, antidepressants, CNS stimulants, or amphetamines if a water-soluble contrast (metrizamide) will be used. These medications should be avoided because they could decrease the seizure threshold.
- Have the patient empty the bladder and bowel before myelography if possible.
- Explain to the patient that he or she must lie very still during the procedure.
- Note that food and fluid restrictions vary according to the type of dye used. Check with the radiology department for specific restrictions.
- Inform the patient that he or she will be tilted into an up-and-down position on the table so that the dye can properly fill the spinal canal and provide adequate visualization in the desired area.

During

- Note the following procedural steps:
  1. A lumbar puncture (see p. 482) or cisternal puncture (see p. 194) is performed.
  2. Fifteen ml of CSF is withdrawn, and 15 ml or more of radiopaque dye or air is injected into the spinal canal. Since the specific gravity of the dye is greater than that of the CSF, the direction of dye flow will depend on the tilt of the table and the patient's position.

M

3. With the needle in place, the patient is placed in the prone position on the tilt table with the head tilted down. A foot support and shoulder brace or harness will keep the patient from sliding.
4. The lights are turned off, and the column of dye is followed in a cephalad direction with fluoroscopy.
5. Representative x-ray films are taken.
6. Obstructions to the flow of the dye are evident, and the level of the lesion is easily detected.
7. After myelography is performed, the needle is removed and a dressing is applied.
8. The patient is returned to the unit on a stretcher and is kept on bed rest.

- Note that this procedure is done by a radiologist in approximately 45 minutes.
- Keep in mind that patient response varies from mild discomfort to severe pain.

After

- Note that nursing interventions after the procedure depend on the type of contrast used.
- Usually, place the patient on bed rest for several hours afterward, as indicated. Position the patient as specifically ordered by the physician in consultation with the radiologist. The head position varies with the dye used. For example, the head is usually elevated after using oil-based and water-soluble contrast agents. After an air-contrast study, the head is positioned lower than the trunk.
- Observe the patient for signs and symptoms of meningeal irritation (e.g., fever, stiff neck, occipital headache, photophobia).
- Observe the patient for seizure activity if metrizamide dye was used.
- If metrizamide was used, do *not* administer medications (e.g., phenothiazines) that may precipitate seizure activity.
- Monitor the patient's vital signs and ability to void.
- Encourage the patient to drink fluids to enhance excretion of the dye and to hasten replacement of CSF.
- Evaluate the patient for delayed reaction to dye (dyspnea, rashes, tachycardia, hives). This usually occurs within the first 2 to 6 hours after the test. Treat with antihistamines or steroids.

Abnormal findings

Cord tumors
Meningeal tumors
Metastatic spinal tumors
Herniated intravertebral
  disks
Arthritic bone spurs
Neurofibromas

Meningiomas
Cervical ankylosing
  spondylosis
Arthritic lumbar stenosis
Avulsion of nerve roots
Cysts
Astrocytomas

Notes

myoglobin

Type of test Blood

Normal findings 0-85 ng/ml or 0-85 nmol/L (SI units)

Test explanation and related physiology

Myoglobin is an oxygen-binding protein found in cardiac and skeletal muscle. Measurement of myoglobin is an index of damage to the myocardium, such as occurs in myocardial infarction or reinfarction. Increased levels indicate cardiac muscle injury or death. Although this test is more sensitive than creatinine phosphokinase (CPK) isoenzymes (see p. 248), it is not as specific because trauma, inflammation, or ischemic changes to the noncardiac skeletal muscles can also cause elevated levels of myoglobin.

Interfering factors

- Recent administration of radioactive substances can affect test results.
- Increased myoglobin levels can occur after IM injections.

Procedure and patient care

Before

- Explain the procedure to the patient.
- Tell the patient that no fasting is required.

During

- Collect approximately 5 ml of venous blood in a red-top tube.

After

- Apply pressure or a pressure dressing to the venipuncture site.
- Observe the venipuncture site for bleeding.

Abnormal findings

Increased levels

Myocardial infarction
Skeletal muscle inflammation (myositis)
Malignant hyperthermia

Muscular dystrophy
Skeletal muscle ischemia
Skeletal muscle trauma
Rhabdomyolysis

Notes

nonstress test (NST, Fetal activity determination)

Type of test Fetal activity study

Normal findings "Reactive" fetus (heart rate acceleration associated with fetal movement)

Test explanation and related physiology

The NST is a noninvasive study that monitors acceleration of the fetal heart rate (FHR) in response to fetal movement. This FHR acceleration is a reflection of the integrity of the central nervous system and fetal well-being. Fetal activity may be spontaneous, induced by uterine contraction, or induced by external manipulation. Oxytocin stimulation is not used. Fetal response is characterized as "reactive" or "nonreactive." The NST indicates a reactive fetus when, with fetal movement, two or more FHR accelerations are detected, each of which must be at least 15 beats per minute for 15 seconds or more within any 10-minute period. The test is 99% reliable in indicating fetal viability and negates the need for the contraction stress test (CST, see p. 229). If the test detects a nonreactive fetus (i.e., no FHR acceleration with fetal movement) within 40 minutes, the patient is a candidate for the CST. A 40-minute test period is used because this is the average duration of the sleep-wake cycle of the fetus. However, the cycle may vary considerably.

The NST is useful in screening high-risk pregnancies and in selecting those patients who may require the CST. An NST is now routinely performed before the CST to avoid the complications associated with oxytocin administration. No complications are associated with the NST.

Procedure and patient care

Before

- Explain the procedure to the patient.
- Encourage verbalization of the patient's fears. The necessity for the study usually raises realistic fears in the expectant mother.
- If the patient is hungry, instruct her to eat before the NST is begun. Fetal activity is enhanced with a high maternal serum glucose level.

During

- After the patient empties her bladder, place her in Sims' position.
- Place an external fetal monitor on the patient's abdomen to record the FHR. The mother can indicate fetal movement by pressing a button on the fetal monitor whenever she feels the fetus move. FHR and fetal movement are concomitantly recorded on a two-channel strip graph.
- Observe the fetal monitor for FHR accelerations associated with fetal movement.
- If the fetus is quiet for 20 minutes, stimulate fetal activity by external methods, such as rubbing the mother's abdomen, compressing the abdomen, ringing a bell near the abdomen, or placing a pan on the abdomen and hitting on the pan.
- Note that a nurse performs the NST in approximately 20 to 40 minutes in the physician's office or in a hospital unit.
- Tell the patient that no discomfort is associated with the NST.

After

- If the results detect a nonreactive fetus, inform the patient that she is a candidate for the CST.

Abnormal finding

Nonreactive fetus

Notes

5'-nucleotidase

Type of test Blood

Normal findings 0-1.6 U or 27-233 nmol/s/L (SI units)

Test explanation and related physiology

5'-Nucleotidase is an enzyme specific to the liver. The 5'-nucleotidase level is elevated in patients with liver diseases, especially those associated with cholestasis. Although levels of other enzymes such as alkaline phosphatase (ALP), alanine aminotransferase (ALT), and aspartate aminotransferase (AST) are elevated with liver diseases, diseases in other organs may also cause elevations of these enzymes. However, when levels of these enzymes *and* 5'-nucleotidase all are elevated, the disease is located specifically within the liver. When the ALT, AST, and ALP levels are elevated and the 5'-nucleotidase level is normal, disease exists in organs that make these enzymes other than the liver (e.g., bone, spleen, kidney).

Interfering factors

- Drugs that may cause increased 5'-nucleotidase levels include hepatotoxic agents.

Procedure and patient care

Before

- Explain the procedure to the patient.
- Tell the patient that no fasting is required.

During

- Collect approximately 7 to 10 ml of venous blood in a red-top tube.
- Indicate on the laboratory slip any medication the patient may be taking to aid in interpretation of test results.

After

- Apply pressure or a pressure dressing to the venipuncture site.
- Assess the venipuncture site for bleeding. Patients with liver dysfunction often have prolonged clotting times.

Abnormal findings
Increased levels

Hepatitis
Cirrhosis
Hepatic necrosis
Hepatic ischemia

Hepatic tumor
Hepatotoxic drugs
Cholestasis

Notes

N

obstetric ultrasonography (Obstetric echography, Pregnant uterus ultrasonography, Pelvic ultrasonography in pregnancy)

Type of test Ultrasound

Normal findings Normal fetal and placental size and position

Test explanation and related physiology

Ultrasound examination of the obstetric patient has proved to be a harmless, noninvasive method of evaluating the female genital tract and fetus. In diagnostic ultrasound, harmless, high-frequency sound waves are emitted from the transducer and penetrate the structure (uterus, placenta, fetus) to be studied. These sound waves are bounced back to a sensor within the transducer and, by electronic conversion, are arranged into a pictorial image of the desired organ. A realistic Polariod picture is taken of the pattern.

Obstetric ultrasonography may be useful in the following circumstances:

1. Making an early diagnosis of normal pregnancy and abnormal pregnancy (e.g., tubal pregnancy)
2. Identifying multiple pregnancies
3. Differentiating a tumor (e.g., hydatidiform mole) from a normal pregnancy
4. Determining the age of the fetus by the diameter of the head
5. Measuring the rate of fetal growth
6. Identifying placental abnormalities such as abruptio placentae and placenta previa
7. Determining the position of the placenta (Ultrasound localization of the placenta is done before amniocentesis.)
8. Making differential diagnoses of various uterine and ovarian enlargements (e.g., polyhydramnios, neoplasms, cysts, abscesses)
9. Determining fetal position

Interfering factors

- Patients who have had recent gastrointestinal contrast studies, since barium creates severe distortion of reflective sound waves
- Patients with air-filled bowels, since gas does not transmit the sound waves well
- Failure to fill the bladder and obesity, which may make the image uninterpretable

Procedure and patient care

Before

- Explain the procedure to the patient.
- Assure the patient that this study has no known deleterious effect on maternal or fetal tissues, even when it is repeated several times.
- Give the patient three to four glasses (200 to 350 ml) of water or other liquid 1 hour before the examination, and instruct her *not* to void until after the procedure is completed. This will permit better transmission of the sound waves and enhance visualization of the uterus.
- Tell the patient that no fasting or sedation is required.

During

- Note the following procedural steps:
  1. The patient is taken to the ultrasound room and placed in the supine position on the examining table.
  2. The ultrasonographer, usually a radiologist, applies a greasy, conductive paste to the abdomen to enhance sound transmission and reception.
  3. A transducer is passed vertically and horizontally over the skin.
  4. Pictures are taken of the reflections.
  5. During the examination the fetal structures are pointed out to the mother.
- Note that this procedure is performed in approximately 20 minutes.
- Inform the patient that no discomfort is associated with this study other than having a full bladder and the urge to void. Some patients may be uncomfortable lying on a hard x-ray table.

O

After

- Remove the lubricant from the patient's skin.
- Provide an opportunity for the patient to void.

Abnormal findings

Tubal pregnancy
Abdominal pregnancy
Hydatidiform mole
Intrauterine growth
  retardation
Multiple fetuses
Fetal death
Abruptio placentae
Abnormal fetal position
  (e.g., breech, transverse)

Placenta previa
Polyhydramnios
Neoplasms of ovaries,
  uterus, or fallopian tubes
Cysts
Abscesses
Hydrocephalus of fetus

Notes

obstruction series (KUB, Flat plate of the abdomen, Plain film of the abdomen, Scout film)

Type of test X-ray

Normal findings

No evidence of bowel obstruction
No abnormal calcifications
No free air

Test explanation and related physiology

The obstruction series is a group of x-ray films performed on the abdomen of patients who have suspected bowel obstruction, paralytic ileus, perforated viscus, abdominal abscess, kidney stones, appendicitis, or foreign body ingestion. This series of films usually consists of at least two x-ray studies. The first is an erect abdominal film that should include visualization of both diaphragms. The film is examined for evidence of free air under either diaphragm, which is pathognomonic for a perforated viscus. This x-ray study is also used to detect air-fluid levels within the intestine. The presence of an air-fluid level is compatible with bowel obstruction or paralytic ileus. Occasionally, patients are too ill to stand erect. In this case an x-ray film can be taken with the patient in the left lateral decubitus position. If free air is present, it will be seen between the liver and the right side of the abdominal wall. As with the erect film, air-fluid levels can also be detected.

The second x-ray film in the obstruction series is usually a supine abdominal x-ray study. This is very similar to the kidney, ureters, and bladder x-ray study (KUB, see p. 448). An abdominal abscess may be seen as a cluster of tiny bubbles within one localized area. A calcification within the course of the ureter could indicate a kidney ureteral stone. A small calcification in the right lower quadrant on the film of a patient complaining of pain in this quadrant may be an appendicolith. A gas-filled, distended bowel is compatible with bowel obstruction or paralytic ileus.

Further, the obstruction series can be used to monitor the clinical course of patients with gastrointestinal (GI) disease. For example, repeated obstruction series on patients who have a partial small bowel obstruction or paralytic ileus can indicate worsening or improvement of the clinical situation.

Frequently a cross-table lateral view of the abdomen is included in an obstruction series to detect abdominal aorta calcification, which often occurs in older patients. The calcification represents the anterior wall of the aorta. If an aortic aneurysm exists, this calcification will be seen to protrude from the spine.

Finally, the supine abdominal x-ray study can be used as a "scout film" before performing GI or abdominal x-ray studies that use contrast, such as a barium enema (BE, see p. 81) or intravenous pyelogram (IVP, see p. 432).

Contraindications

- Patients who are pregnant

Interfering factor

- Previous GI barium contrast study
  Although at times barium within the GI tract can preclude the identification of other important calcifications (e.g., kidney stones), barium can be helpful in outlining the GI anatomy.

Procedure and patient care

Before

- Explain the procedure to the patient.
- Ensure that all radiopaque clothing has been removed.
- Remind the patient that no GI contrast will be used.

During

- Although the procedure varies from facility to facility, note that usually a supine abdominal x-ray film, erect abdominal film, and perhaps a lower erect chest film are taken. Often a cross-table lateral x-ray film is also included.
- Note that the obstruction series is performed in minutes in the radiology department by a radiologic technologist. However, it can be performed at the bedside with a portable x-ray machine. A radiologist interprets the films.
- Tell the patient that no discomfort is associated with this study.

After

▪ Note that no special after-care is needed.

Abnormal findings

Kidney stone
Bowel obstruction
Organomegaly
Presence of foreign body
Bladder distention
Abdominal abscess
Perforated viscus
Abdominal aortic
  calcification

Appendicolithiasis
Paralytic ileus
Abdominal aortic aneurysm
Peritoneal effusion
Abnormal position of the
  kidneys

Notes

O

oculoplethysmography (OPG)

Type of test Manometric

Normal findings Normal and equal blood flow in both carotid arteries

Test explanation and related physiology

OPG is a very important noninvasive study used to measure indirectly blood flow in the ophthalmic artery. Since the ophthalmic artery is the first major branch of the internal carotid artery, its blood flow reflects the carotid blood flow and the alternative blood flow to the brain.

For this study, eye pressures are measured through suction cups placed on the eyes for the recording. OPG is indicated in patients who have symptoms of transient ischemic attacks (TIAs), cardiac bruits, and neurologic symptoms (e.g., dizziness, fainting). If indicated, this procedure may be followed by cerebral angiography. This test is often performed as a follow-up after carotid endarterectomy.

Contraindications

- Patients who have had eye surgery within the last 2 to 6 months
- Patients who have a lens implant
- Patients who have had retinal detachment
- Patients with cataracts
- Patients who are allergic to local anesthetics

Potential complications

- Conjuctival hemorrhage
- Corneal abrasions
  If corneal abrasions occur, the patient's eye is patched and a lubricant (e.g., Dacriose solution) is applied.
- Transient photophobia

Procedure and patient care

Before

- Explain the procedure to the patient.
- Instruct the patient to remove contact lenses, if applicable.

- Inform patients with glaucoma to take their usual medications and eye drops.
- Tell the patient that no fasting or sedation is necessary.

During

- Note the following procedural steps:

  1. The patient is asked to lie on his or her back on a table or bed.
  2. Blood pressure in both arms is taken before the test.
  3. Electrocardiographic (EKG) electrodes are applied to the patient's extremities to detect any abnormal cardiac rhythms.
  4. Anesthetic eye drops are instilled in both eyes to minimize discomfort.
  5. Small detectors are attached to the earlobes to detect blood flow to the ear through the external carotid artery.
  6. Tracings for both ears are taken and compared.
  7. Suction cups resembling contact lenses are applied directly to the eyeball.
  8. Tracings of the pulsations within each eye are recorded.
  9. A vacuum source is applied to the suction cup. This increased pressure causes the pulse in both eyes to disappear temporarily because all blood flow to the eye is stopped.
  10. When the suction source is stopped, the blood flow returns to the eyes. Both pulses should return simultaneously.
  11. The time difference in the pulse rate from one eye to the other, from one ear to the other, and from one ear to the eye on the other side is measured in milliseconds. If internal carotid stenosis is present, blood flow to the eye will be delayed.

- Note that a trained technologist performs this test in approximately 20 to 30 minutes.
- Tell the patient that the eyes usually burn slightly when the ophthalmic drops are applied.
- Inform the patient that when suction is applied, he or she may feel a pulling sensation and vision may temporarily be lost.

After

- Inform the patient that the eye anesthesia usually wears off in about 30 minutes.
- Instruct the patient not to rub the eyes for at least 2 hours. If tears appear, the eye should be blotted dry.
- Inform the patient that contact lenses should not be inserted for at least 2 hours after OPG.
- Tell the patient that the eyes may appear bloodshot for several hours after the test. Artificial tears may be instilled to soothe any irritation in the eyes.
- Inform the patient to wear sunglasses if photophobia is present.

Abnormal finding

Carotid atherosclerotic stenosis

Notes

osmolality, blood (Serum osmolality)

Type of test Blood

Normal findings:

Adult/elderly: 285-295 mOsm/kg H_2O
Child: 275-290 mOsm/kg H_2O

Possible critical values

<265 mOsm/kg H_2O
>320 mOsm/kg H_2O

Test explanation and related physiology

Osmolality measures the concentration of particles in a so-lution. Osmolality increases with dehydration and decreases with overhydration. Increased osmolality will stimulate se-cretion of antidiuretic hormone (ADH). This will result in increased water reabsorption, more concentrated urine, and less concentrated serum. A low serum osmolality will sup-press the release of ADH, resulting in decreased water reab-sorption and large amounts of dilute urine.

The serum osmolality test is useful in evaluating fluid and electrolyte imbalance and in evaluating the presence of or-ganic acids, sugars, or ethanol. The test is very helpful in evaluating seizures, liver disease, hydration status, acid-base balance, ADH function, and liver disease. Osmolality also has an important role in toxicology and workups for coma patients. Values of 385 mOsm/kg of water are associated with stupor in patients with hyperglycemia. When values of 400 to 420 are detected, grand mal seizures can occur. Val-ues greater than 420 can be lethal.

Interfering factors

- Diseases such as cerebrovascular accident (CVA, stroke) or brain tumors may interfere with interpretation of test results.

Procedure and patient care

Before

- Explain the procedure to the patient.
- Tell the patient that no fasting is required.

During

- Collect approximately 5 to 10 ml of venous blood in a red-top tube.
- For pediatric patients, draw blood from a heel stick.

After

- Apply pressure or a pressure dressing to the venipuncture site.
- Observe the venipuncture site for bleeding.

Abnormal findings

Increased levels

Hypernatremia
Dehydration
Hyperglycemia
Mannitol therapy
Azotemia
Uremia
Ingestion of ethanol, methanol, or ethylene glycol
Hyperosmolar nonketotic hyperglycemia
Diabetes insipidus
Hypercalcemia
Renal tubular necrosis
Severe pylonephritis
Ketosis
Shock

Decreased levels

Hyponatremia
Overhydration
Syndrome of inappropriate ADH secretion (SIADH)
Paraneoplastic syndromes associated with lung carcinoma
Excess fluid intake

Notes

osmolality, urine (Urine osmolality)

Type of test Urine

Normal findings:

12- to 14-hour fluid restriction: >850 mOsm/kg H_2O
Random specimen: 50-1400 mOsm/kg H_2O, depending on
fluid intake

Possible critical values

<100 mOsm/kg H_2O in overhydration
>800 mOsm/kg H_2O in dehydration

Test explanation and related physiology

Osmolality is the measurement of the number of dissolved particles in a solution. It is a more exact measurement of urine concentration than specific gravity because specific gravity depends on the number of particles and on the precise nature of the particles in the urine. Specific gravity also requires correction for the presence of glucose or protein as well as for temperature. In contrast, osmolality depends only on the number of particles of solute in a unit of solution. Osmolality can also be measured over a wider range than specific gravity and with greater accuracy.

Osmolality is used in the precise evaluation of the concentrating ability of the kidneys (e.g., in acute and chronic renal failure). This test is used to monitor electrolyte and water balance and to evaluate dehydration. Osmolality is valuable in the workup of patients with renal disease, the syndrome of inappropriate antidiuretic hormone secretion (SIADH), and diabetes insipidus. Osmolality may be used as part of the urinalysis when the patient has glycosuria or proteinuria or has had tests that use radiopaque substances.

Procedure and patient care

Before

- Explain the procedure to the patient.
- Tell the patient that no special preparation is necessary for a random urine specimen.
- Inform the patient that preparation for a fasting urine specimen may require him or her to be on a high-protein

O

diet for 3 days before the test. Instruct the patient to eat a dry supper the evening before the test and drink no fluids until the test is completed the next morning.

During

- Collect a first-voided urine specimen for a random sample.
- For a fasting specimen, instruct the patient to empty the bladder at approximately 6 AM and discard the urine. Then collect the test urine at 8 AM.
- Indicate on the laboratory slip the patient's fasting status.

After

- Send the specimen to the laboratory.
- Provide food and fluids for the patient.

Abnormal findings

Increased levels	Decreased levels
Syndrome of inappropriate ADH secretion (SIADH)	Diabetes insipidus
Acidosis	Hypercalcemia
Shock	Excess fluid intake
Hypernatremia	Renal tubular necrosis
Hepatic cirrhosis	Aldosteronism
Congestive heart failure	Hypokalemia
Addison's disease	Severe pyelonephritis

Notes

oximetry (Pulse oximetry, Ear oximetry, Oxygen saturation)

Type of test Photodiagnostic

Normal findings $\geq 95\%$ or higher

Possible critical values $\leq 75\%$

Test explanation and related physiology

Oximetry is a noninvasive method of monitoring arterial blood oxygen saturation (SaO_2). The SaO_2 is the ratio of oxygenated hemoglobin to the total amount of hemoglobin. The SaO_2 is expressed as a percentage; for example, a saturation of 95% indicates that 95% of the total hemoglobin attachments for oxygen have oxygen attached to them. The SaO_2 is an accurate approximation of oxygen saturation obtained from arterial blood gas study. By correlating the SaO_2 and the patient's physiologic status, a close estimate of the partial oxygen pressure (Po_2) can be obtained.

Oximetry is typically used for monitoring the patient's oxygenation status during the perioperative period and for patients receiving mechanical ventilation. This test is also frequently used in many clinical situations, such as pulmonary rehabilitation programs, stress testing, and sleep laboratories. Oximetry can be used to assess the body's response to various drugs, such as theophylline, which causes bronchodilation, and methacholine, which evokes bronchospasm in people with asthma.

Procedure and patient care
Before

- Explain the procedure to the patient.
- Tell the patient that no fasting is required.

During

- Rub the patient's earlobe, pinna (upper portion of the ear), or fingertip to increase blood flow.
- Clip the monitoring probe or sensor to the ear or finger. The sensor warms and increases blood flow to the tissue. A beam of light passes through the tissue, and the sensor measures the amount of light the tissue absorbs.

O

- Remember that pulse oximetry is constantly monitored during the perioperative period. This test is one of the factors used to determine when the patient is discharged from the recovery room.
- Note that this study is usually performed by a respiratory therapist or nurse at the patient's bedside in a few minutes.
- Tell the patient that no discomfort is associated with this study.

After

- Note that no special after-care is needed.

Abnormal findings

Impaired cardiopulmonary function
Abnormal gas exchange

Notes

Papanicolaou smear (Pap smear, Pap test, Cytologic test for cancer)

Type of test Microscopic examination

Normal findings No abnormal or atypical cells

Test explanation and related physiology

A Pap smear is taken to detect neoplastic cells in cervical and vaginal secretions. This test is based on normal and abnormal cervical and endometrial neoplastic cells being shed into the cervical and vaginal secretions. By examining these secretions microscopically, one can detect early cellular changes compatible with premalignant conditions or an existing malignant condition. The Pap smear is 95% accurate in detecting cervical carcinoma. However, its accuracy in detection of endometrial carcinoma is only approximately 40%. The cells are classified as follows:

Class 1: absence of atypical or abnormal cells (normal)
Class 2: atypical cells, but no evidence of malignancy (worrisome but most frequently caused by inflammation of the cervix)
Class 3: cytologic findings suggestive of but not conclusive concerning malignancy (should be evaluated more extensively)
Class 4: cytologic findings strongly suggestive of malignancy (requires more extensive evaluation)
Class 5: cytologic findings conclusive of malignancy (requires treatment)

Abnormal smears in classes 2 to 4 do not necessarily indicate that the patient has a malignancy. Additional procedures are indicated for these women.

A general movement has occurred over the last 10 years to reclassify Pap smear reporting in terms of cervical intraepithelial neoplasia (CIN). This is a simple designation of the spectrum of intraepithelial dysplasia, which usually occurs before invasive cervical cancer. In contrast to the rigid original classification, CIN reporting recognizes the continuum of cervical dysplasia and allows for some overlap. The subclasses of CIN are defined as follows:

CIN 1: mild and mild-to-moderate dysplasia

CIN 2: moderate and moderate-to-severe dysplasia
CIN 3: severe dysplasia and carcinoma in situ

Basically, CIN 1 includes classes 2 and 3, CIN 2 includes class 3, and CIN 3 comprises classes 4 and 5.

A Pap smear may also be performed to follow some abnormalities (e.g., infertility). An abnormal maturation index is characteristic of an estrogen-progesterone imbalance.

Pap smears should be part of the routine pelvic examination, which is usually performed once a year on women over 18 years of age (or even earlier when the patient is sexually active). Opinions differ regarding the necessity for annual Pap smears. The American Cancer Society recommends that a Pap smear be taken annually for two negative examinations and then repeated once every 3 years until age 65 in asymptomatic women. More frequent testing may be indicated for patients with venereal infections, those with a family history of cervical cancer, and those whose mothers had ingested diethylstilbestrol (DES) during their pregnancies. Usually a routine cervical culture for gonorrhea is obtained during the Pap smear examination.

Contraindications

- Patients presently having routine, normal menses, since this can alter test interpretation

Interfering factors

- A delay in fixing a specimen allows the cells to dry, destroys effectiveness of the stain, and makes cytologic interpretation difficult.
- Using lubricating jelly on the speculum can alter the specimen.
- Douching and tub bathing may wash away cellular deposits and interfere with the test results.
- Menstrual flow can alter test results.
- Infections can interfere with hormonal cytology.
- Drugs such as digitalis and tetracycline can alter the test results by affecting the squamous epithelium.

Procedure and patient care
Before

- Explain the procedure to the patient.
- Instruct the patient not to douche or tub bathe during

the 24 hours before the Pap smear. (Some physicians prefer that patients refrain from sexual intercourse for 24 to 48 hours before the test.)
- Instruct the patient to empty her bladder before the examination.
- Tell the patient that no fasting or sedation is required.

During
- Note the following procedural steps:
  1. The patient is placed in the lithotomy position.
  2. A vaginal speculum is inserted to expose the cervix.
  3. Material is collected from the cervical canal by rotating a moist, saline cotton swab or spatula within the cervical canal and in the squamocolumnar junction.
  4. The cells are immediately wiped across a clean glass slide and fixed either by immersing the slide in equal parts of 95% alcohol and ether or by using a commercial spray (e.g., Aqua Net hair spray). The secretions must be fixed before drying, because drying will distort the cells and make interpretation difficult.
  5. The slide is labeled with the patient's name, age, parity, and date of her last menstrual period.
  6. The patient's medication history (e.g., oral contraceptives) and the reason for the examination should be written on the laboratory request form.

- Note that a Pap smear is obtained by a nurse or a physician in about 10 minutes.
- Tell the patient that no discomfort, except for insertion of the speculum, is associated with this procedure.

After
- Inform the patient that usually she will not be notified unless further evaluation is necessary.

Abnormal findings

Cancer
Infertility
Venereal disease

Inflammatory processes
Fungal conditions
Parasitic conditions

Notes

parathyroid hormone (PTH, Parathormone)

Type of test Blood

Normal findings <2000 pg/ml (vary according to individual laboratory)

Test explanation and related physiology

The serum PTH test measures the quantity of PTH within the blood. PTH is the only hormone secreted by the parathyroid gland and is one of the major factors in calcium metabolism. This test is useful in establishing a diagnosis of hyperparathyroidism and in distinguishing nonparathyroid from parathyroid causes of hypercalcemia. Increased PTH levels are seen in patients with hyperparathyroidism; in patients with nonparathyroid, ectopic PTH-producing tumors; or as a normal compensatory response to hypocalcemia in patients with renal failure or vitamin D deficiency. Decreased levels are seen in patients with hypoparathyroidism or as a compensatory response to hypercalcemia in patients with metastatic bone tumors, sarcoidosis, vitamin D intoxication, or milk-alkali syndrome.

Interfering factors

- Recent injection of radioisotopes may interfere with this test.

Procedure and patient care

Before

- Explain the procedure to the patient.
- Keep the patient NPO except for water after midnight on the day of the test.

During

- Obtain a morning blood specimen because a diurnal rhythm affects PTH levels. (Check with the laboratory if the patient works at night.)
- Collect 5 to 10 ml of venous blood in a red-top tube. Note that some laboratories require 15 ml of blood in an iced plastic syringe.
- Obtain a serum calcium level determination at the same

time, if ordered. The serum PTH and serum calcium levels are important in the differential diagnosis.

After

- Indicate the time the blood was drawn on the laboratory slip because a diurnal rhythm affects test results.
- Apply pressure or a pressure dressing to the venipuncture site.
- Check the venipuncture site for bleeding.

Abnormal findings

Increased levels

Hyperparathyroidism secondary to adenoma or carcinoma of the parathyroid gland
Non-parathyroid PTH-producing tumors (paraneoplastic syndrome)
Lung carcinoma
Kidney carcinoma
Hypocalcemia
Chronic renal failure
Malabsorption syndromes
Vitamin D deficiency
Rickets
Osteomalacia

Decreased levels

Hypoparathyroidism
Hypercalcemia
Metastatic bone tumor
Sarcoidosis
Autoimmune destruction of the parathyroid glands
Vitamin D intoxication
Milk-alkali syndrome
Graves' disease
Hypomagnesemia

Notes

P

partial thromboplastin time, activated
(APTT, Partial thromboplastin time, [PTT])

Type of test Blood

Normal findings

APTT: 30-40 seconds
PTT: 60-70 seconds
Patients receiving anticoagulant therapy: 1.5-2.5 times control value in seconds

Possible critical values

APTT: >70 seconds
PTT: >100 seconds

Test explanation and related physiology

The partial thromboplastin time (PTT) test is used to assess the intrinsic system and the common pathway of clot formation. PTT evaluates factors I (fibrinogen), II (prothrombin), V, VIII, IX, X, XI, and XII. When any of these factors exists in inadequate quantities, as in hemophilia A and B or consumptive coagulopathy, the PTT is prolonged. Because factors II, IX, and X are vitamin K–dependent factors, biliary obstruction, which precludes gastrointestinal absorption of fat and fat-soluble vitamins (e.g., vitamin K) can reduce their concentration and thus prolong the PTT. Since coagulation factors are made in the liver, hepatocellular diseases will also prolong the PTT.

Heparin has been found to inactivate prothrombin (factor II) and to prevent the formation of thromboplastin. These actions prolong the intrinsic clotting pathway for approximately 4 to 6 hours after each dose of heparin. Therefore heparin is capable of providing therapeutic anticoagulation. The appropriate dose of heparin can be monitored by the PTT. PTT test results are given in seconds along with a control value. The control value may vary slightly from day to day because of the reagents used.

Recently, activators have been added to the PTT test reagents to shorten normal clotting time and provide a narrow normal range. This shortened time is called the activated partial thromboplastin time (APTT). The normal APTT is 30 to 40 seconds. Desired ranges for therapeutic anticoagulation are 1½ to 2½ times normal (e.g., 70 seconds). The APTT specimen should be drawn 30 to 60 minutes before the patient's next heparin dose is given. If the APTT is less than 50 seconds, the patient may not be receiving therapeutic anticoagulation and needs more heparin. An APTT greater than 100 seconds indicates that too much heparin is being given. The risk of serious spontaneous bleeding exists when the APTT is this high. The effects of heparin can be reversed immediately by the administration of 1 mg of protamine sulfate for every 100 units of the heparin dose.

Heparin's effect, unlike that of warfarin, is immediate and short-lived. When a thromboembolic episode (e.g., pulmonary embolism, arterial embolism, thrombophlebitis) occurs, immediate and complete anticoagulation is most rapidly and safely achieved by heparin administration. This drug is often given during cardiac and vascular surgery to prevent intravascular clotting during clamping of the vessels. Often, small doses of heparin (5000 U subcutaneously every 12 hours) are given to prevent thromboembolism in high-risk patients. This dose alters the PTT very little, and the risk of spontaneous bleeding is minimal.

Interfering factors

- Drugs that can prolong PTT test values include antihistamines, ascorbic acid, chlorpromazine, heparin, and salicylates.

Procedure and patient care
Before

- Explain the procedure to the patient.
- If the patient is receiving heparin by intermittent injection, plan to draw the blood specimen for the APTT 30 minutes to 1 hour before the next dose of heparin.
- If the patient is receiving continuous heparin, draw the blood at any time.

During

- Collect 5 to 14 ml of venous blood in one or two blue-top tubes.

After

- Apply pressure or a pressure dressing to the venipuncture site.

- Assess the venipuncture site for bleeding. Remember, if the patient is receiving anticoagulants or has coagulopathies, the bleeding time will be increased.
- Assess the patient to detect possible bleeding. Check for blood in the urine and all excretions and assess the patient for bruises, petechiae, and low back pain.
- If severe bleeding occurs, note that the anticoagulant effect of heparin can be reversed by parenteral administration of protamine sulfate.

Abnormal findings
Increased levels

Acquired or congenital clotting factor deficiencies
Cirrhosis of the liver
Vitamin K deficiency
Leukemias
Disseminated intravascular coagulation (DIC)
Heparin administration
Hypofibrinogenemia
von Willebrand's disease
Hemophilia

Decreased levels

Early stages of DIC
Extensive cancer

Notes

pelvic floor sphincter electromyography
(Pelvic floor sphincter EMG, Rectal EMG procedure)

Type of test Electrodiagnostic

Normal findings

Increased EMG signal during bladder filling
Silent EMG signal on voluntary micturition
Increased EMG signal at end of voiding

Test explanation and related physiology

This urodynamic test uses the placement of electrodes in the pelvic floor musculature to evaluate the neuromuscular function of the urinary or anal sphincter. The main benefit of this study is to evaluate external sphincter (skeletal muscle) activity during voiding. This test is also used to evaluate the bulbocavernous reflex and voluntary control of external sphincter or pelvic floor muscles. The pelvic floor sphincter EMG also aids in the investigation of "functional" or "psychologic" disturbances of voiding.

Three electrodes are used for this procedure. Recordings may be made from surface electrodes or needle electrodes within the muscle; surface electrodes are most often used. These electrodes allow for observation of and change in the muscle activity before and during voiding.

Patient cooperation is essential. If the patient does not cooperate, the interpretation of the test results will be difficult.

Contraindications

- Patients who cannot cooperate during the procedure

Procedure and patient care

Before

- Explain the procedure to the patient.
- Inform the patient that cooperation is essential.

During

- Note the following procedural steps:

  1. Two electrodes are placed at the 2 o'clock and 10 o'clock positions on the perianal skin to monitor the pelvic floor muscular during voiding.

2. The third electrode is usually placed on the thigh and serves as a ground.
3. Electrical activity is recorded with the bladder empty and the patient relaxed.
4. Reflex activity is evaluated by asking the patient to cough and by stimulating the urethra and trigone by gently tugging on an inserted Foley catheter (bulbocavernous reflex).
5. Voluntary activity is evaluated by asking the patient to contract and relax the sphincter muscle.
6. The bladder is filled with sterile water at room temperature at a rate of 100 ml/minute.
7. The EMG responses to filling and detrusor hyperreflexia (if present) are recorded.
8. Finally, when the bladder is full and the patient is in a voiding position, the filling catheter is removed and the patient is asked to urinate. In the normal patient the EMG signals build during bladder filling and cease promptly on voluntary micturition, remaining silent until the pelvic floor contracts at the end of voiding.
9. The electrical waves produced are examined for their number and form.

- Note that a urologist performs this study in less than 30 minutes.
- Explain to the patient that this study is slightly more uncomfortable than urethral catheterization.

After

- If needle electrodes were used, observe the needle site for hematoma or inflammation.

Abnormal finding

Neuromuscular dysfunction of lower urinary sphincter

Notes

pelvimetry (Radiographic pelvimetry)

Type of test X-ray

Normal findings Transverse diameter of midpelvis >10.5 cm

Testing explanation and related physiology

Although most abnormalities of the pelvis can be suspected by using clinical measurements, x-ray pelvimetry is the most accurate means of determining adequacy of the pelvic bony structures for a normal vaginal delivery. With pelvimetry, one can compare the capacity of the pelvis with the size of the infant and discover any cephalopelvic disproportion (CPD).

Radiographic pelvimetry is not used often in modern obstetrics because of the risks associated with radiation. However, this study may be indicated in:

1. Patients suspected of having fetuses in abnormal positions when a vaginal delivery is anticipated
2. Patients who have had injury or disease of the bony pelvis or hips that may have caused pelvic distortion
3. Patients with clinically abnormal pelvic measurements
4. Patients who have a debilitating disease and a clinically small or unfavorable pelvis
5. Patients who have a history of difficult delivery
6. Patients in early labor with the fetus's head unengaged
7. Patients admitted for trial labor to rule out a contracted pelvis
8. Patients having dysfunctional labor, especially when the physician is considering oxytocin administration

Although measuring the pelvis clinically is less accurate than x-ray determination, it is adequate for most patients. Radiographic pelvimetry is only important late in pregnancy or during labor. If pelvimetry indicates a difficult or dangerous vaginal delivery, cesarean birth is recommended. Cesarean section is now more frequently performed when vaginal delivery is clinically suspected to be difficult. As a result, x-ray pelvimetry rarely affects the physician's decision concerning the type of delivery. In those rare situations in which vaginal delivery is attempted despite an anticipated difficult de-

P

livery, radiographic pelvimetry is performed more for legal purposes than for medical benefits.

Contraindications

- Patients in early pregnancy, since x-ray films at this time may injure the fetus

Procedure and patient care
Before

- Explain the procedure to the patient.
- Tell the patient that no fasting or sedation is required.
- Instruct the patient to remove all clothing and don a long x-ray gown.

During

- Note the following procedural steps:
  1. In the radiology department a lateral x-ray film is taken with the patient standing (a) to detect the effect of gravity on engagement and (b) to indicate the position of the fetal head when it reaches the lower level of the birth canal.
  2. The patient may then be placed in the supine, lateral, and semirecumbent positions.
  3. During the x-ray exposure the patient is asked to stop breathing.
  4. Generally the patient is instructed to hyperventilate and then stop breathing while the film is taken.
- Note that a radiologic technologist performs this study in approximately 15 minutes.
- Tell the patient that no discomfort is associated with this study.

After

- Provide emotional support for the patient at this difficult time. Most patients are concerned that some problem exists.

Abnormal findings

Cephalopelvic disproportion (CPD)
Abnormal fetal position

Notes

percutaneous transhepatic cholangiography (PTC, PTHC)

Type of test X-ray

Normal findings Normal gallbladder and biliary ducts

Test explanation and related physiology

By passing a needle through the liver and into an intrahepatic bile duct, the biliary system can be directly injected with iodinated x-ray contrast dye. The intrahepatic and extrahepatic biliary ducts and occasionally the gallbladder can be visualized and studied for partial or total obstruction caused by gallstones, benign strictures, malignant tumors, congenital cysts, and anatomic variations. This is especially helpful in jaundiced patients. If the jaundice is found to be result from extrahepatic obstruction, a catheter can be left in the bile duct and used for external drainage of bile.

PTC and endoscopic retrograde cholangiopancreatography (ERCP, see p. 305) are the only methods available to visualize the biliary tree in jaundiced patients. ERCP is used more frequently because of its lower complication rate.

Contraindications

- Patients with allergies to iodine or shellfish
- Patients with evidence of mild cholangitis
  Dye injections increase biliary pressure and cause bacteremia, which may lead to septicemia and shock
- Patients who cannot cooperate and remain still
- Patients with prolonged clotting times

Potential complications

- Allergic reaction to iodinated dye
  Allergic reactions may vary form mild flushing, itching, and urticaria to severe, life-threatening anaphylaxis (evidenced by respiratory distress, drop in blood pressure, shock). In the unusual event of anaphylaxis the patient may be treated with diphenhydramine (Benadryl), steroids, and epinephrine. Oxygen and endotracheal equipment should be on hand for immediate use.
- Peritonitis caused by bile extravasation from the liver after the needle has been removed

P

- Bleeding caused by inadvertent puncture of a large hepatic blood vessel
- Sepsis and cholangitis resulting from injection of the dye into an already infected and obstructed bowel duct
  The pressure of injection pushes the bacteria into the bloodstream, causing a bacteremia.

Interfering factor

- Presence of barium from a previous upper gastrointestinal series or barium enema x-ray study may preclude visualization of the biliary tree.

Procedure and patient care
Before

- Explain the procedure to the patient.
- Obtain informed consent for this procedure.
- Assess the patient for allergies to iodinated dye or shellfish.
- Inform the radiologist if an allergy to iodinated contrast is suspected. The radiologist may prescribe a diphenhydramine (Benadryl) and steroid preparation to be administered before testing. Usually a hypoallergenic, non-ionic contrast will be used during the test.

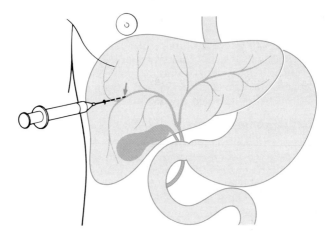

Figure 8 Percutaneous transhepatic cholangiography (PTHC).

- Type and cross-match the patient's blood. The patient may bleed and require a transfusion or surgery.
- Check to make sure that the patient's coagulation studies are within the normal ranges.
- Keep the patient NPO after midnight on the day of the test. A laxative may be ordered.
- Premedicate the patient as indicated, usually with atropine and meperidine.

During

- Note the following procedural steps:

  1. The patient is placed in the supine position on an x-ray table in the radiology department.
  2. The abdominal wall (over the liver) is anesthetized with lidocaine (Xylocaine).
  3. With the use of televised fluoroscopic monitoring, the needle is advanced through the skin and into the liver (see Figure 8).
  4. When bile flows freely through the needle, radiographic dye is injected.
  5. X-ray films are taken immediately.
  6. If an obstruction is found, a catheter is placed over a guide wire and left temporarily in the biliary tract to establish drainage and decompression of the biliary tract.

- Note that PTC is performed by a radiologist in approximately 1 hour, during which the patient must lie completely still.
- Inform the patient that abdominal pain may be felt for several hours after the test. Occasionally, the patient may also have right shoulder-top pain because of diaphragmatic irritation of leaking bile or blood.

After

- Keep the patient on bed rest for several hours.
- If indicated, place a sandbag over the insertion site.
- Observe the patient for hemorrhage or bile leakage. A small amount of bleeding is usually present.
- Keep the patient NPO for a few hours after the test in the event he or she has any intraabdominal bleeding or bile extravasation that requires surgery.

P

- Repeatedly assess the patient's vital signs for evidence of hemorrhage.
- Assess the patient for signs of bacteremia or sepsis.
- If a catheter is left in the biliary tract, establish a sterile, closed drainage system.
- Withhold pain medications to avoid blunting the abdominal signs associated with hemorrhage or bile extravasation.

Abnormal findings

Tumors, strictures, or gallstones of the common bile duct
Sclerosing cholangitis
Biliary sclerosis
Cysts of the common bile duct
Tumors, strictures, inflammation, or pseudocysts of the pancreatic duct
Anatomic biliary or pancreatic duct variations

Notes

pericardiocentesis

Type of test Fluid analysis

Normal findings Minimal amount of clear, straw-colored fluid without evidence of any bacteria, blood, or malignant cells

Test explanation and related physiology

Pericardiocentesis, which involves the aspiration of fluid from the pericardial sac with a needle, may be performed for therapeutic and diagnostic purposes. Therapeutically, the test is performed as a measure to relieve cardiac tamponade by removing fluid and improving diastolic filling. Diagnostically, pericardiocentesis is performed to remove a sample of pericardial fluid for laboratory examination.

Contraindications

- Patients who are uncooperative because of the risk of lacerations
- Patients with a bleeding disorder
  Inadvertent puncture of the myocardium may create uncontrollable bleeding into the pericardial sac, leading to tamponade.

Potential complications

- Laceration of the coronary artery or myocardium
- Needle-induced ventricular arrhythmias (dysrhythmias)
- Myocardial infarction
- Pneumothorax caused by inadvertent puncture of the lung
- Liver laceration by inadvertent puncture
- Pleural infection
- Vasovagal arrest

Procedure and patient care

Before

- Explain the procedure to the patient.
- Obtain informed consent for this procedure.
- Restrict fluid and food intake for at least 4 to 6 hours (if this is an elective procedure).

- Obtain IV access for infusion of fluids and cardiac medications if required.
- Administer pretest medication. Atropine is frequently given to prevent the vasovagal reflex of bradycardia and hypotension.

During

- Note the following procedural steps:

1. The patient is placed in the supine position.
2. An area in the fifth to sixth intercostal space at the left sternal margin (or subxyphoid) is prepared and draped.
3. After skin anesthesia is performed, a large-bore, pericardiocentesis needle is placed on a 50 ml syringe and introduced into the pericardial sac.
4. An electrocardiographic lead is often attached by a clip to the needle to identify any ST segment elevations, which may indicate penetration into the epicardium.
5. Pericardial fluid is aspirated and placed in multiple-specimen containers.
6. Some patients who have recurring cardiac tamponade may require placement of a indwelling pericardial catheter for continuous draining for 1 to 3 days.
7. With certain types of pericarditis, medications (e.g., antibiotics, antineoplastic drugs, corticosteroids) may be instilled during pericardiocentesis.

- Note that a physician usually performs this procedure in the cardiac catheterization laboratory, operating room, or emergency room in approximately 10 to 20 minutes.
- Tell the patient that this procedure is associated with very little discomfort. Most patients feel pressure as the needle is inserted into the pericardial sac.

After

- Closely monitor the patient's vital signs. An increased temperature may indicate infection. Pericardial bleeding would be marked by hypotension or pulsus paradoxus (abnormal decrease in systolic blood pressure during inspiration).
- Label and number the specimen tubes that contain the

pericardial fluid and deliver them to the appropriate laboratories for examination.

1. Usually the fluid is taken to the chemistry laboratory, where the color, turbidity, glucose, albumin, protein, and lactic dehydrogenase (LDH) levels are obtained.
2. A tube of blood often goes to hematology, where the quantity of red and white blood cells are recorded.
3. The bacteriology laboratory performs routine cultures, Gram stains, fungal studies, acid-fast bacilli smears, and cultures.

- Apply a sterile dressing to the catheter if one has been left for continuing pericardial drainage.
- Establish a closed system if continued pericardial drainage is required. This is usually performed via the straight drainage method.
- Note that, to minimize infection, pericardial catheters are usually removed after 2 days, although there are exceptions. After the sutures are cut and the catheter removed, apply a sterile dressing to the puncture site.

Abnormal findings

Pericarditis
Uremia
Hypoproteinemia
Congestive heart failure
Metastatic cancer
Blunt or penetrating cardiac trauma
Rupture of ventricular aneurysm

Notes

phenylketonuria test (PKU test, Guthrie test, Phenylalanine screening)

Type of test Blood; urine

Normal findings
Blood: negative (<2 mg/dl) (Guthrie technique)
Urine: no green coloration

Possible critical values ≥4 mg/dl (Guthrie technique)

Test explanation and related physiology

PKU is an inherited disease characterized by deficiency of the enzyme phenylalanine hydroxylase, which converts phenylalanine to tyrosine. Phenylalanine is an essential amino acid necessary for growth. However, any excess must be degraded by conversion to tyrosine. An infant with PKU lacks the ability to make this necessary conversion to tyrosine. Thus phenylalanine accumulates in the body and spills over into the urine. If the amount of phenylalanine is not restricted in infants with PKU, progressive mental retardation results. Dietary control must begin early to avoid brain damage; therefore diagnosis must be made early.

Routine screening of newborn infants for PKU is now mandatory in most of the United States. The Guthrie blood test is normally done before discharging the newborn from the hospital. It is important to note that this test is not valid until the newborn has ingested an ample amount (for 2 or 3 days) of the amino acid phenylalanine, which is a constitutent of both human and cow's milk. The urine PKU test is normally done after 4 to 6 weeks of age. If the tests are positive, a blood phenylalanine test should be performed.

Interfering factors

- Premature infants may have false positive results because of delayed development of the liver enzymes.
- Ketonuria can produce an altered urine color reaction.
- Infants tested before 24 hours of age may have false negative results.
- Feeding problems (e.g., vomiting) may cause false negative results.

▪ Drugs that may influence screening results include antibiotics, aspirin, and salicylates.

Procedure and patient care

Before

▪ Inform the mother about the purpose of the test and the method of performance.
▪ Assess the infant's feeding patterns before performing the PKU test. An inadequate amount of protein before performing the test can cause false negative results.

During

▪ Place a few drops of a heel stick of blood on filter paper for the *Guthrie test*. This test is performed after the newborn has ingested an ample amount (for 2 to 3 days) of the amino acid phenylalanine.
▪ Indicate on the laboratory slip the present date and time, date and time of birth, and time of first milk feeding.
▪ Note that urine tests can also be used to detect PKU in infants who are at least 6 weeks of age. These tests are usually done at the infant's first checkup.

1. For the *diaper test,* drop 10% ferric chloride on a diaper that contains fresh urine. A green spot indicates probable PKU.
2. For the *Phenistix test,* press a test stick against a diaper containing urine or dip the stick in the urine. A green color reaction indicates probable PKU.

After

▪ If test results are positive, inform the mother that dietary control must begin immediately to prevent brain damage to the infant. This is done by substituting Lofenalac for milk. Later, strained foods low in protein are added to the infant's diet. The dietary treatment is monitored by blood and urine testing.
▪ Instruct women with PKU who wish to have children to begin a low-phenylalanine diet before conception and continue throughout the pregnancy. The risk of producing a mentally retarded infant is very high if the mother remains on a general diet.

Abnormal findings

Phenylketonuria (PKU)
Low-birth-weight infants
Galactosemia
Hepatic encephalopathy

Notes

phosphorus (P, Phosphate, PO$_4$)

Type of test Blood

Normal findings
Adult: 3.0-4.5 mg/dl or 0.97-1.45 mmol/L (SI units)
Elderly: values slightly lower than adult
Child: 4.5-6.5 mg/dl or 1.45-2.1 mmol/L (SI units)
Newborn: 4.3-9.3 mg/dl or 1.4-3.0 mmol/L (SI units)

Possible critical values <1 mg/dl

Test explanation and related physiology
Most of the body's phosphorus is combined with calcium within the skeleton. However, approximately 15% of the phosphorus exists in the blood as a phosphate salt. Dietary phosphorus is absorbed in the small bowel. The absorption is very efficient, and only rarely is hypophosphatemia caused by gastrointestinal malabsorption. Antacids, however, can bind phosphorus and decrease intestinal absorption. Renal excretion of phosphorus should equal dietary intake to maintain a normal serum phosphate level.

Phosphorus levels are determined by calcium metabolism, parathormone (parathyroid hormone, PTH), and, to a lesser degree, by intestinal absorption. Because an inverse relationship exists between calcium and phosphorus, a decrease in one mineral results in an increase in the other. Serum phosphorus levels therefore depend on calcium metabolism, and vice versa.

Regulation of phosphate by PTH is such that PTH tends to decrease phosphate reabsorption in the kidney. However, PTH and vitamin D tend to stimulate phosphate absorption weakly within the gut.

Interfering factors
- Laxatives or enemas containing sodium phosphate can increase phosphorus levels.
- Recent carbohydrate ingestion, including IV glucose administration, causes decreased phosphorus levels because phosphorus enters the cell with glucose.
- Drugs that may cause increased levels include methicillin and vitamin D (excessive).

P

- Drugs that may cause decreased levels include antacids and mannitol.

Procedure and patient care

Before

- Explain the procedure to the patient.
- Keep the patient NPO after midnight on the day of the test.
- If indicated, discontinue IV fluids with glucose for several hours before the test.

During

- Collect approximately 5 to 10 ml of venous blood in a red-top tube.
- Avoid hemolysis. Handle the tube carefully.
- Use a heel stick to draw blood from infants.

After

- Take the specimen to the laboratory immediately.
- Indicate on the laboratory slip the time the blood was obtained.
- Apply pressure or a pressure dressing to the venipuncture site.
- Check the venipuncture site for bleeding.

Abnormal findings

Increased levels (hyperphosphatemia)	Decreased levels (hypophosphatemia)
Hypoparathyroidism	Inadequate dietary ingestion of phosphorus
Renal failure	Chronic antacid ingestion
Increased dietary or IV intake of phosphorus	Hyperparathyroidism
Acromegaly	Hypercalcemia
Hypoparathyroidism	Chronic alcoholism
Bone metastasis	Vitamin D deficiency
Sarcoidosis	Diabetic acidosis
Hypocalcemia	Hyperinsulinism
Liver disease	Rickets (childhood)
Renal failure	Osteomalacia (adult)

Notes

platelet count (Thrombocyte count)

Type of test Blood

Normal findings

Adult/elderly: 150,000-400,000/mm^3 or 150 to 400
 × 10^9/L (SI units)
Premature infant: 100,000-300,000/mm^3
Newborn: 150,000-300,000/mm^3
Infant: 200,000-475,000 mm^3
Child: 150,000-400,000/mm^3

Possible critical values <50,000 or >1 million/mm^3

Test explanation and related physiology

The platelet count is an actual count of the number of platelets (thrombocytes) per cubic milliliter of blood. Platelet activity is essential to blood clotting. Because platelets can clump together, automated counting is subject to at least a 10% to 15% error. Low levels are often hand counted. Counts of 150,000 to 400,000/mm^3 are considered normal. Counts less than 100,000/mm^3 are considered to indicate thrombocytopenia; thrombocytosis is said to exist when counts are greater than 400,000/mm^3. Vascular thrombosis with organ infarction is the major complication of thrombocytosis. Spontaneous hemorrhage may occur with thrombocytopenia.

Spontaneous bleeding is a serious danger when platelet counts fall below 20,000/mm^3. With counts above 40,000/mm^3, spontaneous bleeding rarely occurs. However, prolonged bleeding from trauma or surgery may occur at this level.

Causes of *thrombocytopenia* (decreased number of platelets) include:

1. Reduced production of platelets (secondary to bone marrow failure or infiltration of fibrosis, tumor, etc.)
2. Sequestration of platelets (secondary to hypersplenism)
3. Accelerated destruction of platelets (secondary to antibodies, infections, drugs, prosthetic heart valves)

4. Consumption of platelets (secondary to disseminated intravascular coagulation)
5. Platelet loss from hemorrhage

Thrombocytosis (increased number of platelets) may occur as a compensatory response to severe hemorrhage. Other conditions associated with thrombocytosis include polycythemia vera, leukemia, postsplenectomy syndromes, and various malignant disorders.

Interfering factors

- Living in high altitudes may cause increased platelet levels.
- Strenuous exercise may cause increased levels.
- Decreased levels may be seen before menstruation.
- Drugs that may cause increased levels include oral contraceptives.
- Drugs that may cause decreased levels include acetaminophen, aspirin, chemotherapeutic agents, chloramphenicol, colchicine, H_2-blocking agents (cimetidine, Zantac), hydralazine, indomethacin, isoniazid (INH), quinidine, streptomycin, sulfonamides, thiazide diuretics, and tolbutamide (Orinase).

Procedure and patient care

Before

- Explain the procedure to the patient.
- Tell the patient that no fasting is required.

During

- Collect approximately 5 to 7 ml of peripheral venous blood in a lavender-top tube.
- List on the laboratory slip any drugs or other factors that can affect test results.

After

- Apply pressure or a pressure dressing to the venipuncture site.
- Assess the venipuncture site for bleeding.
- If the results indicate that the patient has a serious platelet deficiency:

  1. Observe the patient for signs and symptoms of bleeding.

2. Check for blood in the urine and all excretions.
3. Assess the patient for bruises, petechiae, bleeding from the gums, epistaxis, and low back pain.

Abnormal findings

Increased levels (thrombocytosis)	Decreased levels (thrombocytopenia)
Malignant disorders	Hypersplenism
Polycythemia vera	Hemorrhage
Leukemia	Idiopathic thrombocyto-penic purpura
Postsplenectomy syndromes	Leukemias
Rheumatoid arthritis	Liver disease
Cirrhosis	Kidney disease
Trauma	Disseminated intravascular coagulation (DIC)
	Systemic lupus erythematosus (SLE)
	Sequela of massive blood transfusion
	Pernicious anemia
	Hemolytic anemia
	Cancer chemotherapy
	Consumption of platelets
	Platelet destruction

Notes

P

plethysmography, arterial

Type of test Manometric

Normal findings

Less than 20 mm Hg difference in systolic blood pressure
  of lower extremity when compared to upper extremity
Normal pulse wave amplitude showing steep upswing,
  acute narrow peak, and more gentle downslope containing dicrotic notch (normal arterial pulse wave)

Test explanation and related physiology

  Plethysmography is usually performed to rule out occlusive disease of the lower extremities. However, it can also
identify arteriosclerotic disease in the upper extremity. This
test does require one normal extremity against which the
other extremities can be compared.

  Arterial plethysmography is performed by applying three
blood pressure cuffs to the extremity. These are then attached to a pulse volume recorder (plethysmograph), and
each pulse wave can be displayed. A reduction in amplitude
of a pulse wave in any of the three cuffs indicates arterial occlusion immediately proximal to the area where the decreased amplitude is noted. Also, a difference in pressure
greater than 20 mm Hg indicates a degree of arterial occlusion in the extremity. A positive result is reliable evidence of
arteriosclerotic peripheral vascular occlusion. A negative result, however, does not definitely exclude this diagnosis,
since extensive vascular collateralization can compensate for
even a complete arterial occlusion.

  Although it is not as accurate as arteriography (see p. 65),
plethysmography is performed without any serious complications and can be done for seriously ill patients who cannot
be transported to the arteriography laboratory.

Interfering factors

- Arterial occlusion proximal to the extremity
- Cigarette smoking because nicotine can cause arterial constriction

Procedure and patient care

Before

- Explain the procedure to the patient.
- Inform the patient that this test is painless.
- Tell the patient that he or she must lie still during the testing procedure.
- Remove all clothing from the patient's extremities.
- Instruct the patient to avoid smoking for at least 30 minutes before the test. Nicotine creates constriction of the peripheral arteries and alters the test results.
- Tell the patient that no fasting is required.

During

- Note the following procedural steps:

    1. The patient is placed in the semirecumbent position.
    2. The cuffs are applied to the extremities and then inflated to 65 mm Hg to increase their sensitivity to pulse waves.
    3. The pulse waves are recorded on the plethysmographic paper.
    4. The amplitudes and form of the pulse wave of each cuff are measured and compared. A marked reduction in wave amplitude indicates arterial occlusive disease.

- Note that this test usually is performed in the noninvasive vascular laboratory or at the patient's bedside by a noninvasive vascular technologist in approximately 30 minutes.
- Inform the patient that results are usually interpreted by a physician and are available in a few hours.
- Remind the patient that no discomfort is associated with this test.

After

- Encourage the patient to verbalize any concerns regarding the test results.

Abnormal findings

Arterial occlusive disease
Arterial trauma
Small vessel diabetic changes
Vascular diseases (e.g., Raynaud's phenomenon)
Arterial embolization

plethysmography, venous (Cuff pressure test)

Type of test Manometric

Normal findings Patent venous system without evidence of thrombosis or occlusion

Test explanation and related physiology

Plethysmography measures changes in the volume of an extremity. Usually, this test is performed on the leg to exclude deep vein thrombosis. During this test, blood pressure cuffs are placed on the leg and attached to a pulse volume recorder. The leg volume can then be recorded as a baseline value. The venous system is occluded by inflating the most proximal cuff *(occlusion cuff)*. The most distal *(recording cuff)* should record a sudden increase in venous volume. When the occlusion cuff is released, the venous volume of the leg should return to preocclusion baseline levels. In patients with venous obstruction, no initial increase in leg volume is recorded. Because venous outflow it obstructed, the venous volume of the leg will not dissipate quickly.

The results of venous plethysmography are less accurate than venography (see p. 779). However, no complications are associated with this noninvasive study. Plethysmography can be done easily and quickly on any patient with suspected venous disease. Further, with the use of portable plethysmography, this test can be performed at the bedside for extremely ill patients.

Interfering factor

- Venous occlusion more proximal to the site of the occlusion cuff

Procedure and patient care

Before

- Explain the procedure to the patient.
- Tell the patient that no fasting is required.
- Assure the patient that no discomfort is associated with the study.
- Instruct the patient to lie still during the testing.
- Remove all clothing from the patient's extremity to be tested.

During

- Note the following procedural steps:

  1. A large inflatable occlusion cuff is placed on the proximal portion of the extremity, usually the leg.
  2. A second, smaller plethysmographic monitor or recording cuff is placed more distal on the leg.
  3. The second cuff is inflated to 10 mm Hg to facilitate recognition of small changes in the leg's venous volume.
  4. The effects of respiration on the leg's venous volume are evaluated. If no significant changes occur with respiration, venous occlusion can be suspected.
  5. The occlusion cuff is inflated to 50 mm Hg. The monitor cuff should demonstrate a rise in venous volume, as displayed on the pulse monitor recorder.
  6. After the highest volume is recorded in the monitor cuff, the occlusion cuff is rapidly deflated. The leg should return to its preocclusion volume within 1 second. If return to preocclusion baseline values is delayed for a long period, venous thrombosis is suspected.
  7. Often, this test is performed concomitantly with Doppler ultrasound of the venous system (see p. 279).

- Note that this test is usually performed in the noninvasive vascular laboratory or at the patient's bedside by a noninvasive vascular technologist in approximately 30 minutes.
- Remind the patient that no discomfort is associated with this test.

After

- Note that no special after-care is needed.

Abnormal findings

Partial venous obstruction
Total venous obstruction

Notes

pleural biopsy

Type of test   Microscopic examination of tissue

Normal findings   No evidence of pathology

Test explanation and related physiology

Pleural biopsy is the removal of pleural tissue for histologic examination. This test is indicated when the pleural fluid obtained by thoracentesis (see p. 706) is exudative fluid, which suggests infection, neoplasm, or tuberculosis. The pleural biopsy is indicated to distinguish between these disease processes.

Pleural biopsy is usually performed through needle biopsy of the pleura. It can also be performed via *pleuroscopy*, which is done by inserting a fiberoptic bronchoscope into the pleural space for inspection and biopsy of the pleura. Pleural tissue may also be obtained by an *open pleural biopsy*, which involves a limited thoracotomy and requires general anesthesia. For this procedure, a small intercostal incision is made, and the biopsy of the pleura is done under direct observation. The advantage of this open procedure is that a larger specimen may be obtained.

Contraindications

- Patients with prolonged bleeding or clotting times

Potential complications

- Bleeding or injury to the lung
- Pneumothorax

Procedure and patient care

Before

- Explain the procedure to the patient.
- Obtain informed consent for this procedure.
- Tell the patient that no fasting or sedation is required.
- Instruct the patient to remain very still during the procedure. Any movement can cause inadvertent needle damage.

During

- Note the following procedural steps:

  1. This procedure is usually performed with the patient in a sitting position with the shoulders and arms elevated and supported by a padded overbed table.
  2. After the presence of the fluid has been determined by the thoracentesis technique, the skin overlying the biopsy site is anesthetized and pierced with a scalpel blade.
  3. A needle is inserted with a cannula until fluid is removed (some fluid is left in the pleural space after the thoracentesis to make the biopsy easier).
  4. The inner needle is removed, and a blunt-tipped, hooked biopsy trocar, attached to a three-way stopcock, is inserted into the cannula.
  5. The patient is instructed to expire all air and then to perform the Valsalva maneuver to prevent air from entering the pleural space.
  6. The cannula and the biopsy trocar are withdrawn while the hook catches the parietal wall and takes a specimen with its cutting edge.
  7. Usually three biopsy specimens are taken from different sites at the same session.
  8. The specimens are placed in a fixative solution and sent to the laboratory immediately.
  9. After the specimens are taken, additional parietal fluid can be removed.

- Note that this procedure is performed by a physician at the patient's bedside, in a special procedure room, or in the physician's office in approximately 30 minutes.
- Because of the local anesthetic, tell the patient that little discomfort is associated with this procedure.

After

- Apply an adhesive bandage to the biopsy site.
- Note that chest x-ray film is usually taken to detect the potential complication of pneumothorax.
- Observe the patient for signs of respiratory distress (e.g., shortness of breath, diminished breath sounds) on the side of the biopsy.
- Observe the patient's vital signs frequently for evidence of bleeding (increased pulse, decreased blood pressure).

- Ensure that the biopsy specimen is sent immediately to the laboratory.

Abnormal findings

Neoplasm
Tuberculosis

Notes

porphyrins and porphobilinogens

Type of test Urine (fresh and 24 hour)

Normal findings

Porphyrins: 50-300 mg/24 hr
Porphobilinogens: 1.5-2 mg/24 hr or no porphobilinogen
  on a random specimen

Test explanation and related physiology

Porphyrins are proteins used in the synthesis of heme in hemoglobin. Porphyrias are hereditary metabolic disorders of heme synthesis.

Abnormalities of porphyrin metabolism may be genetic or drug (usually lead) induced. These abnormalities are marked by increased levels of the heme precursors porphyrin and porphobilinogen. Normally, insignificant amounts of porphyrins are excreted in the urine. In most forms of porphyria, increased levels of porphyrins and porphobilinogen are found in the urine. This test is a quantitative analysis of urinary porphyrins. If porphyrins are present, the urine may be colored amber red or burgundy. The urine may turn even darker after standing in the light.

Interfering factors

- Drugs that may alter test results include aminosalicylic acid (PAS), barbiturates, chloral hydrate, chlorpropamide (Diabinese), ethyl alcohol, griseofulvin, morphine, oral contraceptives, phenazopyridine (Pyridium), procaine, and sulfonamides.

Procedure and patient care

Before

- Explain the procedure to the patient.
- Tell the patient that no fasting is required.

During

Porphobilinogens

- Collect a freshly voided urine specimen.
- Protect the specimen from light.
- For both porphobilinogens and porphyrins, indicate on the laboratory slip any drugs that can affect test results.

Porphyrins

- Instruct the patient to begin a 24-hour urine collection after voiding. Discard the initial specimen and start the 24-hour timing at that point.
- Collect all the urine passed during the next 24 hours.
- Instruct the patient to avoid alcohol ingestion during the collection.
- Show the patient where to store the urine container.
- Keep the specimen on ice or refrigerated during the 24 hours.
- Keep the urine in a light-resistant specimen bottle with a preservative to prevent degradation of the light-sensitive porphyrin.
- Indicate the starting time on the urine container and on the laboratory slip.
- Post the times for the urine collection in a prominent place to prevent accidental discarding of the specimen.
- Instruct the patient to void before defecating so that urine is not contaminated by feces.
- Remind the patient not to put toilet paper in the collection container.
- Encourage the patient to drink fluids during the 24 hours unless contraindicated for medical purposes.
- Collect the last specimen as close as possible to the end of the 24-hour period. Add this urine to the collection.

After

- Transport the urine specimens promptly to the laboratory.

Abnormal findings
Increased levels

Porphyrias
Liver disease
Lead poisoning
Pellagra

Notes

positron-emission tomography (PET)

Type of test Nuclear scan; x-ray

Normal findings Normal patterns of tissue metabolism

Test explanation and related physiology

PET is a unique technique that combines the early biochemical assessment of pathology achieved by nuclear medicine with the precise localization achieved by computed tomography (CT). PET is able to penetrate the body's metabolism by recording tracers of nuclear annihilations in body tissue. The selected tracers are chemically designed to measure body processes (e.g., blood flow and volume, protein metabolism).

A chemical compound with the desired biologic activity is labeled with a radioactive isotope that decays by emitting a positron (or positive electron). The positron combines with an electron, and the two are mutually annihilated with emission of two gamma rays. The gamma rays penetrate the surrounding tissue and are recorded outside the body by a circular array of detectors. Because the gamma rays travel in almost exactly opposite directions, their source can be established with a high degree of accuracy. A computer reconstructs the spatial distribution of the radioactivity for a selected plane within the patient and displays the resulting image on a cathode ray screen. PET provides noninvasive regional assessment of many biochemical processes essential to the functioning of the organ being studied.

The technology of PET is now well developed, and both its capabilities and its limitations are being increasingly understood. Many PET studies are being carried out with results that cannot be obtained by other techniques. These include:

1. Determination of regional metabolism in the heart and brain (e.g., radioactive glucose used to map biochemical activity in the brain)
2. Studies of tissue permeability
3. Measurement of the size of infarcts in the heart from a coronary occlusion
4. Investigation into the physiology of psychosis

5. Assessment of the effects of drugs on diseased or malfunctioning tissues
6. Possibility of measuring the effect of cancer treatment by changes in malignant tissues and by biochemical reactions in surrounding normal tissues

The dose of radioactive material given to the patient, either a gas or injection, produces a radiation exposure comparable to that of other nuclear medicine studies. PET is now being used in more than 40 major medical centers throughout the world. The cost of PET technology is high; it requires a cyclotron, appropriate chemical facilities, computer equipment, and effective group work by physicians, chemists, mathematicians, physiologists, and physicists. This procedure, which was once regarded as exotic, is now on the threshold of becoming a tool of fundamental importance in diagnostic medicine.

Interfering factors

- Recent use (within 24 hours) of caffeine, alcohol, or tobacco can affect test results.
- Excessive anxiety can affect brain function evaluation.
- Drugs that may influence results include tranquilizers and sedatives.

Procedure and patient care
Before

- Explain the procedure to the patient. Because most patients have not heard of this study, they are often anxious and require emotional support.
- Obtain informed consent if required by the institution.
- Inform the patient that he or she may have two IV lines inserted, one for infusion of the radioisotope and the other for serial blood samples.
- Inform the patient that he or she does not need to restrict food or fluids on the day of the test. However, the patient should refrain from alcohol, caffeine, and tobacco for 24 hours.
- Instruct diabetic patients to take their pretest dose of insulin at a meal 3 to 4 hours before the test.
- Tell the patient that no sedatives or tranquilizers should be taken because he or she may need to perform certain mental activities during the test.

- Tell the patient to empty the bladder before the test for comfort.

During

- Note the following procedural steps:

  1. The patient is positioned in a comfortable, reclining chair.
  2. Two IV lines are inserted.
  3. The radioactive material can be infused through an IV line or can be inhaled as a radioactive gas.
  4. The gamma rays that penetrate the tissues are recorded outside the body by a circular array of detectors and are displayed by a computer.
  5. If the brain is being scanned, the patient may be asked to perform different cognitive activities (e.g., reciting the Pledge of Allegiance) to measure brain activity changes during reasoning or remembering.
  6. Extraneous auditory and visual stimuli are minimized by a blindfold and ear plugs.

- Note that this procedure is performed by a physician or trained technologist in approximately 1 to 1½ hours.
- Tell the patient that the only discomfort associated with this study is insertion of the two IV lines.

After

- Instruct the patient to change positions slowly from lying to standing to avoid postural hypotension.
- Encourage the patient to drink fluids and urinate frequently to aid in removal of the radioisotope from the bladder.

Abnormal findings

Myocardial infarction
Cerebrovascular accident
  (CVA, stroke)
Epilepsy
Parkinson's disease
Dementia
Alzheimer's disease

Schizophrenia
Coronary artery disease
Pulmonary edema
Pneumonia
Brain tumor
Breast tumor
Huntington's disease

Notes

potassium, blood (K⁺)

Type of test Blood

Normal findings

Adults/elderly: 3.5-5.0 mEq/L or 3.5-5.0 mmol/L (SI units)
Child: 3.4-4.7 mEq/L
Infant: 4.1-5.3 mEq/L
Newborn: 3.9-5.9 mEq/L

Possible critical values

Adult: <2.5 or >6.5 mEq/L
Newborn: <2.5 or >8.0 mEq/L

Test explanation and related physiology

Potassium is the major cation within the cell. The intracellular potassium concentration is approximately 150 mEq/L, whereas normal serum potassium concentration is about 4 mEq/L. This ratio is the most important determinant in maintaining membrane electrical potential in excitable neuromuscular tissue. Because the serum concentration of potassium is so small, minor changes in concentration have significant consequences. The potassium level should be carefully followed in patients taking potassium-depleting diuretics and in patients with renal failure or acidosis.

Serum potassium concentration depends on many factors, including:

1. *Aldosterone.* This hormone tends to increase renal losses of potassium.
2. *Sodium reabsorption.* As sodium is reabsorbed, potassium is lost.
3. *Acid-base balance.* Alkalotic states tend to lower serum potassium levels by causing a shift of potassium into the cell. Acidotic states tend to raise serum potassium levels by reversing that shift.

Symptoms of hyperkalemia include irritability, nausea, vomiting, intestinal colic, and diarrhea. The electrocardiogram may demonstrate peaked T waves, a widened QRS complex, and depressed ST segment. Signs of hypokalemia are related to a decrease in contractility of smooth, skeletal, and cardiac muscles, which results in weakness, paralysis, hyporeflexia, ileus, increased cardiac sensitivity to digoxin, cardiac arrhythmias (dysrhythmias), flattened T waves, and prominent U waves.

Interfering factors

- Exercise of the forearm with a tourniquet in place may increase potassium levels.
- Hemolysis of blood during venipuncture causes increased levels.
- Drugs that may cause increased potassium levels include aminocaproic acid, antibiotics, antineoplastic drugs, captopril, epinephrine, heparin, histamine, isoniazid (INH), lithium, mannitol, potassium-sparing diuretics, potassium supplements, and succinylcholine.
- Drugs that may cause decreased levels include acetazolamide, aminosalicylic acid (PAS), amphotericin B, carbenicillin, cisplatin, diuretics (potassium wasting), glucose infusions, insulin, laxatives, lithium carbonate, penicillin G sodium (high doses), phenothiazines, salicylates (aspirin), and sodium polystyrene sulfonate (Kayexalate).

Procedure and patient care

Before

- Explain the procedure to the patient.
- Tell the patient that no special diet or fasting is required.

During

- Inform the patient to avoid opening and closing the hand after a tourniquet is applied.
- Collect approximately 5 to 7 ml of venous blood in a red-top or green-top tube.
- Avoid hemolysis.
- Indicate on the laboratory slip any drugs that can affect test results.

After

- Apply pressure or a pressure dressing to the venipuncture site.
- Assess the venipuncture site for bleeding.
- Evaluate the patient with increased or decreased potassium levels for cardiac arrhythmias (dysrhythmias).

- Monitor for hypokalemia in patients taking digoxin and diuretics.
- If indicated, administer resin exchanges (e.g., Kayexalate enema) to correct hyperkalemia.

Abnormal findings

Increased levels (hyperkalemia)

Increased potassium intake
  Excessive dietary intake
  Excessive IV intake
Decreased potassium loss
  Acute or chronic renal failure
  Addison's disease
  Hypoaldosteronism
  Aldosterone-inhibiting diuretics (e.g., spirono-lactone, triamterene)
Shift from intracellular space
  Acidosis
  Infection
  Crush injury to tissues
Pseudohyperkalemia
  Poor venipuncture technique, causing hemolysis
  Transfusion of hemolyzed blood

Decreased levels (hypokalemia)

Decreased potassium intake
  Deficient dietary intake
  Deficient IV intake
Excessive potassium loss
  Gastrointestinal disorders (e.g., diarrhea, vomiting, villous adenomas)
  Diuretics
  Hyperaldosteronism
  Cushing's syndrome
  Renal tubular acidosis
  Licorice ingestion
Shift to intracellular space
  Alkalosis
  Insulin or glucose administration
  Calcium administration

Notes

potassium, urine (K⁺)

Type of test Urine (24 hour)

Normal findings

25-120 mEq/L/day or 25-120 mmol/day (SI units)
Values vary greatly with diet.

Test explanation and related physiology

Potassium is the major cation within the cell. The electrolyte balance of potassium can be measured in both a spot urine and a 24-hour urine collection. A 24-hour collection is especially important to evaluate electrolyte (especially hypokalemia) balance, acid-base balance, and renal and adrenal diseases.

The serum potassium concentration depends on many factors. Aldosterone tends to increase the renal losses of potassium. Also, as sodium is reabsorbed, potassium is lost. Acid-base balance affects potassium concentration as well. Alkalotic states tend to lower serum potassium levels, causing a shift of potassium into the cell. Acidotic states tend to raise serum potassium levels by reversing the shift. Since the kidneys cannot conserve potassium, the balance of potassium in the body is regulated by kidney excretion of potassium through the urine.

Interfering factors

- Dietary intake affects potassium levels.
- Excessive intake of licorice may cause increased levels of potassium in the urine.
- Drugs that may cause increased levels include diuretics, glucocorticoids, and salicylates.

Procedure and patient care

Before

- Explain the procedure to the patient.
- Tell the patient that no special diet is required.

During

- Instruct the patient to begin the 24-hour urine collection after voiding.

- Discard the initial specimen and start the 24-hour timing at that point.
- Collect all urine passed during the next 24 hours.
- Show the patient where to store the urine container.
- Keep the specimen on ice or refrigerated during the entire 24 hours.
- Indicate the starting time on the urine container and the laboratory slip.
- Post the hours for the urine collection in a noticeable place to prevent accidental discarding of the specimen.
- Instruct the patient to void before defecating so that the urine is not contaminated by feces.
- Remind the patient not to put toilet paper in the collection container.
- Encourage the patient to drink fluids during the 24 hours.
- Instruct the patient to collect the last specimen as close as possible to the end of the 24-hour collection. Add this urine to the container.

After

- Transport the urine specimen promptly to the laboratory.

Abnormal findings

Increased levels	Decreased levels
Chronic renal failure	Dehydration
Renal tubular acidosis	Starvation
Dehydration	Vomiting
Starvation	Diarrhea
Cushing's syndrome	Malabsorption
Hyperaldosteronism	Excessive intake of licorice
Alkalosis	Acute renal failure
Excessive intake of licorice	
Vomiting	
Diarrhea	
Diabetic acidosis	
Salicylate toxicity	
Diuretic therapy	

Notes

pregnancy tests

Type of test Blood; urine

Normal findings Negative, unless pregnant

Test explanation and related physiology

All pregnancy tests are based on the detection of human chorionic gonadotropin (HCG), which is secreted by the trophoblast after the ovum is fertilized. HCG will appear in the blood and urine of pregnant women as early as 10 days after conception. Methods of pregnancy testing fall into the following four categories.

Biologic tests

Biologic (animal) tests have been used since the 1920s and are primarily of historical interest today. Urine from the patient is injected into an animal (mice, rabbit, toad, frog). If HCG is present, a specific response will occur in that animal. The exact response varies according to the animal used. These biologic tests have largely been replaced by less expensive, more accurate, and more rapidly performed immunologic tests.

Immunologic tests (agglutination inhibition test, AIT)

Immunologic tests are performed by the use of a commercially prepared reagent and can be completed within 2 minutes or 2 hours, depending on the method used. Immunologic tests are based on the reaction of HCG with antiserum to chorionic gonadotropin.

Radioimmunoassay (RIA)

RIA is a highly sensitive and reliable blood test for the detection of the beta unit of HCG. In this test, maternal serum HCG (unlabeled) and HCG that has been radioactively bound to an antibody (labeled) compete for binding sites. The higher the concentration of HCG in the maternal serum, the greater is the number of binding sites that will be occupied by the unlabeled HCG.

This study requires a blood sample in a red-top tube. However, RIA can also be performed with a urine test. The test can be done in 1 to 5 hours. This test is so sensitive that pregnancy can be diagnosed *before* the first missed menstrual period.

Radioreceptor assay (RRA)

RRA for serum HCG is highly sensitive and accurate. This test can be performed in 1 hour. The major advantage of this study is its reliable diagnosis of early gestation in patients requesting an early termination of pregnancy and in cases where infertile couples are anxious to confirm pregnancy. This study is 90% to 95% accurate 6 to 8 days after conception. Even the minute amounts of HCG secreted in an ectopic pregnancy can be measured with this study. This test is also used in determining early spontaneous abortion in patients who desire to maintain the pregnancy. This test measures the ability of the blood sample to inhibit the binding of radiolabeled-HCG to receptors.

■　■　■

It is important to know that all these pregnancy studies demonstrate the presence of HCG and do not necessarily indicate a normal pregnancy. Hydatidiform mole of the uterus and choriocarcinoma of the uterus, testes, or ovaries can produce HCG. Because HCG is produced by these tumors, determination of HCG can be a valuable test for tumor activity. When HCG levels are elevated in these patients, tumor progression must be suspected. Decreasing HCG levels indicate effective antitumor treatment.

Interfering factors

- Tests performed too early in the pregnancy before a significant HCG level exists can cause false negative results.
- Hematuria and proteinuria in the urine can cause false positive results.
- Hemolysis of blood may interfere with test results.
- Drugs that may cause false negative urine results include diuretics (by causing diluted urine) and promethazine.
- Drugs that may cause false positive results include anticonvulsants, antiparkinsonian drugs, hypnotics, and tranquilizers (especially promazine and its derivatives).

Procedure and patient care

Before

- Explain the procedure to the patient.
- If a urine specimen will be collected, give the patient a urine container the evening before so she can provide a first-voided morning specimen. This specimen generally contains the greatest concentration of HCG.

During

- Collect the first-voided urine specimen for urine testing.
- Collect approximately 7 to 10 ml of venous blood in a red-top tube for serum testing. Avoid hemolysis.

After

- Apply pressure or a pressure dressing to the venipuncture site.
- Assess the venipuncture site for bleeding.
- Emphasize to the patient the importance of antepartal health care.

Abnormal findings

Increased levels

Pregnancy
Ectopic pregnancy
Hydatidiform mole of the uterus
Choriocarcinoma of the uterus, testes, or ovaries
Tumors

Decreased levels

Threatened abortion
Incomplete abortion
Dead fetus

Notes

pregnanediol

Type of test   Urine (24 hour)

Normal findings
Increased excretion after ovulation to >1 mg/24 hr
Values vary according to week of pregnancy.

Test explanation and related physiology

Urinary pregnanediol is measured to evaluate progesterone production by the ovaries and placenta. The main effect of progesterone is on the endometrium. It initiates the secretory phase in anticipation of implantation of a fertilized ovum. Normally, progesterone is secreted by the ovarian corpus luteum following ovulation. Both serum progesterone levels and the urine concentration of progesterone metabolites (pregnanediol and others) are significantly increased during the later half of an ovulatory cycle. Pregnanediol is the most easily measured metabolite of progesterone.

Since pregnanediol levels rise rapidly after ovulation, this study is useful in documenting whether ovulation has occurred and, if so, its exact time. During pregnancy, pregnanediol levels normally rise because of the placental production of progesterone. Repeated assays can be used to monitor the status of the placenta.

Hormone assays for urinary pregnanediol are primarily used today to monitor progesterone supplementation in patients who have an inadequate luteal phase. Urinary assays may be supplemented by plasma assays (progesterone assay, see p. 588), which are quicker and more accurate.

Interfering factors
- Drugs that may cause increased levels include adrenocorticotropic hormone (ACTH).
- Drugs that may cause decreased levels include oral contraceptives and progesterones.

Procedure and patient care
Before
- Explain the procedure to the patient.
- Tell the patient that no special diet is usually required.

- Inform the patient that no sedation or fasting is necessary.

During

- Instruct the patient to begin the 24-hour urine collection. Discard the initial specimen and start the 24-hour timing at that point.
- Collect all urine passed for the next 24 hours.
- Show the patient where to store the urine collection.
- Keep the specimen on ice or refrigerated during the 24 hours. Check with the laboratory to see if a preservative is needed.
- Indicate the starting time on the urine container and the laboratory slip.
- Post the hours for urine collection in a noticeable place to prevent accidental discarding of the specimen.
- Instruct the patient to void before defecating so the urine is not contaminated by feces.
- Remind the patient not to put toilet paper in the collection container.
- Encourage the patient to drink fluids during the 24 hours.
- Instruct the patient to collect the last specimen as close as possible to the end of the 24-hour collection. Add this urine to the container.

After

- Record on the laboratory slip the date of the last menstrual period or the week of gestation during pregnancy.

Abnormal findings

Increased levels	Decreased levels
Ovulation	Threatened abortion
Pregnancy	Fetal death
Luteal cysts of ovary	Toxemia of pregnancy
Arrhenoblastoma of ovary	Amenorrhea
Hyperadrenocorticalism	Ovarian hypofunction
Choriocarcinoma of ovary	Placental failure
Adrenocortical hyperplasia	Preeclampsia
	Ovarian neoplasms
	Breast neoplasms

Notes

progesterone assay

Type of test Blood

Normal findings

Preovulation: 20-150 ng/dl
Midcycle: 300-2400 ng/dl
Pregnancy: >2400 ng/dl

Test explanation and related physiology

Determination of the progesterone level provides evidence to confirm ovulation and to evaluate the function of the corpus luteum. A series of measurements can help define the day of ovulation. Plasma progesterone levels start to rise with the luteinizing hormone (LH) surge and continue to rise for approximately 6 to 10 days and then fall. Normally, blood samples drawn at days 8 and 21 of the menstrual cycle will show a large increase in progesterone levels. Progesterone levels are also very high in early pregnancy. Certain adrenal and ovarian tumors may also produce elevated levels.

Urinary pregnanediol levels (see p. 586) are an indirect measurement of progesterone production. Serum progesterone levels can provide comparable information and are sometimes done in place of endometrial biopsy (see p. 303) to determine the phase of the menstrual cycle.

Interfering factors

- Recent use of radioisotopes may affect test results.
- Hemolysis caused by rough handling of the sample can affect test results.
- Drugs that may interfere with test results include estrogen and progesterone.

Procedure and patient care

Before

- Explain the procedure to the patient.
- Tell the patient that no fasting is required.

During

- Collect approximately 5 to 7 ml of venous blood in a red-top tube.

- Indicate the date of the last menstrual period on the laboratory slip.

After

- Apply pressure or a pressure dressing to the venipuncture site.
- Assess the venipuncture site for bleeding.

Abnormal findings

Increased levels

Pregnancy
Adrenal neoplasms
Ovarian neoplasms

Decreased levels

Amenorrhea
Fetal death
Threatened abortion
Toxemia of pregnancy

Notes

P

prostate-specific antigen (PSA)

Type of test Blood

Normal findings <4 ng/ml

Test explanation and related physiology

PSA is a glycoprotein (part carbohydrate, part protein) normally found in the cytoplasm of prostatic epithelial cells. This antigen can be detected in all males. However, its level is greatly increased in patients who have prostatic cancer. Although PSA was originally measured by histochemical techniques, radioimmunoassay (RIA) techniques have recently increased its accuracy.

Elevated PSA levels are associated with prostate cancer. The higher the levels, the greater is the tumor burden. Further, the PSA assay is a sensitive test for monitoring response to therapy. Successful surgery, radiation, or hormone therapy is associated with a marked reduction in the PSA blood level. Subsequent significant elevation in PSA indicates the recurrence of prostatic cancer.

PSA is more sensitive and specific than other prostatic tumor markers, such as prostatic acid phosphatase (PAP, see p. 539). Also, PSA is more accurate than PAP in monitoring response and recurrence of tumor after therapy. PSA (and PAP) levels may also be elevated in patients with benign prostatic hypertrophy and prostatitis.

Procedure and patient care

Before

- Explain the procedure to the patient.
- Tell the patient that no fasting is required.

During

- Collect approximately 5 ml of blood in a red-top tube.

After

- Apply pressure or a pressure dressing to the venipuncture site.
- Observe the venipuncture site for bleeding.

Abnormal findings
Increased levels

Prostate cancer
Benign prostatic hypertrophy
Prostatitis

Notes

---

protein, blood (Albumin, blood; Serum albumin; Serum globulin; Total protein)

Type of test Blood

Normal findings

Adult/elderly
    Total protein: 6-8 g/dl
    Albumin: 3.2-4.5 g/dl
    Globulin: 2.3-3.4 g/dl
Total protein
    Premature infant: 4.2-7.6 g/dl
    Newborn: 4.6-7.4 g/dl
    Infant: 6.0-6.7 g/dl
    Child: 6.2-8.0 g/dl
Albumin
    Premature infant: 3.0-4.2 g/dl
    Newborn: 3.5-5.4 g/dl
    Infant: 4.4-5.4 g/dl
    Child: 4.0-5.9 g/dl

Test explanation and related physiology

Proteins are constituents of muscle, enzymes, hormones, transport vehicles, hemoglobin, and several other key functional and structural entities within the body. Proteins are the most significant component contributing to the osmotic pressure within the vascular space. This osmotic pressure serves to keep the fluid within the vascular space and thereby minimizes extravasation of fluid.

Albumin and globulin constitute most of the protein within the body and are measured in the total protein. *Albumin* is a protein that is formed within the liver. This makes up approximately 60% of the total protein. The major purpose of albumin within the blood is to maintain colloidal osmotic pressure. Further, albumin transports important blood constituents such as drugs, hormones, and enzymes. *Globulins* are the key building block of antibodies. Their role in maintaining osmotic pressure is far less than that of albumin. Globulins, to a lesser degree, also act as transport vehicles. Both albumin and globulins can be measured separately.

Albumin is synthesized within the liver and is therefore a

measure of hepatocyte function. When disease affects the liver cell, the hepatocyte loses its ability to synthesize albumin. The serum albumin level is greatly decreased. However, because the half-life of albumin is 12 to 18 days, severe impairment of hepatic albumin synthesis may not be recognized until after that period.

Serum albumin and globulin are also measures of nutrition. Malnourished patients have a greatly decreased level of serum proteins. Also, patients who have protein-losing enteropathies and uropathies have low levels of protein despite normal synthesis.

In some diseases, albumin is selectively diminished and globulins are normal or increased to maintain a normal total protein level. For example, in collagen vascular diseases (e.g., lupus erythematosus), capillary permeability is increased. Albumin, a molecule much smaller than globulin, is selectively lost into the extravascular space. Another group of diseases similarly associated with low albumin, high globulin, and normal total protein levels is chronic liver diseases. In these diseases the liver cannot produce albumin, but globulin is adequately made in the reticuloendothelial system. In both these types of diseases the albumin level is low but the total protein level is normal because of increased globulin levels. These changes, however, can be detected if one measures the albumin/globulin ratio. Normally, this ratio exceeds 1.0. The diseases just described that selectively affect albumin levels are associated with lesser ratios.

Interfering factors

- Drugs that may cause increased protein levels include anabolic steroids, androgens, corticosteroids, dextran, growth hormone, insulin, phenazopyridine, and progesterone.
- Drugs that may cause decreased protein levels include ammonium ions, estrogens, hepatotoxic drugs, and oral contraceptives.

Procedure and patient care
Before

- Explain the procedure to the patient.
- Tell the patient that no fasting is usually required.

During

- Collect approximately 5 to 7 ml of blood in a red-top tube.

After

- Apply pressure or a pressure dressing to venipuncture site.
- Observe the venipuncture site for bleeding. Patients with liver dysfunction often have prolonged clotting times.

Abnormal findings
Increased albumin levels

Hemoconcentration

Decreased albumin levels

Liver disease (e.g., hepatitis, extensive metastatic tumor, cirrhosis, hepatocellular necrosis)
Protein-losing enteropathies (e.g., malabsorption syndromes such as Crohn's disease, sprue, Whipple's disease)
Protein-losing nephropathies (e.g., nephrotic syndrome, glomerulonephritis)
Third-space losses (e.g., ascites, third-degree burns)
Malnutrition
Protein dilution secondary to excessive IV fluids
Increased capillary permeability (e.g., collagen vascular diseases such as lupus erythematosus)

Increased globulin levels

Immunologic tumors (e.g., multiple myeloma)

Decreased globulin levels

Malnutrition
Immunologic deficiencies

Increased total protein levels

Hemoconcentration

Decreased total protein levels

See "Decreased albumin levels."

Notes

protein, urine (Albumin, urine; Urine for protein; Urine for albumin)

Type of test Urine

Normal findings
None or up to 8 mg/dl
50-80 mg/24 hr (at rest)
<250 mg/24 hr after strenuous exercise

Test explanation and related physiology

   The urine is evaluated for protein as part of the routine urinalysis. *Proteinuria* is a sensitive indicator of kidney dysfunction. Normally, protein is not present in the urine because the spaces in the normal glomerular filtrate membrane are too small to allow its passage. If, as in glomerulonephritis, the glomerular membrane is injured, the spaces become much larger and protein is allowed to seep out into the filtrate and then into the urine. If this persists at a significant rate, the patient can become hypoproteinemic because of the severe protein loss through the kidneys. This decreases the normal capillary oncotic pressure that holds fluid within the vasculature and causes severe interstitial edema. The combination of proteinuria and edema is known as the *nephrotic syndrome*.

   Proteinuria is probably the most important indicator of renal disease. The urine of all pregnant women is routinely checked for proteinuria, which can be an indicator of preeclampsia. In addition to screening for nephrotic syndrome, urinary protein also screens for complications of diabetes mellitus, glomerulonephritis, amyloidosis, and multiple myeloma.

Interfering factors

- A transient proteinuria may be associated with severe emotional stress, excess exercise, and cold baths.
- Radiopaque contrast media received within the last 3 days may cause false positive results.
- Urine contaminated with vaginal secretions may cause proteinuria.
- Drugs that may cause increased protein levels include ac-

etazolamide, aminoglycosides, amphotericin B, cephalosporins, colistin, griseofulvin, lithium, methicillin, nafcillin, nephrotoxic drugs (e.g., arsenicols, gold salts), oxacillin, penicillamine, penicillin G, phenazopyridine, poly-
mixin B, salicylates, sulfonamides, tolbutamide, and
viomycin.

Procedure and patient care
Before

- Explain the procedure to the patient.
- Tell the patient that no fasting is required.

During

- Collect the first-voided morning urine specimen.
- If indicated, collect a 24-hour urine specimen (see p. 325).

After

- Transport the specimen to the laboratory within 2 hours of collection.
- Mark the container with the date and time of collection.
- If the specimen will not be analyzed immediately, refrigerate it.
- Note that a positive screening test for protein may be confirmed by a 24-hour urine collection (see p. 325).

   1. Fluids are permitted during the 24-hour collection.
   2. The 24-hour urine collection should be refrigerated or preserved with formalin.

Abnormal findings
Increased levels

Nephrotic syndrome
Diabetes mellitus
Multiple myeloma
Preeclampsia
Glomerulonephritis
Congestive heart failure
Malignant hypertension
Polycystic disease
Diabetic glomerulosclerosis

Amyloidosis
Lupus erythematosus
Goodpasture's syndrome
Renal vein thrombosis
Heavy metal poisoning
Galactosemia
Bacterial pyelonephritis
Nephrotoxic drug therapy
Bladder tumors

Notes

protein electrophoresis

Type of test Blood

Normal findings

Total protein: 6-8 g/dl
Albumin: 3.2-4.5 g/dl
Alpha$_1$ globulin: 0.1-0.4 g/dl
Alpha$_2$ globulin: 0.5-1.0 g/dl
Beta globulin: 0.7-1.2 g/dl

Test explanation and related physiology

Total serum protein is a combination of albumin and globulins. *Albumin* is a small protein molecule that is most important in maintaining the oncotic pressure (the pressure that keeps water within the vascular space) of plasma. Albumin also acts as a carrier protein for drugs and hormones. The second type of protein in the blood, *globulins,* are larger molecules and are subclassified into three main groups: alpha, beta, and gamma. *Alpha$_1$ globulins* include alpha antitrypsin and thyroid-binding globulin. *Alpha$_2$ globulins* include serum haptoglobins (bind hemoglobin during hemolysis), ceruloplasmin (carrier for copper), prothrombin, and cholinesterase (an enzyme used in the catabolism of acetylcholine). *Beta$_1$ globulins* include lipoproteins, transferrin, plasminogen, and complement proteins. *Beta$_2$ globulins* include fibrinogen. *Gammaglobulins* are the immune globulins (antibodies) (see p. 427).

Serum protein electrophoresis can separate the various components of blood protein and quantify them according to their electrical charge. Several well-established electrophoretic patterns have been identified and can be associated with specific diseases.

Interfering factors

- Drugs that may alter normal serum electrophoretic patterns include aspirin, bicarbonates, chlorpromazine, corticosteroids, isoniazid, neomycin, phenacemide, salicylates, sulfonamides, and tolbutamide.

P

Procedure and patient care
Before

- Explain the procedure to the patient.
- Tell the patient that no fasting or preparation is required.

During

- Collect approximately 7 to 10 ml of venous blood in a red-top tube.
- Indicate on the laboratory slip any drugs that can affect test results.

After

- Apply pressure or a pressure dressing to the venipuncture site.
- Observe the venipuncture site for bleeding.

Abnormal findings
Decreased albumin levels

Malnutrition
Nephrotic syndrome
Gastrointestinal protein-losing enteropathies

Increased alpha$_1$ globulin levels

Chronic inflammatory disease
Malignancy

Decreased alpha$_1$ globulin levels

Juvenile pulmonary emphysema

Increased alpha$_2$ globulin levels

Nephrotic syndrome
Acute inflammation

Decreased alpha$_2$ globulin levels

Hemolysis

Increased beta$_1$ globulin levels

Lipoprotein disorders

Decreased beta$_1$ globulin levels

Malnutrition
Hypoprotein disorders

Decreased beta$_2$ globulin levels

Consumptive coagulopathy
Disseminated intravascular coagulation (DIC)
Congenital coagulation disorders

Increased gammaglobulin levels

Multiple myeloma
Chronic inflammatory diseases
Malignancy
Hyperimmunization
Dysproteinemias
Acute infection

Notes

prothrombin time (PT, Pro-time)

Type of test Blood

Normal findings
11-12.5 seconds; 85%-100%
Full anticoagulant therapy: 1½-2 times control value; 20%-30%

>20 seconds
Full anticoagulant therapy: >3 times control value

Test explanation and related physiology

The PT is used to evaluate the adequacy of the extrinsic system and common pathway in the clotting mechanism. The PT measures the clotting ability of factors I (fibrinogen), II (prothrombin), V, VII, and X. When these clotting factors exist in deficient quantities, the PT is prolonged. Many diseases and drugs are associated with decreased levels of these factors. These include:

1. *Hepatocellular liver disease* (e.g., cirrhosis, hepatitis, neoplastic invasive processes). Factors I, II, V, VII, IX, and X are produced in the liver. With severe hepatocellular dysfunction, synthesis of these factors will not occur, and serum concentration of these factors will be decreased. Even a small decrease in factor VII will result in marked prolongation of the PT.

2. *Obstructive biliary disease* (e.g., bile duct obstruction secondary to tumor or gallstones or intrahepatic cholestasis secondary to sepsis or drugs). As a result of the biliary obstruction, the bile necessary for fat absorption fails to enter the gut, and fat malabsorption results. Vitamins A, D, E, and K are fat soluble and are also not absorbed. Because the synthesis of factors II, VII, IX, and X depends on vitamin K, these factors will not be adequately produced, and serum concentrations will fall. Factor VII is the first to decrease and will result in prolongation of PT.

Parenchymal (hepatocellular) liver disease can be differentiated from obstructive biliary disease by determination of the patient's response to parenteral vitamin K administration. If the PT returns to normal after 3 days of vitamin K administration (10 mg, IM, twice a day), one can safely assume that the patient has obstructive biliary disease that is causing vitamin K malabsorption. If, on the other hand, the PT does not return to normal with the vitamin K injections, one can assume that severe hepatocellular disease exists and that the liver cells are incapable of synthesizing the clotting factors no matter how much vitamin K is available.

3. *Coumarin ingestion.* The coumarin derivatives, dicumarol and warfarin (Coumadin, Panwarfin) are used to prevent coagulation in patients with thromboembolic disease (e.g., pulmonary embolism, thrombophlebitis, arterial embolism). These drugs interfere with the production of vitamin K–dependent clotting factors, which results in a prolongation of PT, as already described. The adequacy of coumarin therapy can be monitored by following the patient's PT. Appropriate coumarin therapy for full anticoagulation should prolong the PT by one and one-half to two times the control value (or 20% to 30% of the normal value if percentages are used).

Coumarin derivatives are slow acting, but their action may persist for 7 to 14 days after discontinuation of the drug. The action of a coumarin drug can be reversed in 12 to 24 hours by the parenteral administration of vitamin K (phytonadione) given very slowly. The action of coumarin drugs can be enhanced by drugs such as aspirin, quinidine, sulfa, and indomethacin. Barbiturates, chloral hydrate, and oral contraceptives cause increased coumarin drug binding and therefore may decrease the effects of binding coumarin drugs.

■ ■ ■

PT test results are usually given in seconds along with a control value. The control value usually varies somewhat from day to day because the reagents used may vary. The patient's PT should be about equal to the control value. Some laboratories report PT values as percentages of normal activity, since the patient's results are compared with a curve representing normal clotting time. Normally the patient's PT is 85% to 100%.

Interfering factors

- Alcohol intake can increase PT levels.
- A high-fat diet may decrease PT levels.
- Drugs that may cause increased levels include allopurinol, aminosalicylic acid, barbiturates, beta lactam antibiotics, chloral hydrate, cephalothins, chloramphenicol, chlorpromazine (Thorazine), cholestyramine, cimetidine, clofibrate, colestipol, ethyl alcohol, glucagon, heparin, methyldopa (Aldomet), neomycin, oral anticoagulants, propylthiouracil, quinidine, quinine, salicylates, and sulfonamides.
- Drugs that may cause decreased levels include anabolic steroids, barbiturates, chloral hydrate, digitalis, diphenhydramine (Benadryl), estrogens, griseofulvin, oral contraceptives, and vitamin K.

Procedure and patient care

Before

- Explain the procedure to the patient.
- Tell the patient that no fasting is required.
- If the patient is receiving warfarin, obtain the blood specimen before the patient is given the daily dose of warfarin. The daily dose may be increased, decreased, or kept the same depending on the PT test results for that day.

During

- Collect approximately 5 to 7 ml of venous blood in a blue-top tube.
- List on the laboratory slip any drugs that can affect test results.

After

- Apply pressure or a pressure dressing to the venipuncture site.
- Assess the venipuncture site for bleeding. Remember, hemostasis will be delayed if the patient is taking warfarin or if the patient has any coagulopathies.
- If the PT is greatly prolonged, evaluate the patient for bleeding tendencies; that is, check for blood in the urine and all excretions and assess the patient for bruises, petechiae, and low back pain.
- If severe bleeding occurs, the anticoagulant effect of war-

farin can be reversed by the slow parenteral administration of vitamin K (phytonadione).
- Because of drug interactions, instruct the patient not to take any medication unless specifically ordered by the physician.

Abnormal findings
Increased levels

Cirrhosis
Hepatitis
Vitamin K deficiency
Salicylate intoxication

Bile duct obstruction
Coumarin ingestion
Disseminated intravascular
  coagulation (DIC)

Notes

pulmonary angiography (Pulmonary arteriography, Bronchial angiography)

Type of test X-ray with contrast dye

Normal findings Normal pulmonary vasculature

Test explanation and related physiology

Through an injection of a radiographic contrast material into the pulmonary arteries, pulmonary angiography permits visualization of the pulmonary vasculature. Angiography is used to detect pulmonary embolism and a variety of congenital and acquired lesions of the pulmonary vessels.

When pulmonary embolism is suspected, lung scanning should be performed first. If the lung scan is normal, pulmonary embolism is ruled out. However, if the scan is equivocal, the diagnosis of pulmonary embolism is questionable because pathologic parenchymal processes (e.g., emphysema, pneumonia) can also cause abnormalities on the lung scan. Definitive diagnosis for pulmonary embolism may require pulmonary angiography. This may be especially important in elderly patients and patients with peptic ulcers, since the anticoagulant treatment for pulmonary embolism may be associated with significant risks of cerebral or gastrointestinal bleeding. Also, in rare instances, pulmonary embolectomy rather than anticoagulation is considered critical for patient survival. In these cases the angiographic location of the clot is important.

Bronchial angiography is now being done in some facilities to identify bleeding sites in the lungs. For this procedure, catheters are placed transarterially into the orifice of bronchial arteries. Radiopaque material is then injected and the arteries are visualized. If a bleeding site is identified, the site can be injected with a sclerosing agent to prevent further bleeding.

Contraindications

- Patients with allergies to shellfish or iodinated dye
- Patients who are pregnant
- Patients with bleeding disorders

Potential complications

- Allergic reaction to iodinated dye
  Allergic reactions may vary from mild flushing, itching, and urticaria to severe, life-threatening anaphylaxis (evidenced by respiratory distress, drop in blood pressure, shock). In the unusual event of anaphylaxis the patient may be treated with diphenhydramine (Benadryl), steroids, and epinephrine. Oxygen and endotracheal equipment should be immediately available.
- Cardiac arrhythmia (dysrhythmia)
  Premature ventricular contractions (PVCs) during right-sided heart catheterization may lead to ventricular tachycardia and ventricular fibrillation.

Procedure and patient care

Before

- Explain the procedure to the patient.
- Ensure that written and informed consent for this procedure is obtained.
- Inform the patient that a warm flush will be felt when the dye is injected.
- Check the patient for allergies to iodinated dyes and shellfish.
- Inform the radiologist if an allergy to iodine is suspected. The radiologist may prescribe a Benadryl and steroid preparation to be administered before the test. Usually a hypoallergic, non-ionic contrast will be used during the test.
- Determine if the patient has ventricular arrhythmias (dysrhythmias).
- Keep the patient NPO after midnight on the day of the test.
- Administer preprocedural medications as ordered. Atropine is given to decrease secretions. Meperidine is used for sedation and relaxation.

During

- Note the following procedural steps:
  1. The patient is placed on an x-ray table in the supine position.
  2. Electrocardiographic electrodes are attached for cardiac monitoring.

P

3. The catheter is placed into the femoral vein and passed into the inferior vena cava.
4. With fluoroscopic visualization, the catheter is advanced to the right atrium and the right ventricle.
5. The catheter is manipulated into the main pulmonary artery, where the dye is injected.
6. X-ray films of the chest are immediately taken in timed sequence. This allows all vessels visualized by the injection to be photographed. If filling defects are seen in the contrast-filled vessels, pulmonary emboli are present.

- Note that this test is performed by a physician in approximately 1 hour.
- During injection of dye, remind the patient that he or she will feel a burning sensation and flush throughout the body.

After

- Observe the catheter insertion site for inflammation, hemorrhage, and hematoma.
- Evaluate the patient's pulses on the affected extremity.
- Assess the patient's vital signs for evidence of bleeding (decreased blood pressure, increased pulse).
- Apply cold compresses to the puncture site if needed to reduce swelling or discomfort.
- Inform the patient that coughing may occur after this study.
- Educate the patient regarding the need for bed rest for 12 to 24 hours after the test.
- Evaluate the patient for delayed reaction to the dye (dyspnea, rashes, tachycardia, hives). This usually occurs within 2 to 6 hours after the test. Treat with antihistamines or steroids.

Abnormal findings

Pulmonary embolism
Congenital and acquired lesions of the pulmonary vessels (e.g., aneurysms)
Tumors

Notes

pulmonary function tests (PFT)

Type of test Airflow assessment

Normal findings Vary with patient's age, sex, height, and weight

Test explanation and related physiology

Pulmonary function tests are performed to detect abnormalities in respiratory function and to determine the extent of any pulmonary abnormality. The main reasons for pulmonary function include the following:

1. Preoperative evaluation of the lungs and pulmonary reserve. When planned thoracic surgery will result in loss of functional pulmonary tissue, as in lobectomy (removal of part of a lung) or pneumonectomy (removal of an entire lung), a significant risk of pulmonary failure exists if preoperative pulmonary function is already severely compromised by other diseases, such as chronic obstructive pulmonary disease (COPD).
2. Evaluation of response to bronchodilator therapy. Some patients with COPD have a spastic component to their obstructive disease that may respond to long-term use of bronchodilators. Pulmonary function studies performed before and after the use of bronchodilators will identify that group of patients.
3. Differentiation between restrictive and obstructive forms of chronic pulmonary disease. *Restrictive* defects (e.g., pulmonary fibrosis, tumors, chest wall trauma) occur when ventilation is disturbed by a limitation in chest expansion. Inspiration is primarily affected. *Obstructive* defects (e.g., emphysema, bronchitis, asthma) occur when ventilation is disturbed by an increase in airway resistance. Expiration is primarily affected.
4. Determination of the diffusing capacity of the lungs (D_L). Rates are based on the difference in concentration of gases in inspired and expired air.
5. Performance of inhalation tests in patients with inhalant allergies

Pulmonary function tests routinely include determination of the following:

1. Forced vital capacity (FVC)
2. Forced expiratory volume in 1 second (FEV_1)
3. Maximal midexpiratory flow (MMEF)
4. Maximal voluntary ventilation (MVV)
5. Arterial blood gases (see p. 104).

Forced vital capacity. FVC is the amount of air that can be forcefully expelled from a maximally inflated lung position. This volume is decreased below the expected value in obstructive and restrictive pulmonary diseases.

Force expiratory volume in 1 second. FEV_1 is the volume of air expelled during the first second of the FVC. In patients with obstructive disease, airways are narrowed and resistance to flow is high. Therefore not as much air can be expelled in 1 second, and FEV_1 will be reduced below the predicted value. In restrictive lung disease, FEV_1 is decreased not because of airway resistance, but because the amount of air originally inhaled is less. One should therefore measure the FEV_1/FVC ratio. A normal value of 80% is found in patients with restrictive lung disease. In obstructive lung disease this ratio is considerably less than 80%. The FEV_1 measurement will reliably improve with bronchodilator therapy if a spastic component to an obstructive disease exists.

Maximal midexpiratory flow. MMEF is the maximal rate of air flow through the pulmonary tree during forced expiration. This is also called *forced midexpiratory flow.* This test is independent of the patient's effort or cooperation. MMEF is reduced below expected value in obstructive diseases and normal in restrictive diseases.

Maximal volume ventilation. MVV, formerly called "maximal breathing capacity," is the maximal volume of air that the patient can breathe in and out during 1 minute. MVV is decreased below the expected value in both restrictive and obstructive pulmonary disease.

A comprehensive pulmonary functions study may also include evaluation of the following lung volumes and lung capacities, many of which are illustrated in Figure 9.

Tidal volume. TV or VT is the volume of air inspired and expired with each normal respiration.

Inspiratory reserve volume. IRV is the maximal volume of air that can be inspired from the end of a normal inspiration.

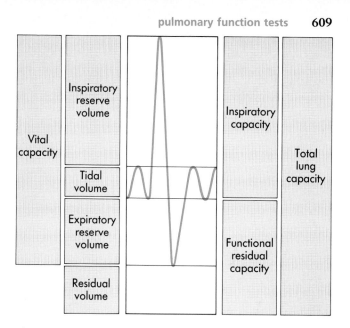

Figure 9 Relationship of lung volumes and capacities.

It represents forced inspiration over and beyond the tidal volume.

Expiratory reserve volume. ERV is the maximal volume of air that can be exhaled after a normal expiration.

Residual volume. RV is the volume of air remaining in the lungs following forced expiration.

Inspiratory capacity. IC is the maximal amount of air that can be inspired after a normal expiration (IC = TV + IRV).

Functional residual volume. FRV is the amount of air left in the lungs after a normal expiration (FRV = ERV + RV).

Vital capacity. VC is the maximal amount of air that can be expired after a maximal inspiration (VC = TV + IRV + ERV).

Total lung capacity. TLC is the volume to which the lungs can be expanded with the greatest inspiratory effort (TLC = TV + IRV + ERV + RV).

Minute volume. MV, sometimes called *minute ventilation,* is the volume of air inhaled and exhaled per minute.

Dead space. Dead space is the part of the tidal volume that does not participate in alveolar gas exchange.

Contraindications

- Patients who are in pain because of inability to cooperate by deep inspiration and expiration
- Patients who are unable to cooperate because of age or mental incapability

Procedure and patient care

Before

- Explain the test to the patient.
- Inform the patient that cooperation is necessary to obtain accurate results.
- Instruct the patient not to use any bronchodilators or to smoke for 6 hours before this test (if requested by physician).
- Withhold the use of small-dose meter inhalers and aerosol therapy before this study.
- Measure and record the patient's height and weight before this study to determine the predicted values.
- List on the laboratory slip any medications the patient is taking.

During

- Note the following procedural steps:

  1. The unsedated patient is taken to pulmonary function laboratory.
  2. The patient breathes into a sterile cylinder, which is connected to a computerized machine to measure and record the desired values.
  3. The patient is asked to inhale as deeply as possible and then to exhale as much air as possible.
  4. From this the machine computes FVC, FEV_1, FEV_1/FVC, and MMEF.
  5. The patient is asked to breathe in and out as deeply and frequently as possible for 15 seconds. The total volume breathed is recorded and multiplied by 4 to obtain the MVV.

Diffusing capacity of the lung
  1. D_L for any gas can be measured as part of pulmonary function studies. The D_L measures the diffusion of gases per minute across the alveolocapillary membrane. Most laboratories employ carbon monoxide (CO) for measuring D_L because CO has a great af-

finity for hemoglobin and only a small concentration of CO is needed in clinical tests. Because of this, the major limiting factor to the transfer of the gas is its rate of diffusion across the alveolocapillary membrane and not pulmonary blood flow.

2. The D_L of CO is usually measured by having the patient inhale a CO mixture.

3. $D_L CO$ is calculated with an analysis of the amount of CO exhaled compared with the amount inhaled. This value is abnormal in patients with adult respiratory distress syndrome (ARDS), congestive heart failure (CHF), collagen vascular disease, Goodpasture's syndrome, and so on.

Inhalation tests

1. These tests may also be performed during pulmonary function studies to establish a cause-and-effect relationship in some patients with inhalant allergies.

2. The *methacholine* or *histamine challenge test* is typically used to detect the presence of hyperactive airway diseases. This test would not be indicated for a patient known to have asthma. A positive methacholine challenge is a greater than 20% reduction in the patient's FEV_1.

3. Care is taken during this challenge test to reverse any severe bronchospasm with prompt administration of an inhalant bronchodilator (e.g., isoproterenol).

After

- Note that occasionally patients with severe respiratory problems are exhausted after the testing and will need rest.

Abnormal findings

Pulmonary fibrosis
Tumors
Chest wall trauma
Emphysema
Chronic bronchitis
Asthma
Inhalant allergy
Interstitial fibrosis
   following pneumonectomy

Bronchiectasis
Airway infections
Pneumonia
Neuromuscular diseases
Scleroderma
Collagen vascular lung diseases

Notes

radioactive iodine uptake (RAIU, Iodine uptake test,[131]I uptake test)

Type of test Nuclear scan

Normal findings

2 hours: 4%-12% absorbed
6 hours: 6%-15% absorbed
24 hours: 8%-30% absorbed

Test explanation and related physiology

The RAIU is a useful guide to thyroid function. This test is based on the ability of the thyroid gland to trap and retain iodine. In this procedure a known quantity of radioactive iodine is given orally to the patient. A gamma ray detector placed over the thyroid gland determines the quantity or percentage of radioactive iodine taken up by the gland over a specific time.

Performing the measurement at different times after the iodine is given allows several aspects of thyroid function to be evaluated. Uptake determination at 30 minutes reflects the ability of the thyroid gland to trap iodine. When uptake is measured at 6 hours, the ability of the thyroid gland to bind iodine organically is evaluated. Maximal iodine uptake is observed within 24 hours. Determinations of iodine uptake after this time measure the ability of the gland to release iodine in the form of thyroid hormone.

Increased thyroid uptake of radioactive iodine is seen in patients with hyperthyroid states. Decreased uptake occurs in patients with hypothyroid conditions. The RAIU tends to be more accurate for diagnosing hyperthyroidism than hypothyroidism.

Contraindications

- Patients who are allergic to iodine or shellfish
- Patients who are pregnant

Potential complication

- Radioactive exposure to the thyroid gland
  This is minimized when ^{123}I or ^{125}I is used instead of ^{131}I.

Interfering factors

- In patients taking exogenous iodine preparations, the iodine will increase the body's iodine pool and decrease uptake by the thyroid gland.
- Iodine-deficient patients will trap increased amounts of iodine, resulting in increased uptake.
- Rebound thyroid stimulation after discontinuation of suppressive doses of thyroid medications results in falsely elevated RAIU levels.
- Recent x-ray studies using iodinated contrast material will decrease uptake.
- Diarrhea caused by decreased absorption of tracer doses in the gastrointestinal tract results in decreased RAIU levels.
- Drugs that may cause increased levels include barbiturates, estrogen, lithium, phenothiazines, and thyroid-stimulating hormone (TSH).
- Drugs that may cause decreased levels include adrenocorticotropic hormone (ACTH), antihistamines, corticosteroids, Lugol's solution, nitrates, saturated solution of potassium iodine (SSKI), thyroid and antithyroid drugs, and tolbutamide.

Procedure and patient care

Before

- Explain the procedure to the patient.
- Assess the patient for allergies to iodine.
- Note that some laboratories prefer to keep the patient NPO after midnight on the day of the test.
- Restrict iodine and thyroid preparations 1 week before testing, if indicated by the institution.
- Evaluate the patient's drug history for interfering factors.

During

- Note the following procedural steps:

  1. A tasteless, dose of radioactive iodine, usually ^{123}I, is given by mouth to the patient. If RAIU is to be determined at 2 hours, the iodine is administered intravenously.
  2. The patient is given written instructions regarding the times to return to the radiology department for scanning.

3. The patient is informed that he or she may usually eat 45 minutes to 1 hour after the dose of iodine has been given.
4. For the scanning, the patient is asked to lie in a supine position.
5. A gamma ray detector is placed over the patient's thyroid gland to determine RAIU.

- List on the laboratory slip the x-ray studies and drugs the patient has received that could affect test results.
- Note that this test is performed in approximately 30 minutes by a radiologic technologist.
- Inform the patient that this test is not uncomfortable.

After

- Inform the patient that the dose of radioactive iodine used in this test is minute and therefore harmless. Tell him or her that no isolation or special urine precautions are necessary.

Abnormal findings

Increased levels

Hyperthyroidism

Decreased levels

Hypothyroidism

Notes

red blood cells and casts (RBCs and casts)

Type of test Urine

Normal findings

RBCs: up to two
RBC casts: none

Test explanation and related physiology

During the routine urinalysis the urine is checked for the presence of blood. Any disruption in the blood-urine barrier, whether at the glomerular or the tubular level, will cause RBCs to enter the urine. This is seen in patients with glomerulonephritis, interstitial nephritis, acute tubular necrosis, pyelonephritis, and renal trauma or renal tumor. Pathologic conditions (e.g., tumors, trauma, stones, infection) involving the mucosa of the collecting system will also cause hematuria. This can easily be detected by routine analysis.

Casts are clumps of material or cells. They are formed in the renal collecting tubule and have the shape of the tubule, thus the term *cast*. RBC casts suggest glomerulonephritis, which may exist in patients with subacute bacterial endocarditis, renal infarct, Goodpasture's syndrome, vasculitis, sickling, and malignant hypertension.

Interfering factors

- Strenuous physical exercise may cause RBC casts.
- Traumatic urethral catheterization may result in RBCs in the urine.

Procedure and patient care

Before

- Explain the procedure to the patient.
- Tell the patient that no fasting is required.

During

- Collect the urine specimen in a plastic urine container.
- If the specimen is contaminated by vaginal discharge or bleeding, a "clean-catch" or "midstream" specimen will be needed. This requires meticulous cleansing of the urinary

R

meatus with an iodine preparation to reduce contamination of the specimen by external organisms. Then the cleaning agent must be completely removed, or it will contaminate the specimen. The midstream collection is obtained by:

1. Having the patient begin to urinate in a bedpan, urinal, or toilet and then stop urinating (This washes the urine out of the distal urethra.)
2. Correctly positioning sterile urine container, into which the patient voids 3 to 4 ounces of urine
3. Capping the container
4. Allowing the patient to finish voiding

After

- Send the urine specimen promptly to the laboratory.
- Note that urine should be checked for casts when it is fresh.

Abnormal findings

Increased RBCs

Gomerulonephritis
Interstitial nephritis
Acute tubular necrosis
Pyelonephritis
Renal trauma
Renal tumor
Cystitis
Prostatitis
Traumatic bladder catheterization

Increased red cell casts

Glomerulonephritis
Subacute bacterial endocarditis
Renal infarct
Goodpasture's syndrome
Vasculitis
Sickling
Malignant hypertension
Systemic lupus erythematosus

Notes

red blood cell count (RBC count, Erythrocyte count)

Type of test Blood

Normal findings

Adult/elderly:
  male, 4.7-6.1 million/mm³
  female, 4.2-5.4 million/mm³
Infant/child: 3.8-5.5 million/mm³
Newborn: 4.8-7.1 million/mm³

Test explanation and related physiology

This test is a count of the number of circulating RBCs in 1 mm³ of peripheral venous blood. The RBC is routinely performed as part of a complete blood count (CBC). Packed within each RBC are molecules of hemoglobin that permit the transport and exchange of oxygen and carbon dioxide. Normally the RBCs exist in the peripheral blood for approximately 120 days. Toward the end of the RBC's life, the cell membrane becomes less pliable; the aged RBC is then hemolyzed and extracted from the circulation by the spleen. Abnormal RBCs have a shorter life span and are extracted earlier. Intravascular RBC trauma, such as that caused by artificial heart valves or peripheral vascular atherosclerotic plaques, also shortens the RBC's life. An enlarged spleen, such as that caused by portal hypertension or leukemia, may inappropriately destroy and remove normal RBCs from the circulation.

Normal RBC values vary according to sex and age. When the value is decreased by more than 10% of the expected normal value, the patient is said to be anemic. Low RBC values are caused by many factors, including:

1. Hemorrhage (as in gastrointestinal bleeding or trauma)
2. Hemolysis (as in glucose-6-phospate dehydrogenase deficiency, spherocytosis, or secondary splenomegaly)
3. Dietary deficiency (as of iron or vitamin B_{12})
4. Genetic aberrations (as in sickle cell anemia or thalassemia)
5. Drug ingestion (as of chloramphenicol, hydantoins, or quinidine)

R

6. Marrow failure (as in fibrosis, leukemia, or antineoplastic chemotherapy)
7. Chronic illness (as in tumor or sepsis)
8. Other organ failure (as in renal disease)

RBC counts greater than normal can be physiologically induced as a result of the body's requirements for greater oxygen-carrying capacity (e.g., at high altitudes). Diseases that produce chronic anoxia (e.g., congenital heart disease) also provoke this physiologic increase in RBCs. Polycythemia vera is a neoplastic condition involving uncontrolled production of RBCs.

Interfering factors

- Normal decreases are seen in the RBC during pregnancy because of normal body fluid increases and dilution of the RBCs.
- Persons living at high altitudes have increased RBCs.
- Dehydration, which results in hemoconcentration, can obscure test interpretation.
- Drugs that may cause increased RBC levels include gentamicin and methyldopa.
- Drugs that may cause decreased RBC levels include chloramphenicol, hydantoins, and quinidine.

Procedure and patient care

Before

- Explain the procedure to the patient.
- Tell the patient that no fasting is required.

During

- Collect approximately 5 to 7 ml of blood in a lavender-top tube.
- Thoroughly mix the blood with the anticoagulant by tilting the tube.
- Avoid hemolysis.
- List on the laboratory slip any drugs or other patient factors that can affect RBC levels.

After

- Apply pressure or a pressure dressing to the venipuncture site.
- Observe the venipuncture site for bleeding.

Abnormal findings
Increased levels

High altitude
Congenital heart disease
Polycythemia vera
Dehydration/
  hemoconcentration
Cor pulmonale
Pulmonary fibrosis
Severe diarrhea

Decreased levels

Hemorrhage
Hemolysis
Anemias
Hodgkin's disease
Hemoglobinopathy
Fibrosis
Leukemia
Antineoplastic chemother-
  apy
Chronic illness
Organ failure (e.g., renal)
Overhydration
Multiple myeloma
Pernicious anemia
Rheumatic diseases
Subacute endocarditis
Pregnancy
Dietary deficiencies

Notes

R

red blood cell indices (RBC indexes, MCV, MCH, MCHC, Blood indices, Erythrocyte indices)

Type of test Blood

Normal findings

Mean corpuscular volume (MCV)
Adult/elderly/child: 80-95 μ^3
Newborn: 96-108 μ^3
Mean corpuscular hemoglobin (MCH)
Adult/elderly/child: 27-31 pg
Newborn: 32-34 pg
Mean corpuscular hemoglobin concentration (MCHC)
Adult/elderly/child: 32-36 g/dl (or 32%-36%)
Newborn: 32-33 g/dl (or 32%-33%)

Test explanation and related physiology

The RBC indices provide information about the size (MCV), weight (MCH), and hemoglobin concentration (MCHC) of RBCs. This test is routinely done as part of a complete blood count (CBC). The results of the RBC, hematocrit, and hemoglobin tests are necessary to calculate the RBC indices. When investigating anemia, it is helpful to categorize the anemia according to the RBC indexes, as shown in Table 8. Cell size is indicated by the terms *normocytic, microcytic,* and *macrocytic*. Hemoglobin content is indicated by the terms *normochromic, hypochromic,* and *hyperchromic*. Additional information about the RBC size, shape, color, and intracellular structure is described in the blood smear study (see p. 109).

Mean corpuscular volume The MCV is a measure of the average volume, or size, of a single RBC and is therefore used in classifying anemias. MCV is derived by dividing the hematocrit by the total RBC count. Normal values vary according to age and sex. When the MCV value is increased, the RBC is said to be abnormally large, or *macrocytic*. This is most frequently seen in megaloblastic anemias (e.g., vitamin B_{12} or folic acid deficiency). When the MCV value is decreased, the RBC is said to be abnormally small, or *microcytic*. This is associated with iron deficiency anemia or thalassemia.

TABLE 8 Categorization of anemia according to RBC indexes

Normocytic,[1] normochromic[2] anemia
Iron deficiency (detected early)
Chronic illness (e.g., sepsis, tumor)
Acute blood loss
Aplastic anemia (e.g., chloramphenicol toxicosis)
Acquired hemolytic anemias (e.g., from a prosthetic cardiac valve)

Microcytic,[3] hypochromic[4] anemia
Iron deficiency (detected late)
Thalassemia
Lead poisoning

Microcytic, normochromic anemia
Renal disease (because of the loss of erythropoietin)

Macrocytic,[5] normochromic anemia
Vitamin B_{12} or folic acid deficiency
Hydantoin ingestion
Chemotherapy

---

[1]Normocytic: normal RBC size.
[2]Normochromic: normal color (normal hemoglobin content).
[3]Microcytic: smaller than normal RBC size.
[4]Hypochromic: less than normal color (decreased hemoglobin content).
[5]Macrocytic: larger than normal RBC size.

Mean corpuscular hemoglobin The MCH is a measure of the average amount (weight) of hemoglobin within an RBC. MCH is derived by dividing the total hemoglobin concentration by the number of RBCs. Because macrocytic cells generally have more hemoglobin and microcytic cells generally have less hemoglobin, the causes for these values closely resemble those for the MCV value.

Mean corpuscular hemoglobin concentration The MCHC is a measure of the average concentration or the percentage of hemoglobin within a single RBC. MCHC is derived by dividing the total hemoglobin concentration by the hematocrit. When values are decreased, the cell has a deficiency of hemoglobin and is said to be *hypochromic* (frequently seen in iron deficiency anemia and thalassemia). When values are normal, the anemia is said be *normocytic* (e.g., hemolytic anemia).

Interfering factors

- Abnormal RBC size can affect indices.
- Extremely elevated white blood cell (WBC) counts can affect RBC indices.

Procedure and patient care

Before

- Explain the procedure to the patient.
- Tell the patient that no fasting is required.

During

- Collect approximately 5 to 7 ml of venous blood in a lavender-top tube.
- Avoid hemolysis.
- Transport the specimen to the hematology laboratory, where the blood is passed through automated machines that calculate the RBC indices.

After

- Apply pressure or a pressure dressing to the venipuncture site.
- Assess the venipuncture site for bleeding.

Abnormal findings

Increased MCV	Decreased MCV
Liver diseases	Iron deficiency anemia
Antimetabolite therapy	Thalassemia
Alcoholism	
Pernicious anemia (vitamin B_{12} deficiency)	
Folic acid deficiency	

Increased MCH

Macrocytic anemia

Increased MCHC

Spherocytosis

Decreased MCH

Microcytic anemia
Hypochromic anemia

Decreased MCHC

Iron deficiency anemia
Thalassemia

Notes

R

red blood cell survival study (RBC survival study,
Splenic sequestration study)

Type of test Nuclear scan

Normal findings
Half-life of RBC = 26-30 days
Spleen/liver ratio = 1:1
Spleen/pericardium ratio < 2:1

Test explanation and related physiology

In patients who have hemolytic anemia the RBCs are destroyed and normally sequestered in the spleen. As a result of this ongoing RBC destruction, the RBC life span will be significantly reduced. This reduction in RBC survival indicates that active hemolysis is occurring and is the cause of the patient's anemia.

Although hemolysis can be identified by determination of the catabolic products of hemoglobin (which are increased) or by measuring the level of circulating haptoglobin—the transport protein that binds hemoglobin (which is decreased)—the nuclear determination of RBC life span can provide a semiquantitative measurement of the degree of hemolysis. This quantitation can be best performed by determining the half-life of the RBC within the circulation. This portion of the test is performed by extracting some of the patient's RBCs, labeling them with chromium-51 (^{51}Cr), and reinjecting them into the patient. Subsequent blood levels of ^{51}Cr indicate the half-life of the labeled RBCs.

The second portion of the test is the imaging of the spleen, liver, and pericardium. In patients who have hemolytic anemia associated with abnormal splenic sequestration, the spleen/liver ratio is in excess of 1:1. However, this abnormally high ratio can occur in patients who have splenomegaly caused by a disease other than hemolytic anemia. Therefore, spleen/pericardium ratios are performed; those greater than 2:1 indicate abnormal splenic sequestration of hemolyzed RBCs. A normal spleen/pericardium ratio with an increased spleen/liver ratio indicates splenomegaly.

This second portion of the splenic sequestration study is also helpful in determining which patients with hemolytic anemia will benefit from splenectomy. Patients who have increased splenic sequestration can be expected to improve greatly as a result of splenectomy. Splenic sequestration is eliminated, and RBC blood cell survival is prolonged.

Contraindications

- Patients who are pregnant, because of the risk of fetal damage

Interfering factors

- Factors that can decrease RBC survival include recent RBC transfusion, increased RBC production, active bleeding, high white blood cell (WBC) counts in excess of 25,000, and high platelet counts greater than 500,000.
- Splenomegaly can increase splenic/pericardium ratios.
- Splenic infarctions can decrease splenic/pericardium ratios.

Procedure and patient care

Before

- Explain the procedure to the patient.
- Assure the patient that he or she will not be exposed to large amounts of radioactivity because only tracer doses of the isotope are used.
- Tell the patient that no preparation or sedation is required.
- Notify the nuclear medicine technologist or physician if blood transfusion or hemorrhage has occurred shortly before or during the study.
- Note that usually a hematocrit, WBC count, platelet count, and reticulocyte count are performed before testing.

During

- Note the following procedural steps:
  1. Approximately 20 ml of blood is withdrawn from the patient, and the RBCs are labeled with ^{51}Cr.
  2. The RBCs are immediately reinjected into the patient.
  3. On the first day of testing, 10 ml of blood is withdrawn by a peripheral venipuncture into a red-top tube.
  4. The RBCs are quantitated for ^{51}Cr counts per minute.
  5. Nuclear imaging of the spleen, liver, and pericardium is carried out.

R

6. This process is repeated three times a week for 3 weeks.
7. The peripheral venous blood ^{51}Cr counts are plotted on a graph, and the half-life is determined.
8. The spleen/liver and spleen/pericardium ratios and nuclear counts are determined.

- Note that this test takes place over 2 to 3 weeks. The results are available on the day after the study is completed. The study is performed by a nuclear medicine technologist or physician.
- Tell the patient that no pain or discomfort is associated with this procedure. The patient must lie still during the nuclear imaging portion of the test.

After

- Inform the patient that because only tracer doses of radioisotopes are used, no precautions need to be taken against radioactive exposure.

Abnormal findings
Increased splenic sequestration

Hemolysis
Splenomegaly

Decreased RBC survival

Hemolysis
Hemorrhage
Abnormally increased erythropoiesis

Notes

renal angiography (Renal arteriography)

Type of test X-ray with contrast dye

Normal findings Normal renal vasculature

Test explanation and related physiology

Through the injection of radiopaque contrast material into the renal arteries, renal angiography permits visualization of the large and small renal vasculature. This permits evaluation of blood flow dynamics, demonstration of abnormal blood vessels, and differentiation of avascular renal cysts from hypervascular cancers. Artherosclerotic narrowing (stenosis) of the renal artery is best demonstrated with this study. The angiographic location of the stenotic area is helpful to the vascular surgeon considering repair. Complete transection of the renal artery by blunt or penetrating trauma will be seen as a total vascular obstruction. Highly vascular renal cancers produce a "blush" of contrast material during angiography.

Contraindications

- Patients with allergies to shellfish or iodinated dye
- Patients who are pregnant
- Patients with bleeding disorders

Potential complications

- Allergic reaction to iodinated dye
  Allergic reactions may vary from mild flushing, itching, and urticaria to severe, life-threatening anaphylaxis (evidenced by respiratory distress, drop in blood pressure, shock). In the unusual event of anaphylaxis the patient may be treated with diphenhydramine (Benadryl), steroids, and epinephrine. Oxygen and endotracheal equipment should be on hand for immediate use.
- Hemorrhage from the puncture site used for arterial access
- Arterial embolism from dislodgement of an atherosclerotic plaque
- Infection

R

Interfering factors

- The presence of gas or feces in the gastrointestinal tract may impair clarity of the x-ray films.

Procedure and patient care

Before

- Explain the procedure to the patient.
- Ensure that informed consent is obtained.
- Inform the patient that a warm flush will be felt when the dye is injected.
- Assess the patient for allergies to iodine dye.
- Inform the radiologist if an allergy to iodine is suspected. The radiologist may prescribe a Benadryl and steroid preparation to be administered before the test. Usually a hypoallergic, non-ionic contrast will be used during the test.
- Determine if the patient has been taking anticoagulants.
- Keep the patient NPO after midnight on the day of the test.
- Note that cathartics may be ordered.
- Mark the patient's peripheral pulses with a pen before catheterization. This will permit quicker assessment of the pulses after the procedure.
- Administer the preprocedural medication as ordered.
- Instruct the patient to void before the study, since the dye acts as an osmotic diuretic.
- Inform the patient that bladder distention may cause discomfort during the study.

During

- Note the following procedural steps:
  1. The patient is usually sedated with meperidine and atropine.
  2. In the angiography room, which is located in the radiology department, the patient is placed on an x-ray table in the supine position.
  3. Since access to the renal arteries is usually achieved through the femoral artery, the groin is prepared and draped in a sterile manner.
  4. The angiocatheter is passed into the femoral artery by percutaneous needle stick and advanced into the aorta.
  5. With fluoroscopic visualization, the catheter is manipulated into the renal artery.

6. Dye is injected and x-ray films are taken in timed sequence over several seconds. This allows all portions of the injection to be photographed.
7. Delayed films may be taken to visualize subsequent filling in the renal vein.
8. After the x-ray films are taken, the catheter is removed and a pressure dressing is applied to the puncture site.

- Note that this procedure is usually performed by an angiographer (radiologist) in about 1 hour.
- Remind the patient that during the dye injection he or she may feel an intense burning flush throughout the body but that this is transient and gone in seconds. The only other discomfort is the groin puncture necessary for arterial access.

After

- Observe the arterial puncture site frequently for hematoma, hemorrhage, or absence of pulse.
- Assess the patient's extremities for signs of ischemia (numbness, tingling, pain, absence of peripheral pulses, loss of function).
- Compare the pulses with the preprocedural baseline values.
- Compare the color and temperature of the involved extremity with that of the uninvolved extremity.
- Assess the patient's pulse and vital signs frequently because embolism or bleeding requires immediate intervention.
- Keep the patient on bed rest for 6 to 8 hours to allow for complete sealing of the arterial puncture.
- Apply cold compresses to the puncture site if needed to reduce discomfort or swelling.
- Encourage the patient to drink fluids after the study to prevent dehydration caused by the diuretic action of the dye. Monitor urine output.
- Evaluate the patient for delayed reaction to the dye (dyspnea, rashes, tachycardia, hives). This usually occurs within the first 2 to 6 hours after the test. Treat with antihistamines or steroids.

R

Abnormal findings

Anatomically aberrant blood vessels
Renal cysts
Renal tumors
Atherosclerotic narrowing of the renal artery
Renovascular causes of hypertension

Notes

renal biopsy (Kidney biopsy)

Type of test Microscopic examination of tissue

Normal findings No pathologic conditions

Test explanation and related physiology

Biopsy of the kidney affords microscopic examination of renal tissue. Renal biopsy is performed for the following purposes:

1. To diagnose the cause of renal disease (e.g., poststreptococcal causes, Goodpasture's syndrome, lupus nephritis)
2. To detect primary and metastatic malignancy of the kidney in patients who may not be candidates for surgery
3. To evaluate the degree of rejection that occurs after kidney transplantation, which enables the physician to determine the appropriate dose of immunosuppressive agents

Renal biopsy is most often obtained percutaneously. During this procedure a needle is inserted through the skin and into the kidney to obtain a sample of kidney tissue. The biopsy needle is more accurately placed when guided by ultrasonography or fluoroscopy. These techniques allow more precise localization of the desired kidney tissue.

Occasionally, open renal biopsy is performed. This involves an incision through the flank and dissection to expose the kidney surgically.

Contraindications

- Patients with coagulation disorders because of the risk of excessive bleeding
- Patients with operable kidney tumors, since tumor cells may be disseminated during the procedure
- Patients with hydronephrosis, since the enlarged renal pelvis can be easily entered and cause a persistent urine leak requiring surgical repair
- Patients with urinary tract infections, since the needle insertion may disseminate the active infection throughout the retroperitoneum

Potential complications

- Hemorrhage from the highly vascular renal tissue
- Inadvertent puncture of the liver, lung, bowel, aorta, and inferior vena cava
- Infection when an open biopsy is performed

Procedure and patient care

Before

- Explain the procedure to the patient.
- Ensure that written and informed consent for this procedure is obtained by the physician.
- Keep the patient NPO after midnight on the day of the test in the event that bleeding or inadvertent puncture of an abdominal organ may necessitate surgical intervention.
- Assess the patient's coagulation studies (prothrombin time [PT], partial thromboplastin time [PTT]).
- Check the patient's hemoglobin and hematocrit values.
- Note that the patient may need to be typed and cross-matched for blood in the event of severe hemorrhage requiring transfusions.
- Tell the patient that no sedative is required.
- Note that the needle stick may be done at the bedside.
- If fluoroscopic or ultrasound guidance is to be used, note that the needle stick is performed in the radiology or ultrasonography department.

During

- Note the following procedural steps:

  1. The patient is placed in a prone position with a sandbag or pillow under the abdomen to straighten the spine.
  2. Under sterile conditions the skin overlaying the kidneys is infiltrated with a local anesthetic (lidocaine).
  3. While the patient holds his or her breath to stop kidney motion, the physician inserts the biopsy needle into the kidney and takes a specimen.
  4. After this procedure is completed, the needle is removed and pressure is applied to the site for approximately 20 minutes.

- Note that this procedure is performed by a physician in approximately 10 minutes.
- Tell the patient that this procedure is uncomfortable, but only minimally if enough lidocaine is used.

After

- After the test, apply a pressure dressing.
- Turn the patient on his or her back and keep on bed rest for about 24 hours.
- Check the patient's vital signs, puncture site, and hematocrit values frequently during this 24-hour period.
- Instruct the patient to avoid any activity that increases abdominal venous pressure (e.g., coughing).
- Assess the patient for signs and symptoms of hemorrhage (e.g., decrease in blood pressure, increase in pulse, pallor, backache, flank pain, shoulder pain, lightheadedness).
- Evaluate the patient's abdomen for signs of bowel or liver penetration (e.g., abdominal pain and tenderness, abdominal muscle guarding and rigidity, decreased bowel sounds).
- Inspect all urine specimens for gross hematuria. Usually the patient's urine will contain blood initially, but this will usually not continue after the first 24 hours. Urine samples may be placed in consecutive chronological order to facilitate comparison for evaluation of hematuria. This is referred to as *rack* or *serial* urine samples.
- Encourage the patient to drink large amounts of fluid to prevent clot formation and urine retention.
- Frequently, obtain blood for a hemoglobin and hematocrit determination after the biopsy specimen to assess for active bleeding. One purple-top tube of blood is needed.
- Instruct the patient to avoid, for at least 2 weeks, strenuous exercise, such as heavy lifting, contact sports, horseback riding, or any activity that could cause jolting of the kidney.
- Teach the patient the signs and symptoms of renal hemorrhage and instruct him or her to call the physician if any of these symptoms occur.
- Instruct the patient to report burning on urination or any temperature elevations. These could indicate a urinary tract infection.

Abnormal findings

Renal disease (e.g., poststreptococcal conditions, Goodpasture's syndrome, lupus nephritis)
Primary and metastatic malignancy of the kidney
Rejection of kidney transplant

Notes

renal scanning (Kidney scan, Radiorenography, Renography, Radionuclide renal imaging, Nuclear imaging of the kidney, DMSA renal scan, DTPA renal scan)

Type of test Nuclear scan

Normal findings Normal size, shape, and function of the kidney

Test explanation and related physiology

This nuclear medicine procedure provides visualization of the urinary tract after the IV administration of a radioisotope. The distribution of the radioactive material is scanned or mapped. Scans do not interfere with the normal physiologic process of the kidney. The resultant image (scan) indicates distribution of the radionuclide within the kidney and ureters.

Each radioactive tracer is handled by the kidney in a different manner. For example, technetium-99m (^{99m}Tc) DTPA is excreted by glomerular filtration. ^{99m}Tc DMSA is taken up by the tubular cells and not appreciably excreted. Iodine-131 (^{131}I) is both filtered by the glomerulus and secreted by the tubules.

Various agents can be used for the scanning. ^{99m}Tc can be tagged to compounds such as DTPA or DSMA to permit static views of the kidney *structures* or to assess dynamic *perfusion* of the kidneys. Orthoiodohippurate can be tagged with ^{131}I to evaluate *excretory function* by measuring the time necessary for the radioisotope to travel through the cortex and pelvis of each kidney. A second injection may be given to evaluate perfusion, structure, and excretory function of the kidney. This is sometimes called a *triple renal study*.

The time of uptake, transit, and excretion of the radioisotope by each kidney is plotted on a graph called a *renogram* curve (isotope renography). This can be compared to a normal reference curve to aid in the detection of abnormalities in either kidney (e.g., tubular disease, urinary obstruction, pyelonephritis, renal vascular hypertension, absence of kidney function).

Renal scanning is used to:

1. Detect renal infarctions. The infarcted area is shown as a nonperfused defect in an otherwise homogeneous renal pattern.
2. Detect renal arterial atherosclerosis or trauma. The renal uptake of the radionucleated material will be delayed or absent on the affected side(s).
3. Monitor rejection of a transplanted kidney. In chronic rejection the uptake and excretion of the nuclear material are delayed.
4. Detect primary renal disease (e.g., glomerulonephritis, acute tubular necrosis). The uptake and excretion of the nuclear material are delayed.
5. Detect pathologic renal or ureteral conditions in patients who cannot have intravenous pyelography (IVP, see p. 432) because of dye allergies
6. Detect renal tumors, abscesses, or cysts. These appear as "cold spots" because of the nonfunctioning tissue.
7. Detect and monitor renovascular hypertension

Contraindications

- Patients who are pregnant because of the risk of fetal damage

Procedures and patient care
Before

- Explain the procedure to the patient.
- Do not schedule a renal scan within 24 hours after an IVP.
- Assure the patient that he or she will not be not exposed to large amounts of radioactivity because only tracer doses of isotopes are used.
- Note that Lugol's solution (10 drops) may be ordered if ^{131}I orthoiodohippurate will be used. This minimizes thyroid uptake of the radioisotope.
- Remind the patient to void before the scan.
- Tell the patient that no sedation or fasting is required but good hydration is essential.
- Instruct the patient to drink two to three glasses of water before the scan.

R

During

- Note the following procedural steps:

  1. The unsedated, nonfasting patient is taken to the nuclear medicine department.
  2. A peripheral IV injection of radionuclide is given. It takes only minutes for the radioisotopes to be concentrated in the kidneys.
  3. While the patient assumes a supine, prone, or sitting position, a gamma ray detector is passed over the kidney area and records the radioactive uptake on either x-ray or Polaroid film.
  4. For a *Lasix renal scan* or a *diuretic renal scan*, the patient is imaged with DTPA. Images are obtained for 20 minutes. Then 40 mg of Lasix is administered intravenously and another 20 minutes of images are obtained.
  5. Scans may be repeated at different intervals after the initial isotope injection.

- Note that the duration of this test varies from 1 to 4 hours depending on the specific information required. Perfusion scans are done in approximately 20 minutes and functional scans in less than 1 hour. Static structure scans require 20 minutes to 4 hours for completion.
- Note that this study is performed by a nuclear medicine technologist or physician.
- Tell the patient that no pain or discomfort is associated with this procedure.
- Inform the patient that he or she must lie still during this study.

After

- Because only tracer doses of radioisotopes are used, inform the patient that no precautions need to be taken against radioactive exposure.
- Tell the patient that the radioactive substance is usually excreted from the body within 6 to 24 hours. Encourage the patient to drink fluids.

Abnormal findings

Urinary obstruction
Pyelonephritis
Renovascular hypertension

Renal tumor
Congenital abnormalities
Renal trauma

Absence of kidney function
Renal infarction
Renal arterial atherosclero-
  sis
Glomerulonephritis

Transplant rejection
Acute tubular necrosis
Tumors
Abscesses
Cysts

Notes

renin assay, plasma (Plasma renin activity [PRA])

Type of test Blood

Normal findings

Adult/elderly: *upright* position, *sodium depleted* (sodium-restricted diet)
           ages 20-39: 2.9-24 ng/ml/hr
           >40: 2.9-10.8 ng/ml/hr

Adult/elderly: *upright* position, *sodium repleted* (normal sodium diet)
           ages 20-39: 0.1-4.3 ng/ml/hr
           >40: 0.1-3.0 ng/ml/hr

Child: 0-3 years: <16.6 ng/ml/hr
       3-6 years: <6.7 ng/ml/hr
       6-9 years: <4.4 ng/ml/hr
       9-12 years: <5.9 ng/ml/hr
       12-15 years: <4.2 ng/ml/hr
       15-18 years: <4.3 ng/ml/hr

Test explanation and related physiology

Renin is an enzyme released by the juxtaglomerular apparatus of the kidney into the renal veins in response to sodium depletion and hypovolemia. Renin activates the renin-angiotensin system, which results in angiotensin II, a powerful vasoconstrictor that also stimulates aldosterone production from the adrenal cortex. Angiotensin and aldosterone increase the blood pressure.

The plasma renin activity (PRA) test is a screening procedure for the detection of essential, renal, or renovascular hypertension. The PRA may be supplemented by other tests such as the renal vein renin assay (see p. 641). A determination of the PRA and a measurement of the plasma aldosterone level (see p. 22) are used in the differential diagnosis of primary versus secondary hyperaldosteronism. Patients with primary hyperaldosteronism will have an increased aldosterone production associated with a decreased renin activity. Patients who have secondary hyperaldosteronism caused by renovascular vascular occlusion or primary renal disease will have increased levels of plasma renin.

Interfering factors

- Renin levels are affected by pregnancy, salt intake, and licorice ingestion.
- Values are higher early in the day, in patients on low-salt diets, and when the patient is in an upright position.
- Drugs that may affect test results include antihypertensives, diuretics, estrogens, oral contraceptives, and vasodilators.

Procedure and patient care

Before

- Explain the procedure to the patient.
- Instruct the patient to maintain a normal diet with a restricted amount of sodium (approximately 3 g/day) for 3 days before the test. A high-sodium diet causes a decrease in renin.
- Inform the patient to discontinue medications (e.g., diuretics, steroids, antihypertensives, vasodilators, oral contraceptives) and licorice for 2 to 4 weeks before the test.
- Usually, draw a fasting blood sample because renin values are higher in the morning.

During

- Usually, perform the test with the patient in an upright position.
- Ensure that the patient stands or sits upright for 2 hours before the blood is drawn.
- If a recumbent sample is ordered, have the patient remain in bed in the morning until the blood sample has been obtained.
- Collect approximately 7 to 12 ml of venous blood and place it in a chilled lavender-top tube with EDTA as an anticoagulant.
- Gently invert the blood tube to allow adequate mixing of the blood sample and the anticoagulant.
- Record the patient's position, dietary status, and time of day on the laboratory slip. Also, note any medication that the patient is currently taking.
- Place the tube of blood on ice and immediately send it to the laboratory.

R

After

- Apply pressure or a pressure dressing to the venipuncture site.
- Observe the venipuncture site for bleeding.
- Tell the patient that usually a normal diet may be resumed.
- Note that medications that were withheld may be reordered.

Abnormal findings

Increased levels

Essential hypertension
Malignant hypertension
Renovascular hypertension
Addison's disease
Renin-producing renal tumors (Bartter's syndrome)
Cirrhosis
Hypokalemia
Hemorrhage

Decreased levels

Salt-retaining steroid therapy
Antidiuretic hormone therapy

Notes

renin assay, renal vein

Type of test Blood

Normal findings Renin ratio of involved kidney to uninvolved kidney <1.4

Test explanation and related physiology

Renin is an enzyme secreted by the kidneys that activates the renin-angiotensin system and causes vasoconstriction and the release of aldosterone. These mechanisms can cause hypertension. Renal vein assays for renin are used to diagnose renovascular hypertension. By injection of a radiopaque dye into the inferior vena cava, the renal veins can be identified. A catheter is placed into each renal vein, and blood is withdrawn from each vein. Radioimmunoassay (RIA) is used to determine the renin quantity in each sample. If hypertension is caused by renal artery stenosis, the renal vein renin level of the affected kidney should be 1.4 or more times greater than that of the unaffected kidney. If the levels are the same, the hypertension is not caused by renal artery stenosis (any stenosis identified on an arteriogram would not be considered severe enough to cause renin-related hypertension). Another cause for the patient's elevated blood pressure must be investigated.

Contraindications

- Patients who are allergic to shellfish or iodinated dye

Potential complications

- Allergic reaction to iodinated dye
  Allergic reactions may vary from mild flushing, itching, and urticaria to severe, life-threatening anaphylaxis (evidenced by respiratory distress, drop in blood pressure, shock). In the unusual event of anaphylaxis the patient may be treated with diphenhydramine (Benadryl), steroids, and epinephrine. Oxygen and endotracheal equipment should be on hand for immediate use.

Procedure and patient care

Before

- Explain the procedure to the patient.

- Ensure that written and informed consent for this procedure is obtained by the physician.
- Assess the patient for allergies to iodine.
- Inform the radiologist if an allergy to iodinated contrast is suspected. The radiologist may prescribe a Benadryl and steroid preparation to be administered before testing. Usually a hypoallergenic, non-ionic contrast will be used during the test.
- Place the patient on a "no added salt" diet and diuretics for 3 days before the examination.
- Keep the patient NPO after midnight on the day of the study.
- Instruct the patient to remain in the upright position for 2 hours before the test.
- Premedicate the fasting patient as ordered. Meperidine and atropine are typically used.

During

- Note the following procedural steps:

  1. The patient is taken to the radiology department and placed on the fluoroscopy table in a supine position.
  2. The patient's groin is prepared and draped in a sterile manner and then anesthetized.
  3. The femoral vein is punctured, and a catheter is placed into the vein and advanced into the inferior vena cava.
  4. Fluoroscopy is used to monitor the catheter placement.
  5. Dye is injected, and the renal veins are identified.
  6. The catheter is placed into one renal vein at a time, and separate blood specimens are withdrawn and labeled.
  7. The catheter is removed, and a pressure dressing is applied to the puncture site.

- Note that this procedure is usually performed by a radiologist in less than 1 hour.
- Inform the patient that the groin puncture needed for this study is uncomfortable.

After

- Usually, place the patient on bed rest for several hours.
- Monitor the patient's vital signs.

- Usually, send the blood to a commercial laboratory for analysis.
- Assess the patient for renal vein thrombosis, which may occur 1 to 7 days after the procedure. This will be manifested by costovertebral tenderness, hematuria, and elevated creatinine levels.
- Observe the venous puncture site frequently for hematoma, hemorrhage, or absence of pulse.
- Compare the color and temperature of the legs.
- Apply cold compresses to the puncture site if needed to reduce discomfort and swelling.
- Evaluate the patient for delayed reaction to the dye (dyspnea, rashes, tachycardia, hives). This usually occurs within the first 2 to 6 hours after the test. Treat with antihistamines or steroids.

Abnormal finding
Increased levels

Renal artery stenosis

Notes

R

reticulocyte count (Retic count)

Type of test Blood

Normal findings

Reticulocyte count
Adult/elderly/child: 0.5%-2%
Infant: 0.5%-3.1%
Newborn: 2.5%-6.5%
Reticulocyte index: 1.0

Test explanation and related physiology

The reticulocyte count is a test for determining bone marrow function and evaluating erythropoietic activity. This test is also useful in identifying anemias. A reticulocyte is an immature red blood cell (RBC) that can be readily identified under the microscope by the staining of a peripheral blood smear with a supravital stain. The reticulocyte count represents a direct measurement of RBC production by the bone marrow. Increased reticulocyte counts are expected as physiologic compensation in patients who are anemic. A normal or low reticulocyte count in an anemic patient indicates that the marrow production of RBCs is inadequate and perhaps is the cause of the anemia (as in aplastic anemia, iron deficiency, vitamin B_{12} deficiency, or depletion of iron stores). An elevated reticulocyte count found in patients with a normal hemogram indicates increased RBC production (compensated hemolysis or hemorrhage). To determine if the increased reticulocyte count indicates adequate erythropoiesis in anemic patients with a decreased hematocrit, one can determine the *reticulocyte index:*

Reticulocyte index =

$$\text{Reticulocyte count (in \%)} \times \frac{\text{Patient's hematocrit}}{\text{Normal hematocrit}}$$

The reticulocyte index in a patient who has a good marrow response to the anemia should be 1.0. If it is below 1.0, even though the reticulocyte count is elevated in the anemic patient, the test indicates that the bone marrow response is inadequate in its ability to compensate (as in iron deficiency, vitamin B_{12} deficiency, or marrow failure).

Interfering factors
- Pregnancy may cause an increased reticulocyte count.

Procedure and patient care
Before
- Explain the procedure to the patient.
- Tell the patient that no fasting is required.

During
- Collect approximately 5 to 7 ml of venous blood in a lavender-top tube.

After
- Apply pressure or a pressure dressing to the venipuncture site.
- Observe the venipuncture site for bleeding.

Abnormal findings

Increased levels	Decreased levels
Hemolytic anemia	Pernicious anemia
Sickle cell anemia	Folic acid deficiency
Hemorrhage (3 to 4 days later)	Adrenocortical hypofunction
Postsplenectomy	Cirrhosis of the liver
Erythroblastosis fetalis	Aplastic anemia
Pregnancy	Radiation therapy
Leukemias	Marrow failure
	Anterior pituitary hypofunction
	Chronic infection

R

Notes

retrograde pyelography

Type of test X-ray with contrast dye

Normal findings Normal outline and size of ureters and bladder

Test explanation and related physiology

Retrograde pyelography refers to radiographic visualization of the urinary tract through ureteral catheterization and the injection of contrast material. The ureters are catheterized during cystoscopy. A radiopaque material is injected into the ureters, and x-ray films are taken. This test can be performed even if the patient has an allergy to IV contrast dye because none of the dye injected into the ureters is absorbed.

Retrograde pyelography is helpful in radiographically examining the ureters in patients when visualization with intravenous pyelography (IVP, see p. 432) is inadequate. Frequently, in patients with unilateral renal disease, the involved kidney and collecting system are not visualized. To rule out ureteral obstruction as a cause of the unilateral kidney disease, retrograde pyelography must be done to examine the ureters. Tumors, benign strictures, tortuous ureters, stones, scarring, and extrinsic compression can cause ureteral obstruction. Retrograde pyelography provides visualization of the ureters when IVP is contraindicated or when the distal portion is not opacified by the IVP ureters.

Potential complications

- Urinary tract infection
  Infections can be caused by the invasive nature of this procedure.
- Sepsis by seeding the bloodstream with bacteria from infected urine
- Perforation of the bladder
- Hematuria
- Temporary obstruction to ureteral urine flow
  Manipulation of the ureters can cause edema, which can result in temporary, partial obstruction to urine flow
- Allergic reaction to iodinated dye

This rarely occurs because the dye is not administered intravenously.

Interfering factor

- Retained barium from previous x-ray studies could obscure visualization.

Procedure and patient care

Before

- Explain the procedure to the patient.
- Ensure that informed consent for this procedure is obtained.
- If enemas are ordered to clear the bowel, assist the patient as needed and record the results.
- If procedure will be done with the patient under local anesthesia, allow the patient to have a liquid breakfast.
- If the procedure will be performed with the patient under general anesthesia, follow the routine general anesthesia precautions. Keep the patient NPO after midnight on the day of the test. Fluids may be given intravenously.
- Administer the preprocedural medications, as ordered, 1 hour before the study. Sedatives decrease the spasm of the bladder sphincter, thus decreasing the patient's discomfort.
- Check the patient for allergies to iodinated dye.

During

- Note the following procedural steps:

    1. The ureteral catheters are passed into the ureters by means of cystoscopy (see p. 261).
    2. Radiopaque contrast material (Hypaque or Renografin) is injected into the ureteral catheters, and x-ray films are taken.
    3. The entire ureter and pelvis are demonstrated.
    4. As the catheters are withdrawn, more dye is injected and more x-ray films are taken to visualize the complete outline of the ureters.

- Note that retrograde pyelography is performed by a urologist in approximately 1 hour in a cystoscopy room or operating room.
- Inform the patient that this study is uncomfortable. If awake, the patient will feel pressure and an urge to void.

R

After

- Check and record the patient's vital signs as ordered. Watch for a decrease in blood pressure and an increase in pulse as an indication of bleeding.
- Observe the patient for signs and symptoms of sepsis (elevated temperature, flush, chills, decreased blood pressure, increased pulse).
- Assess the patient's ability to void for at least 24 hours. Urinary retention may be secondary to edema caused by instrumentation.
- Note the color of the urine; a pink tinge is typically present. Report bright-red blood or clots to the physician.
- Encourage the patient to increase intake of fluids. A dilute urine decreases dysuria. Fluids also maintain a constant flow of urine to prevent stasis and the accumulation of bacteria in the bladder.
- Monitor the patient for bladder spasms. Often, belladona and opium (B&O) suppositories are given to relieve bladder spasms.
- Observe for an allergic reaction to iodine contrast dye by instructing the patient to report symptoms of itching, rash, hives, flushing, shortness of breath, and increased heart rate. Treat with antihistamines or steroids.
- Administer analgesics as needed.

Abnormal findings

Tumors
Strictures
Stones
Ureteral obstruction
Intrinsic and extrinsic tumors affecting the ureters
Congenital anomalies

Notes

rheumatoid factor (RF)

Type of test Blood

Normal findings

Negative (<60 U/ml by nephelometric testing)
Elderly may have slightly increased values.

Test explanation and related physiology

The RF test is useful in the diagnosis of rheumatoid arthritis. Other diseases, such as systemic lupus erythematosus (SLE), may also cause a positive RF test. RF is also occasionally seen in patients with tuberculosis, chronic hepatitis, infectious mononucleosis, and subacute bacterial endocarditis. The elderly often have false positive results.

Rheumatoid arthritis is a chronic inflammatory disease that affects most joints, especially the metacarpal and phalangeal joints, the proximal interphalangeal joints, and the wrists; however, any synovial joint can be involved. In this disease, abnormal immunoglobulin G (IgG) antibodies produced by lymphocytes in the synovial membranes act as antigens. These antigens react with IgG and IgM antibodies to produce immune complexes. These immune complexes can activate the complement system and other inflammatory systems to cause joint damage. The reactive IgM molecule is the RF. Tissues other than the joints, including blood vessels, lungs, nerves, and heart, can be involved in autoimmune inflammation.

Tests for RF are directed toward identification of the IgM antibodies. Approximately 80% of the patients with rheumatoid arthritis have positive RF titers. To be considered positive, RF must be found in a dilution of greater than 1:80. When RF is found in titers less than 1:80, diseases such as SLE, scleroderma, and other autoimmune conditions should be considered. Although the normal value is "no rheumatoid factor identifiable at low titers," a small number of normal patients will have RF present at a very low titer. When the nephelometric testing procedure is used, the normal value is considered to be less than 60 U/ml.

Although there are many ways of detecting RF, the sheep cell agglutination test or the latex fixation test is usually performed. In the *sheep cell agglutination test,* rabbit IgG is placed on the sheep red blood cells (RBCs). When this is mixed with the patient's serum (which has been serially diluted), visual agglutination occurs if any RF is present. In the *latex fixation test,* human IgG is placed on a synthetic latex particle and mixed with the patient's serum. Visual agglutination is then detected if RF is present.

Interfering factors

- Elderly patients often have false positive results.

Procedure and patient care

Before

- Explain the procedure to the patient.
- Tell the patient that no fasting or preparation is required.

During

- Collect approximately 7 ml of venous blood in a red-top tube.

After

- Apply pressure or a pressure dressing to the venipuncture site.
- Observe the venipuncture site for bleeding.

Abnormal findings

Increased levels

Rheumatoid arthritis
Other autoimmune diseases (e.g., systemic lupus erythematosus [SLE])
Chronic viral infections
Subacute bacterial endocarditis
Tuberculosis

Chronic hepatitis
Dermatomyositis
Scleroderma
Infectious mononucleosis
Leukemia
Cirrhosis
Syphilis
Renal disease

Notes

rubella antibody test (German measles test, Hemagglutination inhibition [HAI])

Type of test Blood

Normal findings Lack of susceptibility to rubella if HAI titer is >1:10 to 1:20 or if complement fixation test is negative

Possible critical values Evidence of susceptibility in pregnant women with recent exposure to rubella

Test explanation and related physiology

Screening for rubella antibodies is done to detect immunity to rubella. These tests detect the presence of IgG and IgM antibodies of past and active infections and determine the susceptibility or immunity to the rubella virus, which is the causative agent for German measles. It is vitally important to identify exposure to rubella infection and susceptibility status in pregnant women because infection in the first trimester of pregnancy is associated with congenital abnormalities, abortion, or stillbirth. All pregnant women should be screened for rubella during the first prenatal test.

If the woman's titer is greater than 1:10 to 1:20, she is not susceptible to rubella. If the mother's titer is 1:8 or less, she has little or no immunity to rubella. She should be strongly advised to stay away from any small children, especially those with symptoms of an upper respiratory infection (prodromal symptoms of rubella). In addition, all health care personnel associated with maternal and child care should be screened for rubella. Immunization is not done during pregnancy but should be done after delivery for nonimmune mothers.

A change in the HAI titer activity from the acute to the chronic phase in a patient with a rash is the most useful method of demonstrating a rise in antibody titer levels. With a rubella rash, diagnosis of rubella is confirmed by obtaining an acute sample (taken about 3 days after the onset of the rash) and a convalescent sample (taken about 3 weeks later). A fourfold increase in titer from the acute to the convalescent titer indicates that the rash was caused by rubella.

When pregnant women with an immunity to rubella are

R

exposed to rubella, the HAI test should be repeated. A rise in antibody titer indicates that both the mother and the fetus have been infected by rubella. If the exposure occurred during the first trimester of pregnancy, the fetus is at risk for congenital heart defects, deafness, mental retardation, and cataracts.

Procedure and patient care

Before

- Explain the purpose of the test to the patient.

During

- Collect approximately 7 ml of venous blood in a red-top tube.

After

- Apply pressure or a pressure dressing to the venipuncture site.
- Assess the venipuncture site for bleeding.
- Inform the patient when to return for a follow-up HAI titer, if indicated.

Abnormal finding

Rubella infection

Notes

Schilling test (Vitamin B$_{12}$ absorption test)

Type of test Urine (24-48 hour)

Normal findings Excretion of 8%-40% of radioactive vitamin B$_{12}$ within 24 hours

Test explanation and related physiology

The Schilling test is performed to detect vitamin B$_{12}$ absorption. Normally, ingested vitamin B$_{12}$ combines with intrinsic factor, which is produced by gastric mucosa, and is absorbed in the distal part of the ileum. Pernicious anemia results when absorption of vitamin B$_{12}$ is inadequate. This may be caused by a primary malabsorption problem of the intestinal tract or from lack of intrinsic factor.

The two-stage Schilling test can detect a defect in vitamin B$_{12}$ absorption. With normal absorption of vitamin B$_{12}$, the ileum absorbs more vitamin B$_{12}$ than the body needs and excretes the excess vitamin B$_{12}$ into the urine. However, with impaired vitamin B$_{12}$ absorption, little or no vitamin B$_{12}$ is excreted into the urine.

In the Schilling test, urinary B$_{12}$ levels are measured after the ingestion of radioactive vitamin B$_{12}$. The test can be performed as one stage (without intrinsic factor) or two stage (with intrinsic factor). Patients who have pernicious anemia from lack of intrinsic factor will have an abnormal first-stage and a normal second-stage Schilling test. Patients who have malabsorption from an intestinal source will have an abnormal first- and second-stage Schilling test.

Contraindications

- Patients who are pregnant
- Patients who are lactating

Interfering factors

- Radioactive nuclear material received 10 days before testing can affect results.
- Renal insufficiency may cause reduced excretion of radioactive vitamin B$_{12}$.
- Elderly, diabetic, or hypothyroid patients may have reduced excretion of vitamin B$_{12}$.
- Drugs that may affect test results include laxatives be-

S

cause they could decrease the rate of vitamin B_{12} absorption.

Procedure and patient care
Before

- Explain the procedure to the patient.
- Instruct the patient to remain NPO except for water 8 to 12 hours before the test. Food should not be given until after the patient receives the injections.
- Instruct the patient not to take laxatives during the test period.

During

- Note the following procedural steps:
  1. Radioactive vitamin B_{12} is administered orally to the patient.
  2. Shortly thereafter, nonradioactive vitamin B_{12} is administered to the patient intramuscularly to saturate tissue binding sites and to permit some excretion of radioactive vitamin B_{12} in the urine if it is absorbed.
  3. A 24- to 48-hour urine collection for vitamin B_{12} is obtained.
  4. The patient is encouraged to drink fluids.

Two-stage Schilling test
  1. If indicated, the second stage is performed about 1 week after the first stage.
  2. The fasting patient is provided radioactive vitamin B_{12} combined with human intrinsic factor.
  3. As before, an IM injection of nonradioactive vitamin B_{12} is administered.
  4. Again, 24- to 48-hour urine collections are begun.

Combined one-stage and two-stage Schilling test
  1. The fasting patient receives a capsule of cobalt-57-labeled vitamin B_{12} plus intrinsic factor.
  2. A second capsule of cobalt-58-labeled vitamin B_{12} is also given.
  3. One hour later an IM injection of nonradioactive vitamin B_{12} is administered.
  4. Again, the urine for vitamin B_{12} is collected for 24 to 48 hours.
  5. Percentages of cobalt-57 and cobalt-58 are calculated. Colbalt-57-labeled vitamin B_{12} only will be present in

patients with pernicious anemia secondary to lack of intrinsic factor. No vitamin B_{12} will be present in the urine of patients whose pernicious anemia is caused by primary bowel malabsorption.

After

- Ensure that the urine specimens are promptly transported to the laboratory.

Abnormal findings
Decreased levels

Pernicious anemia
Intestinal malabsorption
Hypothyroidism
Liver disease

Notes

secretin-pancreozymin (Pancreative enzymes)

Type of test Fluid analysis

Normal findings
Volume: 2-4 ml/kg of body weight
HCO_3^- (bicarbonate): 90-130 mEq/L
Amylase: 6.6-35.2 U/kg of body weight

Test explanation and related physiology

Children with cystic fibrosis have mucous plugs that obstruct their pancreatic ducts. The pancreative enzymes (e.g., amylase, lipase, trypsin, chymotrypsin) cannot be expelled into the duodenum and therefore are either completely absent or present only in diminished quantities within the duodenal aspirate. Secretin and pancreozymin are used to stimulate pancreatic secretion of these enzymes. The duodenal contents are aspirated and examined for pH, bicarbonate, and enzyme levels. Amylase is the most frequently measured enzyme. Diminished values are suggestive of cystic fibrosis.

Procedure and patient care

Before

- Explain the procedure to the patient and/or parents.
- Instruct the adult patient to fast for 12 hours before testing.
- Determine pediatric fasting times according to age.

During

- Note the following procedural steps:

  1. With the use of fluoroscopy a Dreiling tube is passed through the patient's nose and into the stomach.
  2. The distal lumen of the tube is placed within the duodenum.
  3. The proximal lumen of the tube is placed within the stomach.
  4. Both lumens are aspirated. The gastric lumen is continually aspirated to avoid contamination of the gastric contents in the duodenum aspirate.
  5. A control specimen of the duodenal juices is collected for 20 minutes.

6. The patient is tested for sensitivity to secretion and pancreozymin by low-dose intradermal injection.
7. If no sensitivity is present, these hormones are administered intravenously. Secretin can be expected to stimulate pancreatic water and bicarbonate secretion. Pancreozymin can be expected to stimulate pancreatic enzyme (lipase, amylase, trypsin, chymotrypsin) secretion.
8. Four duodenal aspirates are collected at 20 minute-intervals and placed in the specimen container.
9. Each specimen is analyzed for pH, volume, bicarbonate, and amylase levels.

- Note that a physician performs this test in approximately 2 hours in the laboratory or at the patient's bedside.
- Tell the patient that he or she may have discomfort and gagging during placement of the Dreiling tube.

After

- Place the aspirated specimens on ice. Send them to the chemistry laboratory as soon as the test is completed.
- Remove the Dreiling tube after completion of the test. Give appropriate nose and mouth care.
- Allow the patient to resume a normal diet.

Abnormal findings

Cystic fibrosis
Sprue

Notes

S

sella turcica x-ray

Type of test X-ray

Normal findings No abnormalities

Test explanation and related physiology

This study involves taking x-ray films of the sella turcica, an area of the bony cranium at the base of the skull. The sella turcica contains the pituitary gland. Pituitary tumors that produce adrenocorticotropic hormone (ACTH) can cause Cushing's syndrome. One can diagnose these tumors easily by detecting erosion and destruction of the normal sella turcica. Computed tomography (CT) is usually done if a pituitary tumor is suspected.

Procedure and patient care

Before

- Explain the procedure to the patient.
- Tell the patient that all objects above the neck must be removed.
- If a glass eye is present, note this on the x-ray examination request because it will present a confusing shadow.

During

- Note that axial (submentovertical), half-axial (Towne), posteroanterior, and lateral views of the skull are usually taken.
- Tell the patient that this test is painless.
- Note that a radiologic technologist performs this test in a few minutes.

After

- Note that no special after-care is needed.

Abnormal findings

Pituitary tumors
Destruction of the sella turcica

Notes

Type of test Fluid analysis

Normal findings

Volume: 2-5 ml
Liquification time: 20-30 minutes after collection
pH: 7.12-8.00
Sperm count (density): 50-200 million/ml
Sperm motility: 60%-80% actively motile
Sperm morphology: 70%-90% normally shaped

Test explanation and related physiology

The semen analysis is one of the most important aspects of the fertility workup, since the cause of a woman's inability to conceive often lies within the man. After 2 to 3 days of sexual abstinence, sperm is collected and examined for volume, sperm count, motility, and morphology.

The freshly collected semen is first measured for volume. After liquification of the white, gelatinous ejaculate, a sperm count is done. Men with very low or very high counts are likely to be infertile. The motility of the sperm is then evaluated. At least 60% of the sperm should show progressive motility. Morphology is studied by staining a semen preparation and calculating the number of normal versus abnormal sperm forms.

A simple sperm analysis, especially if it indicates infertility, is inconclusive because the sperm count varies from day to day. A semen analysis should be done at least twice. Men with *aspermia* (no sperm) or *oligospermia* (20 million/ml) should be evaluated endocrinologically for pituitary, thyroid, adrenal, or testicular aberrations.

A normal semen analysis alone does not accurately assess the male factor, unless the effect of the partner's cervical secretion on sperm survival is also determined (see Sims-Huhner test, p. 668). In addition to its value in infertility workups, semen analysis is also helpful in documenting adequate sterilization after a vasectomy. It is usually performed 6 weeks after the surgery. If any sperm are seen, the adequacy of the vasectomy must be questioned.

Interfering factors

- Drugs that may cause decreased semen levels include antineoplastic agents (e.g., nitrogen mustard, procarbazine, vincristine, methotrexate), cimetidine, estrogens, and methyltestosterone.

Procedure and patient care

Before

- Explain the procedure to the patient.
- Instruct the patient to abstain from sexual activity for 2 to 3 days before collecting the specimen. Prolonged abstinence before the collection should be discouraged, since the quality of the sperm cells and especially their motility may diminish.
- Give the patient the proper container for the sperm collection.
- Instruct the patient to avoid alcoholic beverages for several days before the collection.

During

- Note that semen is best collected by ejaculation into a clean container. For best results the specimen should be collected in the physician's office or laboratory by masturbation.
- Note that less satisfactory specimens can be obtained in the patient's home by coitus interruptus or masturbation.
  1. Instruct the patient to deliver these home specimens to the laboratory within 1 hour after collection.
  2. Tell the patient to avoid excessive heat and cold during transportation of the specimen.

After

- Record the date of the previous semen emission along with the collection time and date of the fresh specimen.
- Tell the patient when and how to obtain the test results. Remember that abnormal results may have a devastating effect on the patient's sexuality.

Abnormal findings

Infertility

Vasectomy (obstruction of vas deferens)

Orchitis

Testicular atrophy

Testicular failure

Hyperpyrexia

sialography

Type of test X-ray

Normal findings No evidence of pathology in salivary ducts and related structures

Test explanation and related physiology

Sialography is an x-ray procedure used to examine the salivary ducts (parotid, submaxillary, submandibular, sublingual) and related glandular structures after the injection of a contrast medium into the desired duct. This procedure is used to detect calculi, strictures, tumors, or inflammatory disease in patients who complain of pain, tenderness, or swelling in these areas.

Contraindications

- Patients with mouth infections

Potential complication

- Allergic reaction to the iodinated dye
  This rarely occurs because the dye is not administered intravenously.

Procedure and patient care
Before

- Explain the procedure to the patient. The thought of a dye injection in the mouth is frightening to many patients. Provide emotional support.
- Obtain informed consent if required by the institution.
- Instruct the patient to remove jewelry, hairpins, and dentures, which could obscure x-ray visualization.
- Instruct the patient to rinse his or her mouth before the procedure with an antiseptic solution to reduce the possibility of introducing bacteria into the ductal structures.

During

- Note the following procedural steps:

  1. X-ray studies are taken before the dye injection is given to ensure that stones are not present, which could prevent the contrast material from entering the ducts.

2. The patient is placed in a supine position on an x-ray table.

3. The contrast medium is injected directly into the desired orifice via a cannula or a special catheter.

4. X-ray films are taken with the patient in various positions.

5. The patient is given a sour substance (e.g., lemon juice) orally to stimulate salivary excretion.

6. Another set of x-ray studies are taken to evaluate ductal drainage.

- Note that a radiologist performs this procedure in the radiology department in less than 30 minutes.
- Tell the patient that he or she may feel a little pressure as the contrast medium is injected into the ducts.

After

- Encourage the patient to drink fluids to eliminate the dye.

Abnormal findings

Calculi
Strictures
Tumors
Inflammatory disease

Notes

sickle cell test (Sickle cell preparation, Sickledex, Hgb S test)

Type of test Blood

Normal findings No sickle cells present

Test explanation and related physiology

Both sickle cell disease (homozygous for hemoglobin [Hgb]S) and sickle cell trait (heterozygous for Hgb S) can be detected by this study. Sickle cell anemia results from a genetic homozygous defect and is caused by the presence of Hgb S instead of Hgb A. When Hgb S becomes deoxygenated, it tends to band in a way that causes the red blood cell (RBC) to assume a sickle shape. These sickled RBCs cannot freely pass through the capillaries and cause plugging of the microvascular tree. This may compromise the blood supply to various organs. Hgb S is found in varying quantities in 8% to 10% of the black population.

The routine peripheral blood smear of patients with sickle cell disease does not contain sickled RBCs unless hypoxemia is present. In the sickle cell test a deoxygenating agent is added to the patient's blood. If 25% or more of the patient's hemoglobin is of the S variation, the cells will assume the crescent (sickle) shape and the test is positive. If no sickling occurs, the test is negative. A negative test indicates that the patient has no or very little Hgb S. Other less common hemoglobin variants can also cause sickling.

This test is only a screening test, and its sensitivity varies according to the method used by the laboratory. The definitive diagnosis is made by hemoglobin electrophoresis (see p. 404), in which Hgb S can be identified and quantified.

Interfering factors

- Any blood transfusions within 3 to 4 months before the sickle cell test can cause false negative results, since the donor's normal hemoglobin may dilute the recipient's abnormal Hgb S.
- Polycythemia can cause false negative results.
- Infants less than 3 months of age can have false negative results.

- Drugs that may cause false negative results include phenothiazines.

Procedure and patient care
Before

- Explain the procedure to the patient.
- Tell the patient that no fasting is required.

During

- Collect approximately 7 ml of venous blood in a lavender-top tube.

After

- Apply pressure or a pressure dressing to the venipuncture site.
- Check the venipuncture site for bleeding.
- If the test is positive, offer the family genetic counseling. A patient with one recessive gene (heterozygous) is said to have sickle cell *trait*. A patient with two recessive genes (homozygous) has sickle cell *anemia*.
- Inform patients with sickle cell anemia that they should avoid situations in which hypoxia may occur (e.g., strenuous exercise, air travel in unpressurized aircraft, travel to high-altitude regions).

Abnormal findings
Sickle cell trait
Sickle cell anemia

Notes

sigmoidoscopy (Proctoscopy, Anoscopy)

Type of test Endoscopy

Normal findings Normal anus, rectum, and sigmoid colon

Test explanation and related physiology

Endoscopy of the lower gastrointestinal (GI) tract allows one to visualize and perform biopsies of tumors, polyps, hemorrhoids, or ulcers of the anus, rectum, and sigmoid colon. *Anoscopy* refers to examination of the anus; *proctoscopy* to examination of the anus and rectum; and *sigmoidoscopy* (the procedure done most frequently) to examination of the anus, rectum, and sigmoid colon. This test can be performed with a rigid or flexible sigmoidoscope. Because the lower GI tract is difficult to visualize radiographically, direct visualization by sigmoidoscopy is helpful.

Further, sigmoidoscopy, as with colonoscopy, can be therapeutic. Reduction of sigmoid volvulus, removal of polyps, and obliteration of hemorrhoids can be performed through the sigmoidoscope.

Contraindications

- Patients who are uncooperative
- Patients with diverticulitis
- Patients with painful anorectal conditions, such as fissures, fistulas, or hemorrhoids
- Patients with severe bleeding
  Blood clots obstruct the view of the scope.
- Patients suspected of having perforated colon lesions

Potential complications˜

- Perforation of the colon
- Bleeding from biopsy sites

Interfering factors

- Poor bowel preparation can obscure visualization of the bowel mucosa.
- Rectal bleeding can obstruct the lens system and preclude adequate visualization.

S

Procedure and patient care
Before

- Explain the procedure to the patient.
- Obtain informed consent for this procedure.
- Assist the patient with the bowel preparation. In most cases, two Fleet enemas are sufficient.
- Instruct the patient to ingest only a light breakfast on the morning of the endoscopy.
- Assure patients that they will be properly draped to avoid unnecessary embarrassment.

During

- Note the following procedural steps:

  1. The patient is placed on the endoscopy table or bed in the left lateral decubitus position. Physicians often prefer the knee-chest position. Many operating and examining tables are easily converted to make the knee-chest position more comfortable. This procedure also can be performed with the patient in the lithotomy position.
  2. Usually, no sedation is required.
  3. The anus is mildly dilated with a well-lubricated finger.
  4. The rigid or flexible sigmoidoscope is placed into the rectum and advanced to its point of maximal penetration.
  5. Air is insufflated during the procedure to distend more fully the lower intestinal tract.
  6. The sigmoid, rectum, and anus are visualized.
  7. Biopsies can be obtained and polypectomy can be performed at the time of sigmoidoscopy.

- Note that a physician trained in GI endoscopy usually performs this procedure in the GI laboratory, operating room, patient's bedside, or outpatient clinic setting in approximately 15 to 20 minutes.
- Tell the patient that he or she probably will feel discomfort and the urge to defecate as the sigmoidoscope is inserted.

After

- Inform the patient that since air has been insufflated into the bowel during the procedure, he or she may have flatulence or gas pains. Ambulation may help.
- Observe the patient for signs of abdominal distention, increased tenderness, or rectal bleeding.
- Tell the patient that slight rectal bleeding may occur if biopsies have been taken.

Abnormal findings

Tumors (benign and malignant)
Polyps
Ulcerative colitis
Pseudomembranous colitis
Crohn's disease (regional enteritis)
Intestinal ischemia
Irritable bowel syndrome

Notes

S

Sims-Huhner test (Postcoital test, Postcoital cervical mucus test, Cervical mucus sperm penetration test)

Type of test   Fluid analysis

Normal findings

Cervical mucus adequate for sperm transmission, survival, and penetration
6 to 20 active sperm per high-power field

Test explanation and related physiology

The Sims-Huhner test consists of a postcoital examination of the cervical mucus to measure the ability of the sperm to penetrate the mucus and maintain motility. This study evaluates the interaction between the sperm and the cervical mucus. It is also a measure of the quality of the cervical mucus. This test can determine the effect of vaginal and cervical secretions on the activity of the sperm. This procedure is only performed after a previously performed semen analysis has been determined to be normal.

This test is performed during the middle of the ovulatory cycle, since at this time the secretions should be optimal for sperm penetration and survival. During ovulation the quantity of cervical mucus is maximal whereas the viscosity is minimal, thus facilitating sperm penetration. The endocervical mucus sample is examined for color, viscosity, and tenacity (spinnbarkheit). The fresh specimen is then spread on a clean glass slide and examined for the presence of sperm. Estimate of the total number and the number of motile sperm per high-power field are reported. Normally, 6 to 20 active sperm cells should be seen in each high-power field. If the sperm are present but not active, the cervical environment is unsuitable (e.g., abnormal pH) for their survival. After the specimen has dried on the glass slide, the mucus can be examined for ferning (see cervical mucus test, p. 169). The Sims-Huhner study is invaluable in fertility examinations; however, it is not a substitute for the semen analysis. If the results of the Sims-Huhner test are less than optimal, the test is usually repeated during the same or next ovulatory cycle.

This analysis is also helpful in documenting cases of suspected rape by testing the vaginal and cervical secretions for sperm.

Procedure and patient care

Before

- Explain the procedure to the patient.
- Inform the patient that basal body temperature recordings should be used to indicate ovulation.
- Tell the patient that no vaginal lubrication, douching, or bathing is permitted until after the vaginal cervical examination because these factors will alter the cervical mucus.
- Inform the patient that this study should be performed after 3 days of sexual abstinence.
- Instruct the patient to remain in bed for 10 to 15 minutes after coitus to ensure cervical exposure to the semen. After resting, the patient should report to her physician for examination of her cervical mucus within 2 hours after coitus.

During

- Note that with the patient in the lithotomy position, the cervix is then exposed by an unlubricated speculum. The specimen is aspirated from the endocervix and delivered to the laboratory for analysis.
- Note that this procedure is performed by a physician in approximately 5 minutes.
- Tell the patient that the only discomfort associated with this study is insertion of the speculum.

After

- Tell the patient how and when she may obtain test results.

Abnormal findings

Infertility
Suspected rape

Notes

S

skull x-ray

Type of test X-ray

Normal findings Normal skull and surrounding structures

Test explanation and related physiology

An x-ray film of the skull allows for the visualization of the bones making up the skull, the nasal sinuses, and any cerebral calcification. The study is indicated for patients in whom a pathologic condition is suspected in any of these structures.

Fractures of the skull are easily seen as abnormal radiolucent lines in an otherwise radiopaque skull bone. Metastatic tumors of the skull can easily be seen as radiolucent spots in an otherwise normal skull. Opacification of the nasal sinuses may indicate sinusitis, hemorrhage, or tumor.

The pineal gland, located in the middle of the brain, is thought to regulate the biorhythms of mammals. This gland may become calcified after puberty. When calcified, the pineal gland is a very useful marker and allows the midline of the brain to be easily identified on the skull x-ray film. Conditions such as unilateral hematoma or tumor will cause a shift of the midline structures (and the calcified pineal gland) to the side opposite the site of the pathologic condition. Simple skull x-ray films, therefore, allow for the easy detection of these unilateral space-occupying lesions.

The sella turcica is the bony structure surrounding and protecting the pituitary gland. Tumors of the pituitary gland may cause an increase in size or an erosion of the sella turcica. These changes can be detected by skull x-ray films.

Procedure and patient care

Before

- Explain the procedure to the patient
- Instruct the patient to remove all objects above the neck, since metal objects and dentures will prevent x-ray visualization of the structures they cover.
- Avoid hyperextension and manipulation of the head if surgical injuries are suspected.
- Tell the patient that no sedation or fasting is required.

During

- Note that the patient is taken to the radiology department and placed on an x-ray table. Axial (submentovertical), half-axial (Towne), posteroanterior, and lateral views of the skull are usually taken.
- Note that a radiologic technologist takes skull films in a few minutes.
- Tell the patient that this test is painless.

After

- If a glass eye is present, note this on the x-ray examination request because it can present a confusing shadow on x-ray film.

Abnormal findings

Skull fractures
Metastatic tumors
Sinusitis
Hemorrhage

Tumor
Hematoma
Congenital anomalies

Notes

S

small bowel follow-through (SBF, Small bowel enema)

Type of test X-ray with contrast dye

Normal findings

Normal positioning, motility, and patency of the small intestine

No evidence of intrinsic obstruction or extrinsic compression

Test explanation and related physiology

An SBF study is performed to identify abnormalities in the small bowel. Usually the patient is asked to drink barium. In patients who cannot drink, barium can be injected through a nasogastric tube. X-ray films are then taken at timed intervals (usually 30 minutes) to follow the progression of barium through the small intestine. Significant delays in transit time of the barium may occur with both benign and malignant forms of obstruction or diminished intestinal motility (ileus). On the other hand, the flow of barium is faster in patients who have hypermotility states of the small bowel (malabsorption syndromes). Failure of the progression of barium through the small bowel can be seen in patients with partial mechanical small bowel obstruction or diminished intestinal motility, as seen in diabetic patients. Further, an SBF series is helpful in identifying and defining the anatomy of small bowel fistulas (abnormal connections between the small bowel and other abdominal organs or skin).

A more accurate radiographic evaluation of the small intestine is provided by the *small bowel enema*. Unlike the SBF, in which the barium is swallowed by the patient, during the small bowel enema the barium is injected into a tube previously passed to the small bowel. This small bowel enema provides better visualization of the entire small bowel because the barium is not diluted by gastric and duodenal juices, as occurs when the patient drinks barium. This test is especially useful in the evaluation of patients with partial small bowel obstruction of unknown etiology. Tumors, ulcers, and small bowel fistulas are more easily identified and defined with the enema.

Contraindications

- Patients who have a complete small bowel obstruction
  The introduction of barium into an obstructed bowel may create a stonelike impaction. However, this is extremely rare.
- Patients suspected of having a perforated viscus
  Barium should not be used in these patients because it may cause prolonged and recurrent abscesses if it leaks out of the bowel. Gastrografin, a water-soluble contrast medium, can be used if perforation is suspected. Unfortunately, Gastrografin becomes diluted very rapidly, thereby minimizing the accuracy of the SBF with this contrast medium.
- Patients who have unstable vital signs
  These patients should be supervised during the time required for this study.

Potential complication

- Barium-induced small bowel obstruction

Interfering factors

- Barium within the intestinal tract from a previous barium x-ray film
  This may obstruct adequate visualization of the small bowel.
- Food or fluid within the gastrointestinal (GI) tract

Procedure and patient care

Before

- Explain the procedure to the patient.
- Instruct the patient not to eat anything for at least 8 hours before the testing. Usually, keep the patient NPO after midnight on the day of the test.
- Inform the patient that the SBF series may take several hours. Suggest that patients bring reading material or some paperwork to occupy their time.
- Accompany the patient to the radiology department if his or her vital signs are not stable.
- Arrange for transportation of the hospitalized patient back to the nursing unit between serial films.

During

▪ Note the following procedural steps:

1. A specially prepared drink containing barium sulfate is mixed as a milkshake, which the patient drinks through a straw.
2. Usually an upper GI series is performed concomitantly (see p. 746).
3. The barium flow is followed through the upper GI tract fluoroscopically.
4. At frequent intervals (15 to 60 minutes), repeat x-ray films are taken to follow the flow of barium through the small intestine. These films are repeated until barium is seen flowing into the right colon. This usually takes 60 to 120 minutes. However, in patients who have delayed progression of the barium, the test may take as much as 24 hours to complete.

Small bowel enema

1. This is usually performed by placing a long, weighted tube transorally. However, a tube can also be placed into the upper small bowel endoscopically.
2. After the tube is in place, a thickened barium mixture is injected through the tube and x-ray films are serially performed, as described for the SBF.

▪ Note that this procedure is performed by a radiologist in the radiology department in approximately 30 minutes.
▪ Tell the patient that this test is not uncomfortable.

After

▪ Inform the patient of the need to evacuate adequately all the barium. Cathartics (e.g., magnesium citrate) are recommended. Initially, stools will be white and should return to normal color with complete evacuation.

Abnormal findings

Small bowel tumors
Small bowel obstruction from intrinsic tumors
Small bowel obstruction from adhesions, extrinsic tumors, or hernia
Inflammatory small bowel disease (e.g., Crohn's disease)
Malabsorption syndromes (e.g., Whipple's disease, sprue)
Congenital anatomic anomalies (e.g., malrotation)

Congenital abnormalities (e.g., small bowel atresia, duplication, Meckel's diverticulum)
Small bowel intussusception
Small bowel perforation

Notes

sodium (Na⁺), blood

Type of test Blood

Normal findings
Adult/elderly: 136-145 mEq/L or 136-145 mmol/L (SI units)
Child: 136-145 mEq/L
Infant: 134-150 mEq/L
Newborn: 134-144 mEq/L

Possible critical values <120 or >160 mEq/L

Test explanation and related physiology

Sodium is the major cation in the extracellular space, where serum levels of approximately 140 mEq/L exist. The concentration of sodium intracellularly is only 5 mEq/L. Therefore sodium salts are the major determinants of extracellular osmolality. The sodium content of the blood is a result of a balance between dietary sodium intake and renal excretion. Normally, individual nonrenal (e.g., sweat) sodium losses are minimal.

Many factors regulate homeostatic sodium balance. For example, aldosterone causes conservation of sodium by decreasing renal losses. Natriuretic hormone, or third factor, increases renal losses of sodium. Antidiuretic hormone (ADH), which controls the reabsorption of water at the distal tubules of the kidney, also affects sodium serum levels.

Water and sodium are physiologically very closely interrelated. As free body water is increased, serum sodium is diluted and the concentration may decrease. The kidney compensates by conserving sodium and excreting water. If free body water were to decrease, the serum sodium concentration would rise. The kidney would then respond by conserving free water. Aldosterone, ADH, and natriuretic factor all assist in these compensatory actions of the kidney.

An average dietary intake of approximately 90 to 250 mEq/day is needed to maintain sodium balance in adults. Symptoms of hyponatremia may include weakness, confusion, lethargy, stupor, and coma. Symptoms of hypernatremia include dry mucous membranes, thirst, agitation, restlessness, hyperreflexia, mania, and convulsions.

Interfering factors

- Recent trauma, surgery, or shock may cause a increase in sodium levels.
- Drugs that may cause increased levels include anabolic steroids, antibiotics, clonidine, corticosteroids, cough medicines, laxatives, methyldopa, nonsteroidal antiinflammatory agents, and oral contraceptives.
- Drugs that may cause decreased levels include carbamazepine, diuretics, sodium-free IV fluids, sulfonylureas, triamterene, and vasopressin.

Procedure and patient care

Before

- Explain the procedure to the patient.
- Tell the patient that no food or fluid is restricted.

During

- Collect 5 to 10 ml of venous blood in a red-top or green-top tube.
- If the patient is receiving an IV infusion, obtain the blood from the opposite arm.
- List on the laboratory slip any drugs that can affect test results.

After

- Apply pressure or a pressure dressing to the venipuncture site.
- Assess the venipuncture site for bleeding.

Abnormal findings

Increased levels (hypernatremia)

Increased sodium intake
   Excessive dietary intake
   Excessive sodium in IV fluids
Decreased sodium loss
   Cushing's syndrome
   Hyperaldosteronism
Excessive free body water loss
   Excessive sweating
   Extensive thermal burns
   Diabetes insipidus
   Osmotic diuresis

S

Decreased levels (hyponatremia)

Decreased sodium intake
   Deficient dietary intake
   Deficient sodium in IV fluids
Increased sodium loss
   Addison's disease
   Diarrhea
   Vomiting or nasogastric aspiration
   Diuretic administration
   Chronic renal insufficiency
Increased free body water
   Excessive oral water intake
   Excessive IV water intake
   Congestive heart failure
   Syndrome of inappropriate secretion of ADH
     (SIADH)
   Osmotic dilution
Third-space losses of sodium
   Ascites
   Peripheral edema
   Pleural effusion
   Intraluminal bowel loss (ileus or mechanical
     obstruction)

Notes

sodium (Na$^+$), urine

Type of test Urine (24 hour)

Normal findings

40-220 mEq/L/day or 40-220 mmol/L (SI units)
Values vary greatly with dietary intake.

Test explanation and related physiology

This test evaluates sodium balance in the body by determining the amount of sodium excreted in the urine in 24 hours. Sodium is the major cation in the extracellular space. Measuring the amount of sodium in the urine is useful for evaluating patients with volume depletion, acute renal failure, adrenal disturbances, and acid-base imbalances. This test is important, especially when the serum sodium concentration is low. For example, in patients with hyponatremia caused by inadequate sodium intake, the urine sodium will be low. However, in patients with hyponatremia caused by chronic renal failure, the urine sodium concentration will be high.

The sodium content in urine is the result of the balance between the dietary sodium and renal excretion of sodium. In the normal individual, nonrenal sodium losses are minimal. Many factors affect this delicate homeostatic sodium balance. For example, aldosterone tends to raise sodium levels by stimulating conservation of sodium by decreasing renal losses. Antidiuretic hormone (ADH), which increases the reabsorption of water in the distal tubules of the kidney, tends to lower sodium levels.

Interfering factors

- Dietary salt intake can increase sodium levels.
- Altered kidney function can affect levels.
- Drugs that may cause increased levels include antibiotics, cough medicines, laxatives, and steroids.
- Drugs that may cause decreased levels include diuretics (e.g., Lasix) and steroids.

Procedure and patient care

Before

- Explain the procedure to the patient.
- Tell the patient that no fasting is required.

During

- Instruct the patient to begin the 24-hour urine collection after urinating. Discard the initial specimen and start the 24-hour timing at that point.
- Collect all urine passed during the next 24 hours.
- Show the patient where to store the urine specimen.
- Keep the specimen on ice or refrigerated during the 24 hours.
- Indicate the starting time on the urine container and on the laboratory slip.
- Post the hours for the urine collection in a noticeable place to prevent accidental discarding of the specimen.
- Instruct the patient to void before defecating so that urine is not contaminated by feces.
- Remind the patient not to put toilet paper in the collection container.
- Encourage the patient to drink fluids during the 24 hours.
- Instruct the patient to collect the last specimen as close as possible to the end of the 24-hour period. Add this urine to the container.

After

- Transport the urine specimen promptly to the laboratory.

Abnormal findings

Increased levels	Decreased levels
Dehydration	Congestive heart failure
Starvation	Malabsorption
Adrenocortical insufficiency	Diarrhea
Diuretic therapy	Renal failure
Hypothyroidism	Cushing's disease
Syndrome of inappropriate ADH secretion (SIADH)	Aldosteronism
	Diaphoresis
Diabetic ketoacidosis	Pulmonary emphysema
Toxemia of pregnancy	

Notes

spinal x-rays (Cervical, thoracic, lumbar, sacral, or coccygeal x-ray studies)

Type of test X-ray

Normal findings Normal spinal vertebrae

Test explanation and related physiology

Spinal x-ray studies can be done to evaluate any area of the spine. They usually include anteroposterior, lateral, and oblique views of these structures. These x-ray films are often done to assess back pain, degenerative arthritic changes, traumatic fractures, tumor invasion, spondylosis (stress fracture of the vertebrae), and spondylolisthesis (slipping of one vertebral disk on the other).

Contraindications

- Patients who are pregnant

Procedure and patient care

Before

- Explain the procedure to the patient.
- Instruct the patient to remove any metal objects covering the area to be visualized.
- Immobilize the suspected fracture site.
- Tell the patient that no fasting or sedation is required. However, if a fracture is suspected, the patient may be kept NPO.

During

- Note that the patient is placed on an x-ray table. Anterior, posterior, lateral, and oblique x-ray films are taken of the desired area on the spinal cord.
- Note that a radiologic technologist takes spinal x-ray films in a few minutes.
- Tell the patient that no discomfort is associated with this study.

After

- Note that positioning and patient activity depend on test results.

S

Abnormal findings

Degenerative arthritic changes
Traumatic fractures
Spondylosis
Spondylolisthesis
Metastatic tumor invasion

Notes

sputum culture and sensitivity (C&S, Culture and Gram stain)

Type of test Sputum

Normal findings Normal upper respiratory tract

Test explanation and related physiology

Sputum cultures are obtained to determine the presence of pathogenic bacteria for patients with respiratory infections, such as pneumonia. *Gram staining* is the first step in the microbiologic analysis of sputum. By staining the sputum, bacteria are classified as gram positive or gram negative. This may be used to guide drug therapy until the C&S report is completed. Determinations of bacterial sensitivity to various antibiotics are done to identify the most appropriate antimicrobial drug therapy. Sputum for C&S should be collected before antimicrobial therapy is initiated, unless the test is being performed to evaluate the effectiveness of the medications already being given. Preliminary reports are usually available in 24 hours. Cultures require at least 48 hours for completion. Sputum cultures for fungus and *Mycobacterium tuberculosis* may take 6 to 8 weeks.

Procedure and patient care

Before

- Explain the procedure for sputum collection to the patient.
- Remind the patient that the sputum must be coughed up from the lungs and that saliva is not sputum.
- Hold antibiotics until after the sputum has been collected.
- Give the patient a sterile sputum container on the night before the sputum is to be collected so that a morning specimen may be obtained on arising.
- Instruct the patient to rinse out his or her mouth with water before the sputum collection to decrease contamination of the sputum by particles in the oropharynx.

During

- Note that sputum specimens are best when the patient awakes in the morning before eating or drinking.

S

- Collect at least 1 teaspoon of sputum in a sterile sputum container.
- Usually, obtain sputum by having the patient cough after taking several deep breaths.
- If the patient is unable to produce a sputum specimen, stimulate coughing by lowering the head of the patient's bed or by giving the patient an aerosol administration of a warm hypertonic solution.
- Note that other methods to collect sputum include endotracheal aspiration, fiberoptic bronchoscopy, and transtracheal aspiration.

After

- Inform the patient to notify the nurse as soon as the sputum is collected.
- Label the sputum and send it to the laboratory as soon as possible.
- Note any current antibiotic therapy on the laboratory slip.

Abnormal findings

Bacterial infections (e.g., pneumonia)
Viral infections
Atypical bacterial infections (e.g., tuberculosis)

Notes

sputum cytology

Type of test Sputum

Normal findings Normal epithelial cells

Test explanation and related physiology

Tumors within the pulmonary system frequently slough cells into the sputum. When the sputum is gathered, the cells are examined. If the cytologic test is positive, malignant cells are seen, indicating a lung tumor. If only normal epithelial cells and no malignant cells are seen, either no malignancy exists or any existing tumor is not shedding cells. Therefore a positive test indicates malignancy and a negative test means nothing.

Procedure and patient care

Before

- Explain the procedure for sputum collection to the patient.
- Remind the patient that the sputum must be coughed up from the lungs and that saliva is not sputum.
- Give the patient a sterile sputum container on the night before the sputum is to be collected so that the morning specimen may be obtained on arising.
- Instruct the patient to rinse out her or his mouth with water to decrease contamination of the sputum by particles in the oropharynx.

During

- Note that sputum specimens are best collected when the patient awakes in the morning.
- Collect at least 1 teaspoon of sputum in the sterile sputum container.
- Usually, obtain sputum by having the patient cough after taking several deep breaths.
- If the patient is unable to produce a sputum specimen, stimulate coughing by lowering the head of the patient's bed or by giving the patient an aerosol administration of a warm hypertonic solution.
- Note that other methods to collect sputum include endo-

tracheal aspiration, fiberoptic bronchoscopy, and transtracheal aspiration.

- Usually, collect sputum for cytology on three separate occasions.

After

- Inform the patient to notify the nurse as soon as the sputum is collected.
- Label the specimen and send it to the laboratory as soon as possible.

Abnormal findings

Malignancies

Notes

stool culture (Stool for culture and sensitivity [C&S], Stool for ova and parasites [O&P])

Type of test Stool

Normal findings Normal intestinal flora

Test explanation and related physiology

Normally, stool contains many bacteria and fungi. The more common bacteria include *Enterococcus, Escherichia coli, Proteus, Pseudomonas, Staphylococcus aureus, Candida albicans, Bacteroides,* and *Clostridia.* Bacteria are indigenous to the bowel. However, several bacteria act as pathogens within the bowel. They include *Salmonella, Shigella, Campylobacter, Yersinia,* pathogenic *E. coli,* and *Staphylococcus.* Parasites can also affect the stool. Common parasites are *Ascaris* (hookworm), *Strongyloides* (tapeworm), and *Giardia* (protozoans). Identification of any of these pathogens in the stool incriminates that bug as the etiology of the infectious enteritis.

Infections of the bowel from bacteria, virus, or parasites usually present as acute diarrhea, excessive flatus, and abdominal discomfort.

Interfering factors

- Urine may inhibit the growth of bacteria. Therefore urine should not be mixed with the feces during collection of a stool sample.
- Recent barium studies can obscure the detection of parasites.
- Drugs that may affect test results include antibiotics, bismuth, and mineral oil.

Procedure and patient care

Before

- Explain the method of stool collection to the patient. Be matter-of-fact to avoid any embarrassment to the patient.
- Instruct the patient not to mix urine or toilet paper with the stool specimen.
- Instruct the patient to use an appropriate collection container.

During

- Ask the patient to defecate into a clean bedpan.
- Place a small amount of stool in a sterile collection container.
- Also, send mucus and blood streaks with the specimen.
- If a rectal swab is to be used, wear gloves and insert the cotton-tipped swab at least 1 inch into the anal canal. Then rotate the swab for 30 seconds and place it into the clean container.

Tape test

- Use this test when pinworms *(Enterobius)* are suspected.
- Place a clear tape in the patient's perianal region. (This is especially helpful in children.)
- Because the female worm lays her eggs at night around the perianal area, apply the tape before bedtime and remove it in the morning before the patient gets out of the bed.
- Press the sticky surface of the tape directly to a glass slide and examine microscopically for pinworm ova.

After

- Handle the stool specimen carefully, as though it is capable of causing infection. Wear gloves when obtaining and handling the specimen.
- Indicate on the laboratory slip any antibiotics that the patient may be taking.
- Promptly send the stool specimen to the laboratory. Delays in transfer of the specimen may affect the viability of the organism. If long delays are necessary, obtain a buffered glycerol-saline solution to be combined to the stool and used as a preservative.
- Note that occasionally, growth of some enteric pathogens take as long as 6 weeks to isolate.
- When pathogens are detected, maintain isolation of the patient's stool until therapy is completed.

Abnormal findings

Bacterial enterocolitis
Protozoan enterocolitis
Parasitic enterocolitis

Notes

stool for occult blood testing (Stool for OB)

Type of test Stool

Normal findings No occult blood within stool

Test explanation and related physiology

Normally, only minimal quantities of occult blood (OB) are passed into the gastrointestinal (GI) tract. Usually, this bleeding is not significant enough to cause a positive result in stool for OB testing. Tumors of the intestine grow into the lumen and are subjected to repeated trauma by the fecal stream. Eventually the friable tumor ulcerates and bleeding occurs. Most often, bleeding is so slight that gross blood is not seen in the stool. The blood can only be detected by chemical assay through the OB testing of the stool.

Benign and malignant GI tumors, ulcers, inflammatory bowel disease, arteriovenous (AV) malformations, diverticulosis, and hematobilia (hemobilia) can all cause OB within the stool. Other more common abnormalities (e.g., hemorrhoids, swallowed blood from oral or nasal pharyngeal bleeding) can also cause OB within the stool.

Recently, it has been well documented that vigorous exercise can create OB within the stool. It is important to note that many drugs and the ingestion of hemoglobin contained in red meats such as beef and pork can cause a false positive OB stool test. The more sensitive the test, the more false positives will be obtained.

When OB testing is properly performed, a positive result should be an indication for a thorough GI evaluation.

Interfering factors

- Bleeding gums following a dental procedure.
- Ingestion of red meat within 3 days before testing.
- Ingestion of fish, turnips, and horseradish.
- Drugs that may cause GI bleeding include anticoagulants, aspirin, colchicine, iron preparations (large doses), non-steroidal antiarthritics, and steroids.
- Drugs that may cause false positive results include colchicine, iron, oxidizing drugs (e.g., iodine, bromides, boric acid), and rauwolfia derivatives.

S

- Drugs that may cause false negative results include vitamin C.

Procedure and patient care

Before

- Explain the procedure to the patient.
- Instruct the patient to refrain from eating any red meat for at least 3 days before the test.
- Instruct the patient to refrain from drugs known to interfere with OB testing.
- Instruct the patient as to method of obtaining appropriate stool specimens. Many procedures are available (e.g., specimen cards, tissue wipes, test paper). Tests can done at home with specimen cards (Hemoccult) and mailed when collected.
- Instruct the patient not to mix urine with the stool specimen.
- Inform the patient as to the need for multiple specimens obtained on separate days to increase the test's accuracy.
- Note that in some centers, a high-residue diet is recommended to increase the abrasive effect of the stool.
- Note on the laboratory slip any anticoagulant medications that the patient may be taking.
- Be gentle in obtaining stool by digital examination. Traumatic digital examination can cause a false positive stool, especially in patients who have prior anorectal disease such as hemorrhoids.

During

Hemoccult slide test
- Place a stool sample on one side of guaiac paper.
- Place two drops of developer on the other side.
- Note that a bluish discoloration indicates OB in the stool.

Tablet test
- Place a stool sample on the developer paper.
- Place a tablet on top of the stool specimen.
- Put two or three drops of tap water on the tablet and allow to flow onto the paper.
- Note that a bluish discoloration indicates OB in the stool.

After

- Inform the patient as to the results.
- If the tests are positive, inquire as to whether the patient had violated any of the previous preparation recommendations.

Abnormal findings

GI tumors
Polyps
Ulcers
Varices
Inflammatory bowel disease
Diverticulosis

Ischemic bowel disease
GI trauma
Recent GI surgery
Hemorrhoids
Esophagitis
Gastritis

Notes

---

sweat electrolytes test (Iontophoretic sweat test)

Type of test Fluid analysis

Normal findings

Sodium values in children
Normal: <70 mEq/L
Abnormal: >90 mEq/L
Equivocal: 70-90 mEq/L
Chloride values in children
Normal: <50 mEq/L
Abnormal: >60 mEq/L
Equivocal: 50-60 mEq/L

Test explanation and related physiology

Patients with cystic fibrosis have increased sodium and chloride contents in their sweat. This fact forms the basis of this test, which is both sensitive and specific for cystic fibrosis. Cystic fibrosis is an inherited disease characterized by abnormal secretion of exocrine glands within the bronchi, small intestines, pancreatic ducts, bile ducts, and skin (sweat glands). Sweat, induced by electrical current *(pilocarpine iontophoresis),* is collected, and its sodium and chloride contents are measured. The degree of abnormality is no indication of the severity of cystic fibrosis; it merely indicates that the patient has the disease.

In children with recurrent respiratory tract infections, malabsorption syndromes, or failure to thrive, this test is indicated to diagnose cystic fibrosis. Almost all patients with cystic fibrosis have sweat sodium and chloride contents two to five times greater than normal values. These levels, in patients with suspicious clinical manifestations, are diagnostic of cystic fibrosis.

The sweat test is not reliable during the first few weeks of life. High serum concentrations of immunoreactive trypsin may be a better test for this age group.

Procedure and patient care

Before

- Explain the procedure to the patient and/or parents.
- Tell the patient and/or parents that no fasting is required.

During

- Note the following procedural steps:

  1. For iontophoresis, a low-level electrical current is applied to the test area (the thigh in infants, the forearm in older children).
  2. The positive electrode is covered by gauze and saturated with pilocarpine hydrochloride, a stimulating drug that induces sweating.
  3. The negative electrode is covered by gauze saturated with a bicarbonate solution.
  4. The electrical current is allowed to flow for 5 to 12 minutes.
  5. The electrodes are removed, and the arm is washed with distilled water.
  6. Paper disks are placed over the test site with the use of clean, dry forceps.
  7. These disks are covered with paraffin to obtain an airtight seal, thereby preventing evaporation of sweat.
  8. After 1 hour the paraffin is removed, and the paper disks are transferred immediately by forceps to a weighing jar and sent for sodium and chloride analysis.
  9. A *screening test* can be done to detect sweat chloride levels. For screening, a test paper containing silver nitrate is pressed against the child's hand for several seconds. The test is positive when the excess chloride combines with the silver nitrate to form white-silver chloride on the paper. That is, the child with cystic fibrosis will leave a "heavy" handprint on the paper.
  10. A positive screening test is usually validated by iontophoresis.

- Note that an experienced technologist performs the sweat test in approximately 1½ hours in the laboratory or at the patient's bedside.
- Inform the patient that the electrical current is small and no discomfort or pain is generally associated with this test.

After

- Initiate extensive education and counseling for the patient and/or parents if the results indicate cystic fibrosis.

Abnormal finding

Cystic fibrosis

Notes

syphilis detection test (Serologic test for syphilis [STS], Veneral Disease Research Laboratory [VDRL], Rapid plasma reagin [RPR], Fluorescent treponemal antibody test [FTA])

Type of test Blood

Normal findings Negative, or nonreactive

Test explanation and related physiology

The serologic tests for syphilis (STS) are used to detect antibodies to *Treponema pallidum,* the causative agent of syphilis. There are two groups of antibodies. The first is a nontreponemal antibody (reagin) directed against a lipoidal agent that results from the *T. pallidum* infection. The second is an antibody directed against the *Treponema* organism itself. The nontreponemal antibody test is relatively nonspecific. These antibodies are most often detected by the *Wassermann test* or the *Venereal Disease Research Laboratory* (VDRL) *test*. A new, more sensitive nontreponemal test is the *rapid plasma reagin* (RPR) *test*. The VDRL and RPR tests, by virtue of their testing for nonspecific antibody, have a high false positive rate. The VDRL test becomes positive about 2 weeks after the patient's inoculation with *Treponema* and returns to normal shortly after adequate treatment is given. The test is positive in nearly all primary and secondary stages of syphilis and in two thirds of patients with tertiary syphilis.

If the VDRL or RPR test is positive, the diagnosis may be confirmed by the *Treponema* test, such as the *fluorescent treponemal antibody absorption test* (FTA-ABS). This second test is much more specific. The FTA test, which tests for a more specific antibody, is more accurate than the VDRL and RPR tests.

False positive and false negative results are rare in all stages of the disease. The FTA test is required before the diagnosis of syphilis can be made with certainty.

Screening for syphilis is usually done during the first prenatal checkup for pregnant women. Syphilis, if untreated, may cause abortion, stillbirth, and premature labor. The effect on the fetus can be central nervous system damage, hearing loss, and possible death.

Interfering factors

- Excessive hemolysis and gross lipemia can affect test results.
- Excess chyle in the blood may interfere with the test results.
- Many conditions cause false positive results when using VDRL and RPR tests. Some of these conditions include *Mycoplasma* pneumonia, malaria, acute bacterial and viral infections, autoimmune diseases, and pregnancy.
- Recent ingestion of alcohol can alter the test results.

Procedure and patient care

Before

- Explain the procedure to the patient.
- Check with the laboratory regarding fasting requirements. Some prefer collecting the specimen before meals. Some laboratories request that the patient refrain from alcohol for 24 hours before the blood test.

During

- Collect approximately 7 ml of blood in a red-top tube.

After

- Apply pressure or a pressure dressing to the venipuncture site.
- Check the venipuncture site for bleeding.
- If the test is positive, instruct the patient to inform recent sexual contacts so they can be evaluated.
- If the test is positive, be sure the patient receives the appropriate antibiotic therapy.

Abnormal finding

Syphilis

Notes

T-tube and operative cholangiogram

Type of test X-ray

Normal findings

Normal common bile duct with no dilation or filling defects

Good runoff of dye through ampulla of Vater and into duodenum

Test explanation and related physiology

In *operative cholangiography* the common bile duct is directly injected with radiopaque material. This is usually performed during cholecystectomy. Stones appear as radiolucent shadows. Gallstones, tumors, or strictures cause partial or total obstruction of the flow of dye into the duodenum. By visualization of the biliary duct structures, the surgeon is provided with the surgical anatomy of the biliary tree. This reduces the possibility of inadvertent common bile duct injury during cholecystectomy. If common duct stones are demonstrated on operative cholangiography, a common duct exploration is performed. Some surgeons perform operative cholangiography on all patients who have cholecystectomy. Other surgeons use specific indications for operative cholangiography, including:

1. Jaundice
2. Abnormal liver enzymes
3. Dilated common bile duct
4. Evidence of pancreatitis
5. Evidence of small stones in the cystic duct during cholecystectomy

T-tube cholangiography is performed postoperatively following a common duct exploration. Its main purpose is to detect retained common bile duct stones and to demonstrate good flow of contrast of bile into the duodenum. This test is performed through the use of a T-shaped rubber tube that is placed into the common bile duct at surgery. This test is usually performed 5 to 10 days after surgery. If no stones are evident, and there is good runoff of bile into the duodenum, the T-tube can be removed. If there are residual stones, the T-tube tract can be used to extract the stones.

Potential complication

- Sepsis caused by increased ductal pressure with dye infusion

Interfering factor

- Barium within the abdomen from a previous upper GI series or barium enema x-ray film precludes visualization of the bile duct.

Procedure and patient care

Before

- Explain the procedure to the patient.
- Tell the patient that no fasting or sedation is required.

During

- Note the following procedural steps:

Operative cholangiogram
1. This is performed through catheterization of the cystic duct during cholecystectomy.
2. A needle or catheter is placed in the common bile duct.
3. The dye is injected directly into the common bile duct.
4. X-ray films are taken while the patient is on the operating table and are immediately reviewed by the surgeon.

T-tube cholangiogram
1. The patient is taken to the radiology department.
2. A sterile dye solution is injected into the T-tube previously placed by the surgeon.
3. X-ray films are taken of the right upper quadrant of the abdomen while the patient is placed in various positions.

- Note that a radiologist or surgeon performs these procedures in approximately 10 minutes.
- Tell the patient that no discomfort is associated with these studies.

After

- Observe the patient for signs of sepsis.
- If a T-tube has been surgically placed, establish a sterile, closed drainage system.

Abnormal findings

Common bile duct stones
Anatomic variations
Stricture or tumor obstructing common bile duct
Bile duct cysts
Bile duct surgical trauma

Notes

therapeutic drug monitoring

Type of test Blood

Normal findings See Table 9.

Test explanation and related physiology

Therapeutic drug monitoring entails taking measurements of blood drug levels to determine effective drug dosages and to prevent toxicity. Drug monitoring is especially important in patients taking medications (e.g., antiarrhythmics, bronchodilators, antibiotics, anticonvulsants, cardiotonics) when the margin of safety between therapeutic and toxic levels is narrow.

Table 9 lists the therapeutic and toxic ranges for most patients. These ranges may not apply to all patients because clinical response is influenced by many factors (e.g., noncompliance, concurrent drug use, other clinical conditions, patient's age and size, extent and rate of drug absorption, metabolism). Also, note that different laboratories use different units for reporting test results and normal ranges. It is important that sufficient time pass between the administration of the medication and the collection of the blood sample to allow for therapeutic levels to occur.

Blood samples can be taken at the drug's *peak level* (the highest therapeutic concentration) or at the *trough level* (the lowest therapeutic concentration). Peak levels are useful when testing for toxicity, and trough levels are useful for demonstrating a satisfactory therapeutic level. Trough levels are often referred to as *residual levels*.

Procedure and patient care

Before

- Explain the procedure to the patient.
- Tell the patient that no food or fluid restrictions are needed.

During

- Collect approximately 7 to 10 ml of venous blood in a tube designated by the laboratory. *Peak* levels are usually obtained 1 to 2 hours after oral intake, approximately 1 hour after IM administration, and about ½ hour after IV administration. *Residual (trough)* levels are usually obtained shortly before (0 to 15 minutes) the next scheduled dose. Consult with pharmacy for specific times.

After

- Apply pressure or a pressure dressing to the venipuncture site.
- Assess the venipuncture site for bleeding.
- Clearly mark all blood samples with the following information: patient's name, diagnosis, name of drug, time of last drug ingestion, time of sample, and any other medications the patient is currently taking.
- Promptly send the specimen to the laboratory.

Abnormal findings

Nontherapeutic levels of drugs
Toxic level of drugs

Notes

T

TABLE 9 Therapeutic drug monitoring data

Drug	Use	Therapeutic level*	Toxic level*
Acetaminophen	Analgesic, antipyretic	Depends on use	>250 μg/ml
Amikacin	Antibiotic	15-25 μg/ml	>25 μg/ml
Aminophylline	Bronchodilator	10-20 μg/ml	>20 μg/ml
Amitriptyline	Antidepressant	120-150 ng/ml	>500 ng/ml
Carbamazepine	Anticonvulsant	5-12 μg/ml	>12 μg/ml
Chloramphenicol	Antiinfective	10-20 μg/ml	>25 μg/ml
Desipramine	Antidepressant	150-300 ng/ml	>500 ng/ml
Digitoxin	Cardiac glycoside	15-25 ng/ml	>25 ng/ml
Digoxin	Cardiac glycoside	0.8-2.0 ng/ml	>2.4 ng/ml
Disopyramide	Antiarrhythmic	2-5 μg/ml	>5 μg/ml
Ethosuximide	Anticonvulsant	40-100 μg/ml	>100 μg/ml
Gentamicin	Antibiotic	5-10 μg/ml	>12 μg/ml
Imipramine	Antidepressant	150-300 ng/ml	>500 ng/ml

Kanamycin	Antibiotic	20-25 μg/ml	>35 μg/ml
Lidocaine	Antiarrhythmic	1.5-5.0 μg/ml	>5 μg/ml
Lithium	Manic episodes of manic-depression psychosis	0.8-1.2 mEq/L	>2.0 mEq/L
Methotrexate	Antitumor agent	>0.01 μmol	>10 μmol/24 hr
Nortriptyline	Antidepressant	50-150 ng/ml	>500 ng/ml
Phenobarbital	Anticonvulsant	10-30 μg/ml	>40 μg/ml
Phenytoin	Anticonvulsant	10-20 μg/ml	>30 μg/ml
Primidone	Anticonvulsant	5-12 μg/ml	>15 μg/ml
Procainamide	Antiarrhythmic	4-10 μg/ml	>16 μg/ml
Propranolol	Antiarrhythmic	50-100 ng/ml	>150 ng/ml
Quinidine	Antiarrhythmic	2-5 μg/ml	>10 μg/ml
Salicylate	Antipyretic, antiinflammatory, analgesic	100-250 μg/ml	>300 μg/ml
Theophylline	Bronchodilator	10-20 μg/ml	>20 μg/ml
Tobramycin	Antibiotic	5-10 μg/ml	>12 μg/ml
Valproic acid	Anticonvulsant	50-100 μg/ml	>100 μg/ml

*Levels vary according to the institution performing the test.

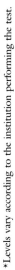

thermography (Mammothermography)

Type of test X-ray

Normal findings No evidence of cancer

Test explanation and related physiology

Thermography is a technique by which differences in heat energy emanating from the skin of the breast are photographed using an infrared detector. The result is a pictorial representation of the breast. Fibrocystic disease, infection, and tumor are all associated with increased blood supply to the affected area. This increased blood supply causes an increase of temperature in the suspicious area, and heat is emitted. That heat is detected by an infrared camera and easily located on a pictorial representation.

Normal tissues and benign tumors are represented as shades of gray. Hot spots are caused by a malignant tumor, fibrocystic changes, or infection and are demonstrated by brighter shades within the red spectrum. Gross breast cysts are occasionally represented as cold or white spots.

Thermography is quite sensitive in detecting breast cancer. However, because other abnormalities (e.g., fibrocystic disease, infection) may be misread as positive, this test is considered nonspecific. The overall accuracy of thermography is far inferior to that of mammography. However, because thermography can be easily and inexpensively performed, it is considered a good screening tool in an attempt to diagnose breast cancer at an early stage. At a time when mammography was expensive and associated with significant amount of radiation exposure, thermography offered a safe and inexpensive alternative to the diagnosis of breast cancer. However, mammography recently has improved greatly in its accuracy, minimal radiation exposure, and accessibility to the public. As a result, thermography is rarely used today.

Contraindications

- Premenstrual patients who have severe engorgement of their breasts
- Patients who have recently been exposed to excessive sunlight causing sunburn

- Patients who have recently had acute infection of the breast

Interfering factors

- Pregnancy because of the increased vascularity of the breasts

Procedure and patient care

Before

- Explain the procedure to the patient.
- Instruct the patient to disrobe from the waist up.
- Provide the patient with a suitable x-ray gown.

During

- Note the following procedural steps:
  1. The patient is taken to the thermography room, which is usually in the radiology department.
  2. After a short period of heat equilibration, a thermo-scope is placed over a small area of the breast to determine normal breast temperatures.
  3. The infrared scanning unit is adjusted to establish a baseline normal temperature.
  4. The unit is placed in position to scan both breasts from frontal and lateral views.
- Note that a radiologic technologist usually performs this test in approximately 20 minutes and that a radiologist interprets the results.
- Tell the patient that no discomfort is associated with this test.

After

- Take this opportunity to instruct the patient in breast self-examination.

Abnormal findings

Cancer
Fibrocystic changes
Acute suppurative infection
Gross cysts

Notes

thoracentesis and pleural fluid analysis
(Pleural tap)

Type of test Fluid analysis

Normal findings Normal pleural fluid

Test explanation and related physiology

Thoracentesis is an invasive procedure that entails the insertion of a needle into the pleural space for removal of fluid (or rarely air). Pleural fluid is removed for both diagnostic and therapeutic purposes. Therapeutically, it is done to relieve pain, dyspnea, and other symptoms of pleural pressure. Removal of this fluid also permits better radiographic visualization of the lung.

Diagnostically, thoracentesis is performed whenever a pleural effusion (abnormal accumulation of fluid in the pleural space) of unknown etiology is recognized. A decubitus chest x-ray film is obtained before thoracentesis to ensure that the pleural fluid is mobile and therefore accessible to a needle placed within the pleural space.

The pleural fluid is usually evaluated for gross appearance; cell counts; protein, lactic dehydrogenase (LDH), glucose, and amylase levels; Gram stain and bacteriologic cultures; *Mycobacterium tuberculosis* and fungus; cytology; carcinoembryonic antigen (CEA) levels; and sometimes for other specific tests. Each is discussed separately.

Gross appearance. The color, optical density, and viscosity are noted as the pleural fluid appears in the aspirating syringe. Empyema is characterized by the presence of a foul odor and the presence of thick, puslike fluid. An opalescent, pearly fluid is characteristic of chylothorax (chyle in the pleural cavity).

Cell counts. The white blood cell (WBC) and differential counts are determined. A WBC count exceeding $1000/mm^3$ is suggestive of an exudate. The predominance of polymorphonuclear leukocytes (PMNs) usually is an indication of an acute inflammatory condition (e.g., pneumonia, pulmonary infarction, early tuberculosis effusion). When more than one half of the WBCs are small lymphocytes, the effusion is usually caused by tuberculosis or tumor.

Protein content. Levels greater than 3 g/dl are characteristic of exudates, whereas transudates usually have a protein content of less than 3 g/dl. *Transudates* are most frequently caused by congestive heart failure, cirrhosis, nephrotic syndrome, myxedema, peritoneal dialysis, and acute glomerulonephritis. *Exudates* are most often found in infectious disease and in neoplastic conditions. However, collagen vascular disease, pulmonary infarction, gastrointestinal diseases, trauma, and drug hypersensitivity are also causes of exudative effusions.

Lactic dehydrogenase. A pleural fluid/serum LDH ratio greater than 0.6 is typical of an exudate. An exudate is identified with a high degree of accuracy if the pleural fluid/serum protein ratio is greater than 0.5 and the pleural fluid/serum LDH ratio is greater than 0.6.

Glucose. Usually, pleural glucose levels approximate serum levels. Low values appear to be a combination of glycolysis by the extra cells and impairment of glucose diffusion because of damage to the pleural membrane. Values less than 60 mg/dl are occasionally seen in tuberculosis or malignancy and typically occur in rheumatoid arthritis and empyema.

Amylase. In a malignant effusion the amylase concentration is slightly elevated. Very high amylase levels are seen when the effusion is caused by pancreatitis or rupture of the esophagus associated with leakage of salivary amylase.

Gram stain and bacteriologic culture. These tests are routinely performed when bacterial pneumonia or empyema is a possible cause of the effusion. If possible, these should be done before the initiation of antibiotic therapy.

Cultures for Mycobacterium tuberculosis and fungus. Tuberculosis is less often a cause for pleural effusion in the United States today than it was in the past. Fungus may be a cause of pulmonary effusion in patients with compromised immunologic defenses.

Cytology. A cytologic study is performed to detect tumor cells in approximately 50% to 60% of patients with malignant effusions. Breast and lung are the two most frequent tumors; lymphoma is the third.

Carcinoembryonic antigen. Pleural fluid CEA levels are elevated in various malignant (gastrointestinal, breast) conditions.

Special tests. The pH of pleural fluid is usually 7.4 or greater. The pH is typically less than 7.2 when empyema is present. The pH may be 7.2 to 7.4 in tuberculosis or malignancy.

A total lipid and cholesterol count should be done if chylothorax is suspected by the opalescent, pearly appearance of the fluid.

In some instances the rheumatoid factor (RF, see p. 649) and the complement levels (see p. 21) are also measured in pleural fluid.

Pleural fluid antinuclear antibody (ANA) and pleural fluid/ANA ratios are often used to evaluate pleural effusion secondary to systemic lupus erythematosus (SLE).

Contraindications

- Patients with significant thrombocytopenia

Potential complications

- Pneumothorax because of puncture of the visceral pleura or entry of air into the pleural space
- Interpleural bleeding because of puncture of tissue or a blood vessel
- Hemoptysis caused by needle puncture of a pulmonary vessel or by inflammation
- Reflex bradycardia and hypertension
- Pulmonary edema
- Seeding of the needle tract with tumor

Procedure and patient care

Before

- Explain the procedure to the patient.
- Obtain informed consent for this procedure.
- Tell the patient that no fasting or sedation is necessary.
- Inform the patient that movement or coughing should be minimized to avoid inadvertent needle damage to the lung or pleura during the procedure.
- Administer a cough suppressant before the procedure if the patient has a troublesome cough.
- Note that an x-ray film or ultrasound scan is often used to assist in location of the fluid. Fluoroscopy may also be used.

During

- Note the following procedural steps:
  1. The patient is usually placed in an upright position

with the arms and shoulders raised and supported on an padded overhead table. This position spreads the ribs and enlarges the intercostal space for insertion of the needle.

2. Patients who cannot sit upright are placed in a side-lying position on the unaffected side with the side to be tapped uppermost.

3. The thoracentesis is performed under strict sterile technique.

4. The needle insertion site, which is determined by percussion, auscultation, and examination of a chest x-ray film, ultrasound scanning, or fluoroscopy, is aseptically cleansed and anesthetized locally.

5. The needle is positioned in the pleural space, and the fluid is withdrawn with a syringe and a three-way stopcock.

6. A spring or Kelly clamp may be placed on the needle at the chest wall to stabilize the needle depth during the fluid collection.

7. A short polyethylene catheter may be inserted into the pleural space for fluid aspiration; this decreases the risk of puncturing the visceral pleural and inducing a pneumothorax.

8. Also, large volumes of fluid may be collected by connecting the catheter to a gravity-drainage system.

- Note that this procedure is performed by a physician at the patient's bedside, in a procedure room, or in the physician's office in less than ½ hour.
- Monitor the patient's pulse for reflex bradycardia and evaluate the patient for diaphoresis and the feeling of faintness during the procedure.
- Although local anesthetics eliminate pain at the insertion site, tell the patient that he or she may feel a pressurelike pain when the pleura is entered and the fluid is removed.

After

- Place a small bandage over the needle site. Usually, turn the patient on the unaffected side for 1 hour to allow the pleural puncture site to heal.
- Label the specimen with the patient's name, date, source of fluid, and diagnosis. Send promptly to the laboratory.
- Obtain a chest x-ray study as indicated to check for the complication of pneumothorax.

- Monitor the patient's vital signs.
- Observe the patient for coughing or for the expectoration of blood (hemoptysis), which may indicate trauma to the lung.
- Evaluate the patient for signs and symptoms of pneumothorax, tension pneumothorax, subcutaneous emphysema, and pyogenic infection (e.g., tachypnea, dyspnea, diminished breath sounds, anxiety, restlessness, fever).
- Assess the patient's lung sounds for diminished breath sounds, which could be a sign of pneumothorax.
- If the patient has no complaints of dyspnea, normal activity usually can be resumed 1 hour after the procedure.

Abnormal findings

Empyema
Chylothorax
Infection
Pneumonia
Pulmonary infarction
Tuberculosis effusion
Cirrhosis
Nephrotic syndrome
Myxedema
Peritoneal dialysis
Acute glomerulonephritis
Collagen vascular disease

Pulmonary infarction
Gastrointestinal disease
Trauma
Drug hypersensitivity
Tuberculosis
Rheumatoid arthritis
Pancreatitis
Ruptured esophagus
Tumors
Lymphoma
Systemic lupus erythematosus

Notes

throat culture and sensitivity (C&S)

Type of test Microscopic examination

Normal findings Negative

Test explanation and related physiology

Because the throat is normally colonized by many organisms, culture of this area serves only to isolate and identify a few particular pathogens (e.g., streptococci, meningococci, gonococci, *Bordetella pertussis, Corynebacterium diphtheriae*). Recognition of these organisms requires treatment. Streptococci are most often sought because a beta-hemolytic streptococcal pharyngitis may be followed by rheumatic fever or glomerulonephritis. This type of streptococcal infection most frequently affects children between the ages of 3 and 15 years. Therefore all children who have a sore throat and fever should have a throat culture done to attempt to identify streptococcal infections. In adults, however, fewer than 5% of patients with pharyngitis have a streptococcal infection. Therefore, throat cultures in adults are only indicated when the patient has severe or recurrent sore throat often associated with fever and palpable lymphadenopathy. These adults often have a history of streptococcal infections.

All cultures should be performed before antibiotic therapy is initiated. Otherwise the antibiotic may interrupt the growth of the organism in the laboratory. More often than not, however, the physician will want to institute antibiotic therapy before the culture results are reported. In these instances a *Gram stain* of the specimen smeared on a slide is most helpful and can be reported in less than 10 minutes. All forms of bacteria are grossly classified as gram positive (blue staining) or gram negative (red staining). Knowledge of the shape of the organism (e.g., spheric [coccus], rod shaped [bacillus]) can also be very helpful in the tentative identification of the infecting organism. With knowledge of the Gram stain results, the physician can institute a reasonable antibiotic regimen based on past experience as to the organism's possible identity. Most organisms take approximately 24 hours to grow in the laboratory, and a preliminary report can be given at that time. Occasionally, 48 to 72 hours are required for growth and identification of the organism. Cul-

T

tures may be repeated on completion of appropriate antibiotic therapy to identify resolution of the infection.

Interfering factors

- Drugs that can affect test results include antibiotics and antiseptic mouthwashes.

Procedure and patient care

Before

- Explain the procedure to the patient.

During

- Obtain a throat culture by depressing the tongue with a wooden tongue blade and touching the posterior wall of the throat and areas of inflammation, exudation, or ulceration with a sterile cotton swab.
- Avoid touching any other part of the mouth.
- Wear gloves and handle the specimen as if it were capable of transmitting disease.
- Place the swab in a sterile container and send to the microbiology laboratory within 30 minutes.
- Indicate on the laboratory slip any medications that the patient may be taking that could affect test results.

After

- Notify the physician of any positive results so appropriate antibiotic therapy can be initiated.

Abnormal findings

Bacterial pathogens (e.g., streptococci)

Notes

thyroid scanning (Thyroid scintiscan)

Type of test Nuclear scan

Normal findings

Normal size, shape, position, and function of the thyroid gland

No areas of decreased or increased uptake

Test explanation and related physiology

Thyroid scanning allows the size, shape, position, and anatomic function of the thyroid gland to be determined with the use of radionuclear scanning. A radioactive substance such as iodine-131 (^{131}I) is given to the patient to visualize the thyroid gland. A scanner is passed over the neck area, and an image is recorded.

Thyroid nodules are easily detected by this technique. Nodules are classified as functioning (warm/hot) or nonfunctioning (cold), depending on the amount of radionuclide taken up by the nodule. A functioning nodule could represent a benign adenoma or a localized toxic goiter. A nonfunctioning nodule may represent a cyst, carcinoma, nonfunctioning adenoma or goiter, lymphoma, or localized area of thyroiditis.

Scanning is useful in:

1. Patients with a neck mass or substernal mass
2. Patients who have a thyroid nodule. Thyroid cancers are usually nonfunctioning (cold) nodules.
3. Patients who have hyperthyroidism. Scanning will assist in differentiating Graves' disease (diffusely enlarged hyperfunctioning thyroid gland) from Plummer's disease (nodular hyperfunctioning gland).
4. Patients who have metastatic tumors without a known primary site. A normal scan excludes the thyroid gland as a possible primary site.
5. Patients who have a well-differentiated form of thyroid cancer. Areas of metastasis may show up on subsequent whole-body nuclear scans.

Contraindications

- Patients who are allergic to iodine or shellfish
- Patients who are pregnant

Potential complication

- Radiation-induced oncogenesis
  This complication is eliminated if technetium or low-radioactive iodine isomers are used instead of ^{131}I.

Interfering factors

- Drugs that may affect test results include cough medicines, multiple vitamins, oral contraceptives (some), and thyroid drugs
- Iodine-containing foods
- Recent administration of x-ray contrast agents

Procedure and patient care

Before

- Explain the procedure to the patient.
- Check the patient for allergies to iodine.
- Instruct the patient about medications that need to be restricted for weeks before the test (e.g., thyroid drugs, medications containing iodine).
- Obtain a history concerning previous contrast x-ray studies, nuclear scanning, or intake of any thyroid-suppressive or antithyroid drugs.
- Tell the patient that fasting is usually not required. Check with the laboratory.

During

- Note the following procedural steps:

  1. A standard dose of radioactive iodine or technetium is usually given to the patient by mouth. The capsule is tasteless.
  2. Scanning is usually performed 24 hours later. If technetium is used, scanning may be performed 2 hours later.
  3. At the designated time the patient is placed in a supine position and a detector is passed over the thyroid area.
  4. The radioactive counts are recorded and displayed.

- Note that this study is performed by a radiologic technologist in less than 30 minutes.
- Tell the patient that no discomfort is associated with this study.

After

- Assure the patient that the dose of radioactive iodine used in this test is minute and therefore harmless. No isolation and no special urine precautions are needed.

Abnormal findings

Adenoma
Toxic and nontoxic goiter
Cyst
Carcinoma
Lymphoma
Thyroiditis

Graves' disease
Plummer's disease
Metastasis
Hyperthyroidism
Hypothyroidism
Hashimoto's disease

Notes

T

thyroid-stimulating hormone (TSH, Thyrotropin)

Type of test Blood

Normal findings

Adult: 2-10 μU/ml or 2-10 mU/L (SI units)
Newborn: 3-18 μU/L or 3-18 mU/L
Cord: 3-12 μU/L or 3-12 mU/L
Values vary between laboratories.

Test explanation and related physiology

The TSH concentration aids in differentiating *primary* from *secondary* hypothyroidism. Pituitary TSH secretion is stimulated by hypothalamic TRH. Low levels of triiodothyronine and thyroxine (T_3, T_4) are the underlying stimuli for thyroid-releasing hormone (TRH) and TSH. Therefore a compensatory elevation of TRH and TSH occurs in patients with primary hypothyroid states, such as surgical or radioactive thyroid ablation; patients with burned-out thyroiditis, thyroid agenesis, or congenital cretinism; or patients taking antithyroid medications.

In secondary hypothyroidism the function of the hypothalamus or pituitary gland is faulty because of tumor, trauma, or infarction. Therefore TRH and TSH cannot be secreted, and plasma levels of these hormones are near 0 despite low T_3 and T_4 levels.

The TSH test is also used to evaluate and monitor exogenous thyroid replacement. This test is also done to detect primary hypothyroidism in newborns who have low screening T_4 levels. TSH and T_4 levels are frequently measured to differentiate pituitary from thyroid dysfunction. A decreased T_4 and normal or elevated TSH level can indicate a thyroid disorder. A decreased T_4 with a decreased TSH can indicate a pituitary disorder.

Interfering factors

- Recent radioisotope administration can affect test results.
- Severe illness can cause decreased TSH levels.
- Drugs that may cause increased levels include antithyroid medications, lithium, potassium iodide, and TSH injection.

- Drugs that may cause decreased levels include aspirin, dopamine, heparin, steroids, and T_3.

Procedure and patient care

Before

- Explain the procedure to the patient.
- Tell the patient that no food or drink restrictions are necessary.

During

- Collect approximately 5 ml of venous blood in a red-top tube.
- Use a heel stick to obtain blood from newborns.

After

- Apply pressure or a pressure dressing to the venipuncture site.
- Assess the venipuncture site for bleeding.

Abnormal findings

Increased levels

Primary hypothyroidism
    (thyroid dysfunction)
Thyroiditis
Thyroid agenesis
Congenital cretinism

Decreased levels

Secondary hypothyroidism
    (pituitary dysfunction)
Hyperthyroidism
Pituitary hypofunction

Notes

thyroid-stimulating hormone stimulation test (TSH stimulation test)

Type of test   Blood

Normal findings   Increased thyroid function with administration of exogenous TSH

Test explanation and related physiology

The TSH stimulation test is used to differentiate *primary* (or thyroidal) hypothyroidism from *secondary* (or hypothalamic-pituitary) hypothyroidism. Normal people and patients with hypothalamic-pituitary hypothyroidism are capable of increasing thyroid function when exogenous TSH is given. However, patients with primary thyroidal hypothyroidism are not; their thyroid gland is inadequate and cannot function no matter how much stimulation it receives. Patients with less than a 10% increase in radioactive iodine uptake (RAIU) or less than a 1.5 µg/dl rise in thyroxine (T_4) are considered to have a primary cause for their hypothyroid state. If the initially low uptake is caused by inadequate pituitary stimulation of an intrinsically normal thyroid gland, the RAIU should increase at least 10% and the T_4 level should rise 1.5 µg/dl or more. This is characteristic of secondary hypothyroidism.

Procedure and patient care

Before

- Explain the procedure to the patient.
- Obtain baseline levels of RAIU (see p. 612) or T_4 (see p. 724) as indicated.
- Tell the patient that no fasting is required.

During

- Administer 5 to 10 units of TSH intramuscularly for 3 days.
- Repeat the levels of RAIU or T_4 as indicated.

After

- Apply pressure or a pressure dressing to the venipuncture site.
- Assess the venipuncture site for bleeding.

Abnormal findings

Primary (thyroidal) hypothyroidism
Secondary (hypothalamic-pituitary) hypothyroidism

Notes

thyroid ultrasound (Thyroid echogram, Thyroid sonogram)

Type of test Ultrasound

Normal findings Normal size, shape, and position of thyroid gland

Test explanation and related physiology

Ultrasound examination of the thyroid gland is valuable for distinguishing cystic from solid thyroid nodules. If the nodule is found to be purely cystic (fluid filled), the fluid can simply be aspirated. Surgery is avoided. However, if the nodule has a mixed or solid appearance, tumor may be present and surgery is usually required for diagnosis and treatment.

This study may be repeated at intervals to determine the response of a thyroid mass to medical therapy. This test is also the procedure of choice for studying the thyroid gland of pregnant patients, since no radioactive iodine is used.

Procedure and patient care

Before

- Explain the procedure to the patient.
- Tell the patient that breathing or swallowing will not be affected by the placement of a transducer on the neck.
- Inform the patient that a liberal amount of lubricant will be applied to the neck to ensure effective transmission and reception of sound waves.
- Tell the patient that no fasting or sedation is required.

During

- Note the following procedural steps:
    1. The patient is taken to the ultrasonography department (usually in the radiology department) and placed in the supine position with the neck hyperextended.
    2. Gel is applied to the patient's neck.
    3. A sound transducer is passed over the nodule.
    4. Photographs are taken of the image displayed.
- Note that an ultrasound technologist usually performs

this study in approximately 15 minutes and that a radiologist evaluates the results.

- Tell the patient that no discomfort is associated with this study.

After

- Assist the patient in removing the lubricant from his or her neck.

Abnormal findings

Cysts
Tumors
Thyroid adenoma
Thyroid carcinoma
Goiters

Notes

thyrotropin-releasing hormone test (TRH test, Thyrotropin-releasing factor test [TRF test])

Type of test Blood

Normal findings Prompt rise in serum TSH level to approximately twice the baseline value in 30 minutes after an IV bolus of TRH (response normally greater in women)

Test explanation and related physiology

The TRH test assesses the responsiveness of the anterior pituitary gland via its secretion of thyroid-stimulating hormone (TSH) to an IV injection of TRH. After the TRH injection, the normally functioning pituitary gland should secrete TSH. In hyperthyroidism, either a slight increase or no increase in the TSH level is seen, since pituitary TSH production is suppressed by the direct effect of excess circulating thyroxine and triiodothyronine (T_4, T_3) on the pituitary gland. A normal result is considered reliable evidence for excluding the diagnosis of thyrotoxicosis. The TRH test is one of the most reliable confirmatory procedures for hyperthyroidism. Other tests are often compared to it to detect their accuracy.

In addition to assessing the responsiveness of the anterior pituitary gland, this test aids in the detection of primary, secondary, and tertiary hypothyroidism. In primary hypothyroidism (thyroid gland failure), the increase in the TSH level is two or more times the normal result. With secondary hypothyroidism (anterior pituitary failure), no TSH response occurs. Tertiary hypothyroidism (hypothalamic failure) may be diagnosed by a delayed rise in the TSH level. Multiple injections of TRH may be needed to induce the appropriate TSH response in this case.

The TRH test may be useful in differentiating primary depression from manic-depressive psychiatric illness and from secondary types of depression. In primary depression the TSH response is blunted in most patients, whereas patients with other types of depression have a normal TRH-induced TSH response.

Interfering factors

- Pregnancy can increase the TSH response to TRH.
- Drugs that can modify the TSH response include antithyroid drugs, aspirin, corticosteroids, estrogens, levodopa, and T_4.

Procedure and patient care

Before

- Explain the procedure to the patient.
- Instruct the patient to discontinue thyroid preparations for 3 to 4 weeks before the TRH test.
- Assess the patient for medications currently being taken.
- Tell the patient that no fasting or sedation is required.

During

- Administer a 500 μg bolus of thyrotropin-releasing hormone (TRH) intravenously.
- Obtain venous blood samples at intervals and measured for thyroid-stimulating hormone (TSH) levels.

After

- Apply pressure or a pressure dressing to the venipuncture site.
- Assess the venipuncture site for bleeding.
- Indicate on the laboratory slip if the patient is pregnant.
- List any medications that the patient is taking.

Abnormal findings

Hyperthyroidism
Hypothyroidism
Psychiatric primary depression
Acute starvation
Old age (especially in men)
Pregnancy

Notes

T

thyroxine (T$_4$, Thyroxine screen)

Type of test   Blood

Normal findings

Murphy-Pattee technique
Neonate: 10.1-20.0 µg/dl
1-4 months: 7.5-16.5 µg/dl
4-12 months: 5.5-14.5 µg/dl
1-6 years: 5.6-12.6 µg/dl
6-10 years: 4.9-11.7 µg/dl
Over 10 years: 4-11 µg/dl
Radioimmunoassay: 5-10 µg/dl

Possible critical values

Newborn: <7.0 µg/dl
Adult: <2.0 µg/dl if myxedema coma possible;
    >20 µg/dl if thyroid storm possible

Test explanation and related physiology

The serum thyroxine study is a direct measurement of the total amount of T$_4$ present in the patient's blood. Greater-than-normal levels indicate hyperthyroid states, and subnormal values are seen in hypothyroid states. Newborns are screened by T$_4$ tests to detect hypothyroidism. Mental retardation can be prevented by early diagnosis.

This is a very reliable test of thyroid function. However, results are affected by thyroid-binding globulin (TBG). Because T$_4$ is bound by serum proteins such as TBG, any increase in these proteins (as in pregnant women and in patients taking oral contraceptives) will cause fictitious elevated levels of T$_4$ and to some extent triiodothyronine (T$_3$). Therefore the levels of these carrier proteins (e.g., TBG) are concomitantly measured by T$_3$ resin uptake studies (see p. 740). T$_3$ resin results must be considered in interpreting the T$_4$ test results.

Interfering factors

- T$_4$ levels may be increased after x-ray iodinated contrast studies.

- Pregnancy will cause increased levels.
- Drugs that may cause increased levels include clofibrate, estrogens, heroin, methadone, and oral contraceptives.
- Drugs that may cause decreased levels include anabolic steroids, androgens, antithyroid drugs (e.g., propylthiouracil), lithium, phenytoin (Dilantin), and propranolol (Inderal).

Procedure and patient care
Before

- Explain the procedure to the patient.
- Evaluate the patient's medication history.
- If indicated, instruct the patient to stop exogenous T_4 medication 1 month before testing.
- Tell the patient that no fasting is required.

During

Adult
- Collect a venous blood specimen in a red-top tube.
- List on the laboratory slip any drugs that can affect test results.

Newborn
- Perform a heel stick to obtain blood.
- Thoroughly saturate the circles on the filter paper with blood.
- Note that prompt collection and processing are crucial to the early detection of hypothyroidism.
- Note that optimal collection time is 2 to 4 days after birth. However, all newborns should be screened before discharge (regardless of age) because of the consequences of delayed diagnosis.

After

- Apply pressure or a pressure dressing to the venipuncture site.
- Assess the venipuncture site for bleeding.

T

Abnormal findings
Increased levels

Hyperthyroid states (e.g., Graves' disease, Plummer's disease, toxic thyroid adenoma)
Acute thyroiditis
Pregnancy

Decreased levels

Hypothyroid states (e.g., cretinism, myxedema)
Protein malnutrition
Renal failure

Notes

thyroxine index, free (FTI, FT$_4$ index)

Type of test Blood

Normal findings 0.8-2.4 ng/dl or 10-31 pmol/L (SI units)

Test explanation and related physiology:

The FTI study measures the amount of free T$_4$, which is only a fraction of the total T$_4$. The free T$_4$ is the unbound T$_4$ that enters the cell and is metabolically active. The diagnostic value of measuring the FTI is that it is not affected by thyroid-binding globulin (TBG) abnormalities; therefore it correlates more closely with the true hormonal status than do total T$_4$ or triiodothyronine (T$_3$) determinations. To determine the FTI, the T$_3$ uptake (see p. 740) is measured and multiplied by the measured T$_4$ (see p. 724). This simple mathematic computation corrects the estimated total T$_4$ assay for the effects of TBG protein alterations.

This index is useful in diagnosing hyperthyroidism and hypothyroidism, especially in patients with abnormalities in TBG levels. High FTI calculations suggest hyperthyroidism; low FTI values suggest hypothyroidism. The FTI study also aids in the evaluation of the thyroid status of pregnant women and patients who have abnormal TBG levels and are being treated with certain drugs (e.g., estrogen, phenytoin, salicylates).

Interfering factor

- Recent radionuclear scan

Procedure and patient care

Before

- Explain the procedure to the patient.
- Obtain the T$_4$ value and T$_3$ uptake ratio.

During

- Multiply the T$_3$ uptake value by the T$_4$ value to obtain the FTI.

After

- Apply pressure or a pressure dressing to the venipuncture site.
- Check the venipuncture site for bleeding.

Abnormal findings
Increased levels

Hyperthyroidism

Decreased levels

Hypothyroidism

Notes

TORCH test

The term *TORCH* (*t*oxoplasmosis, *o*ther, *r*ubella, *c*yto-megalovirus, *h*erpes) has been applied to infections with recognized detrimental effects on the fetus. The effects on the fetus may be direct or indirect (e.g., precipitating abortion or premature labor). Included in the category of *other* are infections (e.g., syphilis). All these tests are discussed separately.

T

toxicology screening

Type of test Blood; urine

Normal findings See Tables 10 and 11 for blood toxicology and urine toxicology.

Test explanation and related physiology

Toxicology screening is done to determine the cause of acute drug toxicity, to monitor drug dependency, and to detect the presence of narcotics in the body for medicolegal purposes. Toxicology screening is especially important in patients with a drug overdose or poisoning.

Procedure and patient care
Before

- Explain the procedure to the patient or significant others.
- If the specimen is obtained for medicolegal testing, ensure that the patient or family member has signed a consent form.
- Obtain as much information as possible about the drug type, amount, and ingestion time.
- Carefully assess the patient for respiratory distress (a common adverse reaction of drug overdosage).

During

- Collect blood as designated by the laboratory or urine specimens as indicated. Urine specimens are usually collected in the presence of the nurse.
- Collect gastric contents for analysis if indicated.
- Note that hair and nail samples can be used to detect or document exposure to arsenic and mercury.

After

- Apply pressure or a pressure dressing to the venipuncture site.
- Assess the venipuncture site for bleeding.
- Assess the patient for respiratory distress (a common adverse reaction of drug overdosage).
- Refer the patient for appropriate drug and psychiatric counseling.

TABLE 10 Blood toxicology screening

Drug	Type	Therapeutic level*	Toxic level*
Acetaminophen	Analgesic, antipyretic	Depends on the use	>250 µg/ml
Alcohol	—	None	80-200 mg/dl (mild to moderate intoxication)
			250-400 mg/dl (marked intoxication)
			>400 mg/dl (severe intoxication)
Amobarbital	Sedative, hypnotic	0.5-3.0 µg/ml	>10 µg/ml
Butabarbital	Sedative, hypnotic	0.5-3.0 µg/ml	>10 µg/ml
Carboxyhemoglobin (COHb, carbon monoxide)	Gas	None	>30% COHb (beginning of coma)

*Levels vary according to the institution performing the test.

Continued.

T

TABLE 10 Blood toxicology screening—cont'd

Drug	Type	Therapeutic level*	Toxic level*
Dilantin	Anticonvulsant	10-20 µg/ml	>20 µg/ml
Glutethimide	Sedative	0.5-3.0 µg/ml	>10 µg/ml
Lead	—	None	>40 µg/dl
Lithium	Manic episodes of manic-depression psychosis	0.8-1.2 mEq/L	>2.0 mEq/L
Meprobamate	Antianxiety agent	0.5-3.0 µg/ml	>10 µg/ml
Methyprylon	Hypnotic	0.5-3.0 µg/ml	>10 µg/ml
Phenobarbital	Anticonvulsant	15-30 µg/ml	>40 µg/ml
Salicylate	Antipyretic, antiinflammatory, analgesic	100-250 µg/ml	>300 µg/ml

TABLE 11 Urine toxicology screening for amphetamines

Drug	Therapeutic level*	Toxic level*
Amphetamine	2-3 μg/ml	>3 μg/ml
Dextroamphetamine	0.1-1.5 μg/ml	>15 μg/ml
Methamphetamine	3-5 μg/ml	>40 μg/ml
Phenmetrazine	5-30 μg/ml	>50 μg/ml

*Levels vary according to the institution performing the test.

Abnormal finding

Toxicity

Notes

T

toxoplasmosis antibody titer

Type of test Blood

Normal findings

Titers <1:16 indicate no previous infection.
Titers 1:16-1:256 are usually prevalent in general population.
Titers >1:256 suggest recent infection.
Rising titers are of great significance.

Test explanation and related physiology

Toxoplasmosis is a protozoan disease caused by *Toxoplasma gondii*, which is found in poorly cooked or raw meat and in the feces of cats. This disease is characterized by central nervous system lesions, which may lead to blindness, brain damage, and death. The condition may occur congenitally or postnatally. Because about one quarter to one half of the adult population are asymptomatically affected with toxoplasmosis, the Centers for Disease Control recommends that pregnant patients be serologically tested for this disease.

The presence of antibodies before pregnancy probably ensures protection against congenital toxoplasmosis in the child. Chronic toxoplasmosis, which affects a large percentage of adults, will not cause spontaneous abortion or infection of the infant. Fetal infection occurs only if the mother acquires toxoplasmosis after conception. Repeat testing of the pregnant patient with high or negative titers may be done before the 20th week and before delivery to identify antibody converters and to determine appropriate therapy (e.g., therapeutic abortion at 20 weeks, treatment during the remainder of the pregnancy, or treatment of the newborn). Hydrocephaly, microcephaly, and chronic retinitis and convulsions are complications of congenital toxoplasmosis. Congenital toxoplasmosis is diagnosed when the test levels are persistently elevated or when a rising titer is found in the infant 2 to 3 months after birth.

Procedure and patient care
Before

- Explain the procedure to the patient.

During

- Collect approximately 5 ml of blood in a red-top tube.
- Indicate on the laboratory slip if the patient is pregnant or has been exposed to cats.

After

- Apply pressure or a pressure dressing to the venipuncture site.
- Assess the venipuncture site for bleeding.

Abnormal finding

Toxoplasmosis infection

Notes

T

triglycerides (TGs)

Type of test Blood

Normal findings

Adult/elderly: male, 40-160 mg/dl or 0.4-1.6 g/L (SI units)
female, 35-135 mg/dl or 0.35-1.35 g/L (SI units)

		Male	*Female*
Child:	0-5 years:	30-86 mg/dl	32-99 mg/dl
	6-11 years:	31-108 mg/dl	35-114 mg/dl
	12-15 years:	36-138 mg/dl	41-138 mg/dl
	16-19 years:	40-163 mg/dl	40-128 mg/dl

Test explanation and related physiology

TGs are a form of fat that exist within the bloodstream. They are transported by very low-density lipoproteins (VLDLs) and low-density lipoproteins (LDLs). TGs are produced in the liver by using glycerol and other fatty acids as building blocks. The purpose of a TG is to act as a storage source for energy. When TG levels in the blood are in excess, TGs are deposited into the fatty tissues. TGs are a part of a lipid profile that also evaluates cholesterol (see p. 190) and lipoproteins (see p. 464). A lipid profile is performed to assess the risk of coronary and vascular disease.

Interfering factors

- Ingestion of fatty meals can cause elevated TG levels.
- Ingestion of alcohol can cause elevated levels.
- Pregnancy can cause increased levels.
- Drugs that may cause increased TG levels include cholestyramine, estrogens, and oral contraceptives.
- Drugs that may cause decreased levels include ascorbic acid, asparaginase, clofibrate, and colestipol.

Procedure and patient care

Before

- Explain the procedure to the patient.
- Instruct the patient to fast for 12 to 14 hours before the test. Only water is permitted.
- Tell the patient not to drink alcohol for 24 hours before the test.

- Inform the patient that dietary indiscretion for as much as 2 weeks before this test will influence results.

During

- Collect 5 to 10 ml of venous blood in a red-top tube.

After

- Apply pressure or a pressure dressing to the venipuncture site.
- Assess the venipuncture site for bleeding.
- Mark the patient's age and sex on the laboratory slip.
- Instruct the patient with increased TG levels regarding diet, exercise, and appropriate weight.

Abnormal findings
Increased levels

Glycogen storage disease
Hyperlipidemias
Hypothyroidism
High-carbohydrate diet
Poorly controlled diabetes
Risk of arteriosclerotic occlusive coronary disease and peripheral vascular disease
Nephrotic syndrome
Hypertension
Alcoholic cirrhosis
Pregnancy
Myocardial infarction

Decreased levels

Malabsorption syndrome
Malnutrition
Hyperthyroidism

Notes

triiodothyronine (T_3 radioimmunoassay [T_3 by RIA])

Type of test   Blood

Normal findings

Adult/elderly: 110-230 ng/dl or 1.2-1.5 nmol/L (SI units)
Newborn: 90-170 ng/dl
Child (6-12 years): 115-190 ng/dl

Test explanation and related physiology

As with the thyroxine (T_4) test, the serum T_3 test is an accurate measure of thyroid function. T_3 is less stable than T_4 and occurs in minute quantities in the active form. Generally, when the T_3 level is below normal, the patient is in a hypothyroid state. An elevated T_3 determination is clinically important in the patient who has a normal T_4 level but has all the symptoms of hyperthyroidism. In this patient the test may identify T_3 thyrotoxicosis. This test is not the same as the T_3 uptake test (see p. 740) and should not be confused with it.

Interfering factors

- Radioisotope administration before the test can alter the results.
- T_3 values are increased in pregnancy.
- Drugs that may cause increase levels include estrogen, methadone, and oral contraceptives.
- Drugs that may cause decreased levels include anabolic steroids, androgens, phenytoin (Dilantin), propranolol (Inderal), reserpine, and salicylates (high dose).

Procedure and patient care

Before

- Explain the procedure to the patient.
- Determine whether the patient is taking any exogenous T_3 medication because this will affect test results.
- Withhold drugs that may affect results (with physician's approval).
- Tell the patient that no fasting is required.

During

- Collect approximately 5 to 10 ml of venous blood in a red-top tube.
- List on the laboratory slip any medications the patient is currently taking.

After

- Apply pressure or a pressure dressing to the venipuncture site.
- Observe the venipuncture site for bleeding.

Abnormal findings

Increased levels

Hyperthyroidism
T_3 thyrotoxicosis
Thyroiditis
Toxic adenoma

Decreased levels

Hypothyroidism
Starvation
Chronic illness

Notes

T

triiodothyronine uptake test (T_3 resin uptake test, Resin triiodothyronine uptake test [RT_3U, T_3RU])

Type of test Blood

Normal findings 25%-35% (varies with different laboratories)

Test explanation and related physiology

The T_3 resin uptake test indirectly quantifies *thyroid-binding globulin* (TBG) and *thyroid-binding prealbumin* (TBPA) in the blood. Pregnancy, oral contraceptives, and some genetic disorders tend to raise inappropriately the quantity of these carrying proteins. As a result, thyroxine (T_4) and T_3 levels may be artificially elevated, but the patient may be euthyroid. Similarly, androgenic hormones, intercurrent serious illness, and nephrotic syndromes tend to lower the quantity of these proteins, thereby causing falsely low T_3 and T_4 levels in euthyroid patients. Therefore accurate assessment of the patient's thyroid status requires measurement of the TBG and TBPA levels, as done by RT_3U testing. Because this is an exchange resin test, high results indicate low TBG and TBPA levels and low results indicate high TBG and TBPA levels.

The T_3 uptake test is useful for the diagnosis of hypothyroidism or hyperthyroidism. This test is also used with the T_4 to provide the free T_4 index (see p. 727). It is important to note that the RT_3U test is *not* a measurement of serum T_3.

Interfering factors

- Recent radioisotope scans before the blood collection can affect test results.
- Drugs that may cause elevated TBG and TBPA levels include anabolic steroids, heparin, phenytoin (Dilantin), salicylates (high dose), thyroid agents, and warfarin (Coumadin).
- Drugs that may cause decreased levels include antithyroid agents, clofibrate, estrogen, oral contraceptives, and thiazides.

Procedure and patient care

Before

- Explain the procedure to the patient.
- Tell the patient that no fasting is required.

During

- Collect approximately 5 to 7 ml of venous blood in a red-top tube.
- List on the laboratory slip any drugs that can affect test results.

After

- Apply pressure or a pressure dressing to the venipuncture site.
- Assess the venipuncture site for bleeding.

Abnormal findings

Increased levels

Hyperthyroidism
Protein malnutrition
Nephrotic syndrome
Malnutrition
Renal failure

Decreased levels

Hypothyroidism
Pregnancy
Acute hepatitis

Notes

tuberculin test

Type of test Skin

Normal findings Negative; reaction <5 mm

Test explanation and related physiology

Although this test is used to detect tuberculosis infection, it is unable to indicate whether the infection is active or dormant. For this test a *purified protein derivative* (PPD) of the tubercle bacillus is injected intradermally. If the patient is infected with tuberculosis (whether active or dormant), lymphocytes will recognize the PPD antigen and cause a local reaction. If the patient is not infected by tuberculosis, no reaction will occur. If the test is negative and the physician strongly suspects tuberculosis, a "second-strength" PPD can be used. If this test is then negative, the patient does not have tuberculosis.

The PPD test can also be used as part of a series of skin tests done to assess the immune system. If the immune system is nonfunctioning because of poor nutrition or chronic illness (e.g., neoplasia, infection), the PPD test will be negative despite the patient having had an active or dormant tuberculosis infection. It has been well established that surgery is associated with greater mortality in these patients (with immunoincompetence) than in patients whose immune systems are intact.

Laboratory testing for tuberculosis is usually performed as part of the routine prenatal evaluation in pregnant women. Often, this may be the mother's first contact with the health care system in several years.

When a patient known to have active tuberculosis receives a PPD test, the local reaction may be so severe as to cause a complete skin slough requiring surgical care. When these patients are eliminated from PPD testing, the test has no complications. The PPD test will not cause active tuberculosis because no live organisms exist in the test solution.

Contraindications

- Patients with known active tuberculosis
- Patients who have received *bacille Calmette-Guérin* (BCG) immunization against PPD, since these patients will dem-

onstrate a positive reaction to the PPD vaccination even though they have never had tuberculosis infection

Procedure and patient care
Before

- Explain the procedure to the patient.
- Assure the patient that she or he will not develop tuberculosis from this test.
- Assess the patient for previous history of tuberculosis. Report a positive history to the physician.
- Evaluate the patient's history for previous PPD results and BCG immunization.

During

- Prepare the patient's forearm with alcohol and allow it to dry.
- Intradermally inject the PPD. A skin wheal will occur.
- Circle the area with indelible ink.
- Record the time at which the PPD was injected.

After

- Read the results in 48 to 72 hours.
- Examine the test site for induration (hardening). Measure the area of induration (*not* redness) in millimeters.
- If the test is positive, ensure that the physician is notified and the patient is treated appropriately.
- If the test is positive, check the patient's arm 4 to 5 days after the test to be certain that a severe skin reaction has not occurred.

Abnormal findings
Positive results

Tuberculosis infection

Negative results

Possible immunoincompetence in chronically ill patients

Notes

tubular phosphate reabsorption (TPR, Tubular reabsorption of phosphate [TRP])

Type of test Blood; urine (hourly or 24 hour)

Normal findings 80%-90%

Test explanation and related physiology

The TPR test indirectly measures parathyroid hormone (PTH) by estimating its effects on renal phosphate reabsorption. TPR is primarily done to detect primary hyperparathyroidism. This test value is calculated using the serum creatinine level (see p. 243), the serum phosphate concentration (see p. 561), and the creatinine clearance rate (see p. 245). Results are based on the ratio of creatinine clearance to phosphate clearance. Values less than 80% indicate diminished renal tubular reabsorption of phosphate and suggest primary hyperparathyroidism. Decreased values may also be associated with sarcoidosis, myeloma, and hypercalcemia caused by malignancy.

Interfering factors

- Low-phosphate diet raises TPR values.
- High-phosphate diet lowers TPR values.

Procedure and patient care

Before

- Explain the procedure to the patient.
- Instruct the patient concerning the method that will be used (24-hour urine sample or hourly samples).
- Instruct the patient that he or she should have a normal phosphate diet (greater than 500 mg per day and less than 3000 mg per day).

During

24-hour urine test

- Keep the patient NPO, except for water, for 8 hours before drawing the blood sample.
- Collect 24-hour urine sample using a preservative.
- Draw blood early in the urine collection.

Hourly urine test
- Instruct the patient to drink several 8-ounce glasses of water and empty the bladder. (This marks the beginning of the test.)
- One hour later, draw a blood specimen for phosphorus and creatinine measurements.
- One hour later (2 hours after beginning the test), instruct the patient to void for determination of the urine volume and urine concentration of creatinine and phosphorus.
- Note that urine may be collected again 1 hour later.

After

- Mark each specimen with the time it was collected.
- Send the specimen to the laboratory as soon as it is collected.

Abnormal findings
Decreased values

Primary hyperparathyroidism
Sarcoidosis
Myeloma
Hypercalcemia caused by malignancy

Notes

T

upper gastrointestinal x-ray study (Upper GI series, UGI)

Type of test X-ray with contrast dye

Normal findings Normal size, contour, patency, filling, positioning, and transit of barium through the lower esophagus, stomach, and upper duodenum

Test explanation and related physiology

The upper GI study consists of a series of x-ray films of the lower esophagus, stomach, and duodenum, usually using barium sulfate as the contrast medium. However, when there is concern for leakage of x-ray contrast through a perforation of the GI tract, Gastrografin (a water-soluble contrast) is used. The purpose of this examination is to detect ulcerations, tumors, inflammations, or anatomic malpositions (e.g., hiatal hernia) within these organs. Obstruction of the upper GI tract is also easily detected.

In this test the patient is asked to drink barium. As the contrast descends, the lower esophagus is examined for position, patency, and filling defects (e.g., tumors, scarring, varices). As the contrast enters the stomach, the gastric wall is examined for benign or malignant ulcerations, filling defects (most often in cancer), and anatomic abnormalities (e.g., hiatal hernia). As the contrast leaves the stomach, patency of the pyloric channel and the duodenum is evaluated. Benign peptic ulceration is the most common pathologic condition affecting these areas. Extrinsic compression caused by tumors, cysts, or enlarged pathologic organs (e.g., liver) near the stomach can also be identified by anatomic distortion of the outline of the upper GI tract.

Contraindications

- Patients with complete bowel obstructions
- Patients suspected of upper GI perforation
  Water-soluble Gastrografin should be used instead of barium.
- Patients whose vital signs are unstable
  These patients should be supervised during the time required for this test.

- Patients who are uncooperative because of the necessity of frequent position changes

Potential complications

- Aspiration of barium
- Constipation or partial bowel obstruction caused by inspissated barium in the small bowel or colon

Interfering factors

- Previously administered barium
  This may block visualization of the upper GI tract.
- Poor performance status of the patient
  Incapacitated patients cannot assume the multiple positions required for the study.
- Food and fluid in the stomach
  This gives the false impression of filling defects within the stomach, precluding adequate evaluation of the gastric mucosa.

Procedure and patient care

Before

- Explain the procedure to the patient. Allow the patient to verbalize concerns.
- Instruct the patient to abstain from eating for at least 8 hours before the test. Usually, keep the patient NPO after midnight on the day of the test.
- Assure the patient that the test will not cause any discomfort.

During

- Note the following procedural steps:

  1. The patient is asked to drink about 16 ounces of barium sulfate. This is a chalky substance usually suspended in milkshake form and drunk through a straw. Usually the drink is flavored to increase the palatability.
  2. After drinking the barium, the patient is moved through several position changes (e.g., prone, supine, lateral) to promote filling of the entire upper GI tract.
  3. Films are taken at the discretion of the radiologist who is observing the flow of barium fluoroscopically.
  4. The flow of barium is followed through the lower esophagus, stomach, and duodenum.

U

5. Several films are taken throughout the course of the test.
6. In an *air-contrast upper GI,* the patient is asked to swallow rapidly some carbonated power. This creates carbon dioxide in the stomach, thereby providing air contrast to the barium within the stomach and increased visualization of the gastric mucosa.

- Note that a radiologist performs this procedure in approximately 30 minutes.
- Tell the patient that he or she may be uncomfortable lying on the hard x-ray table and occasionally may experience the sensation of bloating or nausea during the test.

After

- Inform the patient that if Gastrografin was used, he or she may have significant diarrhea. Gastrografin is an osmotic cathartic.
- Instruct the patient to use a cathartic (e.g., milk of magnesia) if barium sulfate was used as the contrast medium. Water absorption may cause the barium to harden and create a fecal impaction if catharsis is not carried out.
- Instruct the patient to watch his or her stools to ensure that all the barium has been removed. The stools should return to normal color after completely expelling the barium, which may take as much as a day and a half.

Abnormal findings

Esophageal cancer
Esophageal varices
Hiatal hernia
Esophageal diverticula
Gastric cancer
Gastric inflammatory diseases (e.g., Ménétrièr's disease)
Benign gastric tumors (e.g., leiomyomas)
Extrinsic compression by pancreatic pseudocysts, cysts, pancreatic tumors, or hepatomegaly
Perforation of the esophagus, stomach, or duodenum
Congenital abnormalities (e.g., duodenal web, pancreatic rest, malrotation syndromes)
Gastric ulcer (benign and malignant)
Gastritis
Duodenal ulcers
Duodenal cancer
Duodenal diverticulum

urea nitrogen blood test (Blood urea nitrogen [BUN], Serum urea nitrogen)

Type of test Blood

Normal findings

Adult: 10-20 mg/dl or 3.6-7.1 mmol/L (SI units)
Elderly: may be slightly higher than those of adults
Child: 5-18 mg/dl
Infant: 5-18 mg/dl
Newborn: 3-12 mg/dl
Cord: 21-40 mg/dl

Possible critical values >100 mg/dl (indicates serious impairment of renal function)

Test explanation and related physiology

The BUN measures the amount of urea nitrogen in the blood. Urea is formed in the liver as the end product of protein metabolism. During digestion, protein is broken down into amino acids. In the liver, these amino acids are catabolized and free ammonia is formed. The ammonia is combined to form urea. The urea is then deposited into the blood and transported to the kidneys for excretion. Therefore the BUN is directly related to the metabolic function of the liver and the excretory function of the kidney. It serves as an index of the function of these organs.

Nearly all renal diseases cause an inadequate excretion of urea, which causes the blood concentration to rise above normal. The BUN also increases in conditions other than primary renal disease. For example, when excess amounts of protein are available for hepatic catabolism (from the diet or in gastrointestinal bleeding), large quantities of urea are made. BUN levels may also vary according to the state of hydration, with increased levels seen in dehydration and decreased levels seen in overhydration. Finally, one must be aware that the synthesis of urea depends on the liver. Patients with severe primary liver disease will have a decreased BUN. With combined liver and renal disease (as in hepatorenal syndrome), the BUN can be normal not because renal excretory function is good, but rather because poor hepatic functioning resulted in decreased formation of urea.

U

The BUN is interpreted in conjunction with the creatinine test (see p. 243). These tests are referred to as *renal function studies.*

Interfering factors

- Changes in protein intake may affect BUN levels.
- Advanced pregnancy may cause increased levels.
- Overhydration and underhydration will affect levels.
- Drugs that may cause increased BUN levels include allopurinol, aminoglycosides, cephalosporins, chloral hydrate, cisplatin, furosemide, guanethidine, indomethacin, methotrexate, methyldopa, nephrotoxic drugs (e.g., aspirin, amphotericin B, bacitracin, carbamazepine, colistin, gentamicin, methicillin, neomycin, penicillamine, polymyxin B, probenecid, vancomycin), propranolol, rifampin, spironolactone, tetracyclines, thiazide diuretics, and triamterene.
- Drugs that may cause decreased levels include chloramphenicol and streptomycin.

Procedure and patient care

Before

- Explain the procedure to the patient.
- Tell the patient that no fasting is required.

During

- Collect approximately 5 ml of blood in a red-top tube.
- Avoid hemolysis.

After

- Apply pressure or a pressure dressing to the venipuncture site.
- Observe the venipuncture site for bleeding.

Abnormal findings

Increased levels

Renal disease (e.g., glomerulonephritis, pyelonephritis, acute tubular necrosis)
Urinary obstruction (e.g., from tumors, stones, prostatic hypertrophy)
Hypovolemia
Shock
Congestive heart failure

Burns
Excessive protein catabolism
Gastrointestinal bleeding
Myocardial infarction
Renal failure
Nephrotoxic drugs
Excessive protein ingestion
Dehydration
Starvation

Decreased levels

Liver failure
Overhydration
Negative nitrogen balance (e.g., malnutrition)
Pregnancy

Notes

urethral pressure profile (UPP, Urethral pressure measurements)

Type of test   Manometric

Normal findings   Maximal urethral pressures in normal patients (cm H_2O):

Age	Male	Female
<25 years	37-126	55-103
25-44 years	35-113	31-115
45-64 years	40-123	40-100
>64 years	35-105	35-75

Test explanation and related physiology

The UPP indicates the intraluminal pressure along the length of the urethra with the bladder at rest. Indications for this urodynamic investigation include the following:

1. Assessment of prostatic obstruction
2. Assessment of stress incontinence in females
3. Assessment of postprostatectomy sequelae of incontinence
4. Assessment of the adequacy of external sphincterotomy
5. Analysis of the effects of drugs on the urethra
6. Analysis of the effects of stimulation on urethral flow
7. Assessment of adequacy of implanted artificial urethral sphincter devices

Contraindications

- Patients with urinary tract infections

Procedure and patient care

Before

- Explain the procedure to the patient.
- Since many patients are embarrassed by this procedure, assure the patient that he or she will be draped to ensure privacy.
- Tell the patient that no fasting or sedation is required.

During

- Note the following procedural steps:
  1. A catheter is placed into the bladder.
  2. Fluids (or gas) are instilled through the catheter, which is withdrawn while the pressures along the urethral wall are obtained.
  3. A constant infusion of the fluids or gas is maintained by a motorized syringe pump.
  4. The catheter is removed, and the test is completed.
- Note that this test is usually performed by a urologist in less than 15 minutes.
- Explain to the patient that this test is slightly more uncomfortable than urethral catheterization.

After

- Give the patient a sitz bath if requested.

Notes

U

uric acid, blood

Type of test Blood

Normal findings

Adult: male, 2.1-8.5 mg/dl or 0.15-0.48 mmol/L
        female, 2.0-6.6 mg/dl or 0.09-0.36 mmol/L
Elderly: values may be slightly increased.
Child: 2.5-5.5 mg/dl or 0.12-0.32 mmol/L
Newborn: 2.0-6.2 mg/dl

Possible critical values >12 mg/dl

Test explanation and related physiology

Uric acid is a nitrogenous compound that is a product of purine (a deoxyribonucleic acid [DNA] building block) catabolism. Uric acid is excreted to a large degree by the kidney and to a smaller degree by the intestinal tract. When the uric acid levels are elevated (hyperuricemia), the patient may have gout. Causes of hyperuricemia can be overproduction or decreased excretion of uric acid (e.g., kidney failure). Overproduction of uric acid may occur in patients who have a catabolic enzyme deficiency that stimulates purine metabolism or in patients with cancer in whom purine and DNA turnover is great. Other causes of hyperuricemia may include alcoholism, leukemias, metastatic cancer, multiple myeloma, hyperlipoproteinemia, diabetes mellitus, renal failure, stress, lead poisoning, and dehydration caused by diuretic therapy. Ketoacids (as occur in diabetic or alcoholic ketoacidosis) may compete with uric acid for tubular excretion and can cause decreased uric acid excretion. Many causes of hyperuricemia production are undefined and therefore labeled as *idiopathic*.

Interfering factors

- Stress may cause increased uric acid levels.
- Recent use of x-ray contrast agents may cause decreased levels.
- Drugs that may cause increased levels include alcohol, ascorbic acid, aspirin (low dose), caffeine, cisplatin, diazoxide, diuretics, epinephrine, ethambutol, levodopa,

methyldopa (Aldomet), nicotinic acid, phenothiazines, and theophylline.
- Drugs that may cause decreased levels include allopurinol, aspirin (high dose), azathioprine (Imuran), clofibrate, corticosteroids, estrogens, glucose infusions, guaifenesin, mannitol, probenecid, and warfarin.

Procedure and patient care
Before

- Explain the procedure to the patient.
- Follow the facility's requirements regarding fasting. (Some institutions recommend that the patient fast.)

During

- Collect approximately 5 to 7 ml of venous blood in a red-top tube.
- List on the laboratory slip any drugs that can affect test results.

After

- Apply pressure or a pressure dressing to the venipuncture site.
- Assess the venipuncture site for bleeding.

Abnormal findings

Increased levels (hyperuricemia)

Gout
Arthritis
Soft tissue deposits of uric acid (tophi)
Uric acid kidney stones
Lead poisoning
Hypothyroidism
Multiple myeloma
Metastatic cancer
Acidosis
Toxemia of pregnancy
Alcoholism
Leukemias
Hyperlipoproteinemia
Diabetes mellitus
Renal failure

Decreased levels

Wilson's disease
Fanconi's syndrome
Yellow atrophy of the liver

U

Stress
Cancer chemotherapy
Shock
Strenuous exercise
Starvation

Notes

uric acid, urine

Type of test Urine (24 hour)

Normal findings Adult/elderly/child: 250-750 ml/24 hr

Test explanation and related physiology

Uric acid is a nitrogenous compound that is a product of purine (a deoxyribonucleic acid [DNA] building block) catabolism. Uric acid is excreted to a large degree by the kidney and to a smaller degree by the intestinal tract. When the uric acid levels are elevated, the patient may have gout. Uric acid levels can be measured in both the blood and the urine. Urine levels of uric acid are helpful in evaluating uric acid metabolism in gout and for assessing in hyperuricosuria in patients with renal calculus formation. This test also helps to identify people at risk for stone formation.

Interfering factors

- Recent use of x-ray contrast agents can increase uric acid levels in the urine.
- Drugs that may interfere with test results include alcohol, antiinflammatory preparations, salicylates, thiazide diuretics, vitamin C, and warfarin.

Procedure and patient care

Before

- Explain the procedure to the patient.
- Tell the patient that no special diet is usually required.

During

- Instruct the patient to begin the 24-hour urine collection after voiding. Discard the initial specimen and start the 24-hour timing at that point.
- Collect all the urine passed during the next 24 hours. A preservative may be used.
- Show the patient where to store the urine container.
- Keep the specimen on ice or refrigerated during the entire 24 hours. (Note that some laboratories do not require refrigeration.)
- Indicate the starting time on the urine container and laboratory slip.

U

- Post the hours for the urine collection in a noticeable place to prevent accidental discarding of the specimen.
- Instruct the patient to void before defecating so the urine is not contaminated by feces.
- Remind the patient not to put toilet paper in the collection container.
- Encourage the patient to drink fluids during the 24 hours.
- Instruct the patient to collect the last specimen as close as possible to the end of the 24-hour period. Add this urine to the container.

After

- Transport the urine specimen promptly to the laboratory.

Abnormal findings

Increased levels (uricosuria)

Gout
Chronic myelogenous leukemia
Polycythemia vera
Ulcerative colitis
Febrile illness
Liver disease
Toxemia of pregnancy
High purine diet

Decreased levels

Kidney disease (chronic glomerulonephritis, urinary obstruction)
Eclampsia
Lead toxicity
Chronic alcohol ingestion

Notes

urinalysis

Type of test Urine

The urinalysis usually includes the following, all of which are discussed separately:

pH (see p. 771)
Appearance (see p. 760)
Color (see p. 760)
Odor (see p. 769)
Specific gravity (see p. 773)
Protein (see p. 595)
Glucose (see p. 384)
Ketones (see p. 441)
Blood (see p. 615)
Leukocyte esterase (see p. 460)
Microscopic examination
   Red blood cell (see p. 615)
   White blood cell (see p. 792)
   Casts (see pp. 309, 336, 417, 615, 785, and 792)
   Crystals (see p. 253)
   Bacteria (see p. 764)

U

urine appearance and color

Type of test Urine

Normal findings
Appearance: clear
Color: amber yellow

Test explanation and related physiology
The urine appearance and color are obtained as part of a routine urinalysis. The appearance of a normal urine specimen should be clear. Cloudy urine may be caused by the presence of pus, red blood cells (RBCs), or bacteria. However, normal urine may also be cloudy because of ingestion of certain foods (e.g., large amounts of fat), urates, or phosphates.

The color of the urine ranges from pale yellow to amber because of the pigment *urochrome*. The color indicates the concentration of the urine and varies with the specific gravity. Dilute urine is straw colored, and concentrated urine is deep amber.

Abnormally colored urine can result from a pathologic condition or from the ingestion of certain foods or medicine. For example, bleeding from the kidney produces dark-red urine, whereas bleeding in the lower urinary tract produces bright-red urine. Dark-yellow urine may indicate the presence of urobilinogen or bilirubin. *Pseudomonas* organisms usually produce green urine. Beets may cause red urine. Rhubarb can color the urine brown. Many frequently used drugs also can affect urine color (Table 12).

Interfering factors
- Certain foods affect urine color. Carrots can cause a dark-yellow color. Beets can cause a red-colored urine. Rhubarb may cause a red or brown discoloration.
- Urine color darkens with prolonged standing.
- Many drugs affect urine color and appearance (see Table 12).

Procedure and patient care
Before

- Explain the procedure to the patient.
- Tell the patient that no fasting is required.

During

- Collect a voided specimen in a urine container.
- If the specimen is likely to be contaminated by vaginal discharge or bleeding, collect a "clean-catch" or "midstream" specimen. This requires meticulous cleansing of the urinary meatus with an iodine preparation to reduce contamination of the specimen by external organisms. Then the cleansing agent must be completely removed, or it will contaminate the specimen. The midstream collection is obtained by:

  1. Having the patient begin to urinate in a bedpan, urinal, or toilet and then stop urinating (This washes the urine out of the distal urethra.)
  2. Correctly positioning a sterile urine container, into which the patient voids 3 to 4 ounces of urine
  3. Capping the container
  4. Allowing the patient to finish voiding

After

- Transport the urine specimen to the laboratory promptly.

Abnormal findings

Bacteria
Pus
Red blood cells
Certain foods (e.g., beets, carrots)
Drug therapy (see Table 12)
Pathologic conditions (e.g., bleeding from kidney)

Dehydration
Overhydration
Diabetes insipidus
Fever
Excessive sweating
Jaundice

U

Notes

TABLE 12 Frequently used drugs that can affect urine color

Generic and brand names	Drug classification	Urine color
Anisindione (Miradon)	Oral anticoagulant	Red-orange in alkaline urine
Cascara sagrada	Stimulant laxative	Red in alkaline urine; yellow-brown in acid urine
Chloroquine (Aralen)	Antimalarial	Rusty yellow or brown
Chlorzoxazone (Paraflex)	Skeletal muscle relaxant	Orange or purple-red
Danthron (Modane)	Stimulant laxative	Pink or red in alkaline urine
Dioctyl calcium sulfosuccinate (Doxidan, Surfak)	Laxative	Pink to red to red-brown
Furazolidone (Furoxone)	Antiinfective, antiprotozoal	Brown
Iron preparations (Ferotran, Imferon)	Hematinic	Dark brown or black on standing

Levodopa	Antiparkinsonian	Dark brown on standing
Methylene blue (Urolene Blue)	Antimethemoglobinemic	Blue-green
Nitrofurantoin (Macrodantin, Ni-trodan)	Antibacterial	Brown
Phenazopyridine (Pyridium)	Urinary tract analgesic	Orange to red
Phenindione (Eridione)	Anticoagulant	Red-orange in alkaline urine
Phenolphthalein (Ex-Lax)	Contact laxative	Red or purplish pink in alkaline urine
Phenothiazines (e.g., prochlorpera-zine [Compazine])	Antipsychotic, neuroleptic, anti-emetic	Red-brown
Phenytoin (Dilantin)	Anticonvulsant	Pink, red, red-brown
Riboflavin (vitamin B)	Vitamin	Intense yellow
Rifampin	Antibiotic	Red-orange
Sulfasalazine (Azulfidine)	Antibacterial	Orange-yellow in alkaline urine
Triamterene (Dyrenium)	Diuretic	Pale blue fluorescence

U

urine culture and sensitivity (C&S)

Type of test Urine

Normal findings Negative

Test explanation and related physiology

Urine cultures and sensitivities are obtained to determine the presence of pathogenic bacteria in patients with suspected urinary tract infections. All cultures should be performed before antibiotic therapy is initiated. Otherwise the antibiotic may interrupt the growth of the organism in the laboratory. More often than not, however, the physician will want to institute antibiotic therapy before the culture results are reported. In these instances a *Gram stain* of the specimen smeared on a slide is most helpful and can be reported in less than 10 minutes. All forms of bacteria are grossly classified as gram positive (blue staining) or gram negative (red staining). Knowledge of the shape of the organism (e.g., spheric, rod-shaped) can also be very helpful in the tentative identification of the infecting organism. With knowledge of the Gram stain results, the physician can institute a reasonable antibiotic regimen based on past experience as to the organism's possible identity. Most organisms require about 24 hours to grow in the laboratory, and a preliminary report can be given at that time. Occasionally, 48 to 72 hours are required for growth and identification of the organism. Cultures may be repeated after appropriate antibiotic therapy to assess for complete resolution of the infection (especially in urinary tract infections).

In some institutions, to save money, urine cultures are only done if the urinalysis suggests a possible infection. In these institutions, urine is collected and "split." One half is sent for urinalysis, and the other half is held in the laboratory refrigerator and evaluated only if the urinalysis indicates a possible infection.

Interfering factors

- Drugs that may affect test results include antibiotics.

Procedure and patient care

Before

- Explain to the patient the procedure for collecting a clean-catch (midstream) urine collection.
- Hold antibiotics until after the urine specimen has been collected.
- Provide the patient with the necessary supplies for the collection.

During

- Note that a *clean-catch* or *midstream* urine collection is required for C&S testing. This requires meticulous cleansing of the urinary meatus with an iodine preparation to reduce contamination of the specimen by external organisms. Then the cleansing agent must be completely removed, or it will contaminate the urine specimen. The midstream collection is obtained by:

  1. Having the patient begin to urinate in a bedpan, urinal, or toilet and then stop urinating (This washes the urine out of the distal urethra.)
  2. Correctly positioning a sterile urine container, into which the patient voids 3 to 4 ounces of urine
  3. Capping the container
  4. Allowing the patient to finish voiding

- Note that *urinary catheterization* may be needed for patients unable to void. However, this procedure is not usually performed because of the risk of inducing organisms and because of patient discomfort.
- For inpatients with an *indwelling urinary catheter,* obtain a specimen by attaching a small-gauge (e.g., 25) needle to a syringe and aseptically inserting the needle into the catheter at a point distal to the sleeve leading to the balloon. Urine is aspirated and then placed in a sterile urine container. (Usually the catheter tubing distal to the puncture site needs to be clamped for 15 to 30 minutes before the aspiration of urine to allow urine to fill the tubing. After the specimen is withdrawn, the clamp is removed.)
- Note that *suprapubic aspiration* of urine is a safe method of obtaining urine in neonates and infants. The abdomen is prepared with an antiseptic, and a 25-gauge needle is inserted into the suprapubic area 1 inch above the sym-

U

physis pubis. Urine is aspirated into the syringe and then transferred to a sterile urine container.

- Collect specimens from infants and young children in a disposable pouch called a *U bag*. This bag has an adhesive backing around the opening to attach to the child.
- Note that for patients with a *urinary diversion* (e.g., an ileal conduit), catheterization should be done through the stoma. Urine should *not* be collected from the ostomy pouch.
- Indicate on the laboratory slip any medications that can affect test results.

After

- Transport the specimen to the laboratory immediately (at least within 30 minutes). If unable to do so, the specimen may be refrigerated up to 2 hours.
- Notify the physician of any positive results so that appropriate antibiotic therapy can be initiated.

Abnormal finding

Urinary tract infection

Notes

urine flow studies (Uroflowmetry, Urodynamic studies)

Type of test Urodynamic

Normal findings Depend on the patient's age, sex, and volume voided

Test explanation and related physiology

Uroflowmetry is the simplest of the urodynamic techniques, being noninvasive and requiring simple and relatively inexpensive equipment. This study measures the volume of urine expelled from the bladder per second. This test is indicated to investigate dysfunctional voiding or suspicious outflow tract obstruction. It is also done before and after any procedure designed to modify the function of the urologic outflow tract.

The urine flow depends greatly on the volume of urine voided. The flow rates are highest and most predictable in the urine volume range of 200 to 400 ml. Over 400 ml the efficiency of the bladder muscle is greatly decreased. Nomograms of maximal flow versus voided volume can be used for accurate test result interpretation, taking into account the patient's sex and age. If the flow rates are abnormally low, the test should be repeated to check for accuracy.

Modern urine flowmeters provide a permanent graphic recording. If flowmeters are not available, the patient can time the urinary stream with a stopwatch and record the voided volume. From this the average flow is calculated.

In some cases it is more valuable to analyze several voided volumes and flow rates rather than a single flow rate. If this is to be done, the patient is taught to use a flowmeter. A graph of flow versus volume can be plotted. This, together with clinical observation, provides very valuable information on the severity of outflow obstruction, the likelihood of urinary retention, and the state of compensation or decompensation of the detrusor muscle.

U

Procedure and patient care

Before

- Explain the procedure to the patient.
- Instruct the patient how to void into the urine flowmeter.
- Determine the number of flow rates that will be needed.

During

- Note that this test should be performed when the patient has a normal desire to void and in conditions suitable for privacy. The bladder should be adequately full. Essentially, all the patient must do is urinate into the flowmeter. Several different types of flowmeters are available.
- Tell the patient no discomfort is associated with this test.
- Note that the duration of this test is several seconds.

After

- Record the position of the patient, the method of filling the bladder (it should be natural), and whether or not this study was part of another evaluation.

Abnormal findings

Dysfunctional voiding
Outflow tract obstruction caused by urethral stricture, prostatic cancer, or hypertrophy

Notes

urine odor

Type of test Urine

Normal findings Aromatic

Test explanation and related physiology

Determination of urine odor is part of a routine urinalysis. The aromatic odor of fresh, normal urine is caused by the presence of volatile acid. The urine of patients with diabetic ketosis has a strong, sweet smell of acetone. In infected persons, urine has a very foul odor. Patients with a fecal odor to their urine may have a rectal fistula.

Interfering factors

- Some foods (e.g., asparagus) produce characteristic urine odors.
- When urine stands for a long time and begins to decompose, it has an ammonia-like smell.
- Drugs that may affect urine odor include antibiotics and vitamins.

Procedure and patient care

Before

- Explain the procedure to the patient.
- Tell the patient that no fasting is required.

During

- Collect a voided specimen in a urine container and cover it.
- If the specimen is likely to be contaminated by vaginal discharge or hemorrhage, collect a "clean-catch" or "midstream" specimen. This requires meticulous cleansing of the urinary meatus with an iodine preparation to reduce contamination of the specimen by external organisms. Then the cleansing agent must be completely removed, or it will contaminate the specimen. The midstream collection is obtained by:

  1. Having the patient begin to urinate in a bedpan, urinal, or toilet and then stop urinating (This washes the urine out of the distal urethra.)

U

2. Correctly positioning a sterile urine container, into which the patient voids 3 to 4 ounces of urine
3. Capping the container
4. Allowing the patient to finish voiding

After

- Transport the specimen to the laboratory as soon as possible.

Abnormal findings

Infection
Ketonuria
Urinary tract infection
Rectal fistula

Maple sugar urine disease
Phenylketonuria
Hepatic failure

Notes

urine pH

Type of test Urine

Normal findings 4.6-8.0 (average = 6.0)

Test explanation and related physiology

The urinary pH is part of a routine urinalysis. The analysis of the pH of a freshly voided urine specimen indicates the acid-base balance of the patient. An *alkaline* pH is obtained in a patient with alkalemia. Also, bacteriura, urinary tract infection, or a diet high in citrus fruits or vegetables can cause increased urine pH. Certain medications (e.g., streptomycin, neomycin, kanomycin) are effective in treating urinary tract infections when the urine is alkaline. *Acidic* urine is generally obtained in patients with acidemia, which can result from metabolic or respiratory acidosis, starvation, diarrhea, or a diet high in meat products or cranberries.

The urine pH is useful in identifying crystals in the urine and determining the predisposition to form a given type of stone. Acidic urine is associated with xanthine, cystine, uric acid, and calcium oxalate stones. To treat or prevent these urinary calculi, the urine should be kept alkaline. Alkaline urine is associated with calcium carbonate, calcium phosphate, and magnesium phosphate stones. To prevent or treat these stones, the urine should be kept acidic.

Interfering factors

- The urine pH becomes alkaline on standing because of the action of urea-splitting bacteria, producing ammonia.
- The urine pH of an uncovered specimen will become alkaline because carbon dioxide will vaporize from the urine into the air.
- Dietary factors affect urine pH. Alkaline urine is observed in people who eat large quantities of citrus fruits, dairy products, and vegetables. Acidic urine is observed with a diet high in meat and certain fruits (e.g., cranberries).
- Drugs that may cause an acidic urine include ammonium chloride, chlorothiazide diuretics, and methenamine mandelate.
- Drugs that may cause an alkaline urine include acetazolamide, potassium citrate, and sodium bicarbonate.

U

Procedure and patient care

Before

- Explain the procedure to the patient.
- Tell the patient that no fasting is required.

During

- Collect a voided specimen in a urine container and cover.
- If the specimen is contaminated by vaginal discharge or bleeding, collect a "clean-catch" or "midstream" specimen. This requires meticulous cleansing of the urinary meatus with an iodine preparation to reduce contamination of the specimen by external organisms. Then the cleansing agent must be completely removed, or it will contaminate the specimen. The midstream collection is obtained by:
  1. Having the patient begin to urinate in a bedpan, urinal, or toilet and then stop urinating (This washes the urine out of the distal urethra.)
  2. Correctly positioning a sterile urine container, into which the patient voids 3 to 4 ounces of urine
  3. Capping the container
  4. Allowing the patient to finish voiding

After

- Transport the specimen to the laboratory as soon as possible.
- If the specimen cannot be processed immediately, refrigerate it.

Abnormal findings

**Increased levels
  (alkaline urine)**

Respiratory alkalosis
Metabolic alkalosis
Urea-splitting bacteria
Vegetarian diet
Renal failure with inability
  to form ammonia
Gastric suction
Vomiting
Diuretic therapy
Renal tubular acidosis
Urinary tract infection

**Decreased levels
  (acidic urine)**

Metabolic acidosis
Diabetes mellitus
Diarrhea
Starvation
Respiratory acidosis
Emphysema
Sleep
Pyrexia

urine specific gravity (Specific gravity of urine)

Type of test Urine

Normal findings
Adult: 1.005-1.030 (usually 1.010-1.025)
Elderly: values decrease with advancing age.
Newborn: 1.001-1.020

Test explanation and related physiology

The specific gravity is a measure of the concentration of particles (including wastes and electrolytes) in the urine. A high specific gravity indicates a concentrated urine; a low specific gravity indicates a dilute urine. Determination of specific gravity is part of a routine urinalysis.

The specific gravity is used to evaluate the concentrating and excretory power of the kidney. The specific gravity must be interpreted in light of the presence or absence of glycosuria and/or proteinuria. The measurement of urine specific gravity is easier and more convenient than the measure of osmolality (see p. 535). The specific gravity correlates roughly with osmolality. Knowledge of the specific gravity is needed for interpreting the results of most parts of a urinalysis. Specific gravity is usually evaluated by using a refractometer or a dipstick.

Interfering factors

- Recent use of radiographic dyes in the urine increase the specific gravity.
- Drugs that may cause increased levels include dextran and sucrose.

Procedure and patient care
Before

- Explain the procedure to the patient.
- Tell the patient that no fasting is usually required.

During

- Place the first-voided AM specimen in a urine container.
- Mark the container with the date and time of collection.

U

After

- Transport the specimen to the laboratory within 2 hours.
- If the test is not run immediately, refrigerate the specimen.

Abnormal findings
Increased levels

Dehydration (because kidneys are reabsorbing all available free water; thus excreted urine is very concentrated)

Pituitary tumor or trauma that causes syndrome of inappropriate release of excessive antidiuretic hormone (SIADH), resulting in excessive water reabsorption

Decrease in renal blood flow (as in heart failure, renal artery stenosis, or hypotension)

Glycosuria and proteinuria

Water restriction

Fever

Excessive sweating

Vomiting

Diarrhea

X-ray contrast dye

Decreased levels

Overhydration

Diabetes insipidus (because of the inadequate ADH secretion, which causes a decrease in water reabsorption)

Renal failure (because the kidney has lost its ability to concentrate urine through water reabsorption)

Diuresis

Hypothermia

Glomerulonephritis

Pyelonephritis

Notes

vanillylmandelic acid and catecholamines
(VMA and epinephrine, Norepinephrine, Metanephrine,
Normetanephrine, Dopamine)

Type of test Urine (24 hour)

Normal findings
VMA

Adult/elderly: 2-7 mg/24 hr or 10-35 μmol/24 hr
Newborn: <1.0 mg/24 hr
Infant: <2.0 mg/24 hr
Child: 1-3 mg/24 hr
Adolescent: 1-5 mg/24 hr

Catecholamines

Epinephrine
Adult/elderly: 0.5-20 μg/24 hr
Child: 0-1 years: 0-2.5 μg/24 hr
      1-2 years: 0-3.5
      2-4 years: 0-6.0
      4-7 years: 0.2-10
      7-10 years: 0.5-14
Norepinephrine
Adult/elderly: 15-80 μg/24 hr
Child: 0-1 years: 0-10 μg/24 hr
      1-2 years: 0-17
      2-4 years: 4-29
      4-7 years: 8-45
      7-10 years: 13-65
Dopamine
Adult/elderly: 65-400 μg/24 hr
Child: 0-1 years: 0-85 μg/24 hr
      1-2 years: 10-140
      2-4 years: 40-260
      Over 4 years: 65-400
Metanephrine: 24-96 μg/24 hr
Normetanephrine: 75-375 μg/24 hr

Test explanation and related physiology

This 24-hour urine test for VMA and catecholamines is
primarily performed to diagnose hypertension secondary to

pheochromocytoma. This test is also used to detect the presence of neuroblastomas and rare adrenal tumors.

A *pheochromocytoma* is an adrenal tumor that frequently secretes abnormally high levels of epinephrine and norepinephrine. These hormones cause episodic or persistent hypertension by causing peripheral arterial vasoconstriction. Dopamine is the precursor of epinephrine and norepinephrine. Metanephrine and normetanephrine are catabolic products of epinephrine and norepinephrine, respectively. VMA is the product of catabolism of both metanephrine and normetanephrine. In patients with pheochromocytoma, one or all of these substances will be present in excessive quantities in a 24-hour collection of urine.

Interfering factors

- Increased levels of VMA can be caused by certain foods (e.g., tea, coffee, cocoa, vanilla, chocolate).
- Vigorous exercise, stress, and starvation can cause increased VMA levels.
- Drugs that may cause increased *VMA* levels include caffeine, epinephrine, levodopa, lithium, and nitroglycerin.
- Drugs that may cause decreased *VMA* levels include clonidine, disulfiram (Antabuse), guanethidine, imipramine, monoamine oxidase (MAO) inhibitors, phenothiazines, and reserpine.
- Drugs that may cause increased *catecholamine* levels include alcohol (ethyl), aminophylline, caffeine, chloral hydrate, clonidine (chronic therapy), contrast media (iodine containing), disulfiram, epinephrine, erythromycin, insulin, methenamine, methyldopa, nicotinic acid (large doses), nitroglycerin, quinidine, riboflavin, and tetracyclines.
- Drugs that may cause decreased *catecholamine* levels include guanethidine, reserpine, and salicylates.
- Falsely decreased levels of VMA can be caused by uremia, alkaline urine, and radiographic iodine contrast agents.

Procedure and patient care
Before

- Explain the dietary restrictions and the 24-hour urine collection procedure to the patient.
- For 2 or 3 days before the 24-hour collection for VMA and throughout the collection, place the patient on a

VMA-restricted diet. Generally, instruct the patient to avoid coffee, tea, bananas, chocolate, cocoa, licorice, citrus fruit, all foods and fluids containing vanilla, and also aspirin. Obtain specific restrictions from the laboratory.

- Restrict the patient from taking antihypertensive medications, and sometimes all medications, during this period and possibly even longer.

During

- Collect the 24-hour urine specimen using a preservative.
- Instruct the patient to begin the 24-hour urine collection after voiding. Discard the initial specimen and note the time; this is the starting time.
- Collect all urine passed during the next 24 hours. Refrigerate or keep on ice during the collection period.
- Post the hours for the urine collection in a prominent place to avoid accidental discarding of the specimen.
- Remind the patient to void before defecating so that the urine is not contaminated by feces.
- Instruct the patient not to put toilet paper in the collection container.
- Encourage the patient to drink fluids during the 24 hours unless contraindicated for medical purposes.
- Collect the last specimen as close as possible to the end of the 24-hour period. Add this urine to the container.
- Indicate the time of the last specimen collected on the laboratory slip or urine container.
- Identify and minimize factors contributing to patient stress and anxiety. Excessive physical exercise and emotion can alter catecholamine test results by causing an increased secretion of epinephrine and norepinephrine.

After

- Send the specimen to the laboratory as soon as the test is completed.
- Allow the patient to have foods and drugs that have been restricted in preparation for the test.

Abnormal findings
Increased levels

Pheochromocytomas
Neuroblastomas
Ganglioneuromas

Ganglioblastomas
Severe stress
Strenuous exercise
Acute anxiety

Notes

venography of lower extremities
(Phlebography, Venogram)

Type of test X-ray with contrast dye

Normal findings No evidence of venous thrombosis or obstruction

Test explanation and related physiology

Venography is an x-ray study designed to identify and locate thrombi within the venous system of the lower extremities. During this study, dye is injected into the venous system of the affected extremity. X-ray films are then taken at timed intervals to visualize the venous system. Obstruction to the flow of dye or a filling defect within the dye-filled vein indicates that thrombosis exists. A positive study accurately confirms the diagnosis of venous thrombosis. A normal study, however, although not as accurate, does make the diagnosis of venous thrombosis very unlikely. Often, both extremities are studied, even though only one leg is suspected to contain deep vein thrombosis. The normal extremity is used for comparison with the involved extremity.

Contraindications

- Patients who have severe edema of the legs, making venous access impossible
- Patients who are uncooperative
- Patients who are allergic to iodinated dye or shellfish
- Patients with renal failure because the iodinated dye is nephrotoxic

Potential complications

- Allergic reaction to iodinated dyes
  Allergic reactions vary from flushing, itching, and urticaria to severe, life-threatening anaphylaxis (evidenced by respiratory distress, drop in blood pressure, shock). In the event of anaphylaxis the patient may be treated with diphenhydramine (Benadryl), steroids, and epinephrine. Oxygen and endotracheal equipment should be on hand for immediate use.
- Renal failure, especially in the elderly who are chronically

V

dehydrated or who may have a mild degree of renal failure
- Subcutaneous infiltration of the dye, causing cellulitis and pain
- Venous thrombophlebitis caused by the dye
- Bacteremia caused by a break in sterile technique
- Venous embolism caused by dislodgement of a deep vein clot induced by the dye injection

Procedure and patient care

Before

- Explain the procedure to the patient.
- Obtain informed consent for this procedure.
- Assess the patient for allergies to iodinated dyes and shellfish. If a suspected allergy exists and the venogram is absolutely necessary, the patient should receive a steroid and antihistamine preparation. Notify the radiologist of the potential for allergic reaction so that hypoallergenic, non-ionic contrast can be used.
- If needed, provide appropriate pain medication so the patient is able to lie still during the procedure.
- Ensure that the patient is appropriately hydrated before testing. Injection of the iodinated contrast can cause renal failure, especially in the elderly.

During

- Note the following procedural steps:
  1. The patient is taken to the radiology department and placed in a supine position on the x-ray table.
  2. Catheterization of a superficial vein on the foot is performed. This may require a surgical cutdown.
  3. An iodinated, radiopaque dye is injected into the vein.
  4. X-ray films are taken to follow the course of the dye up the leg.
  5. Frequently a tourniquet is placed on the leg to prevent filling of the superficial saphenous vein. All the dye therefore goes to filling the deep venous system, which contains the most clinically significant thrombosis that can embolize.
- Note that a radiologist performs this study in approximately 30 to 90 minutes.
- Tell the patient that the venous catheterization is only as

uncomfortable as a cutaneous heel stick or a small incision in the foot.
- The dye may cause the patient to feel a warm flush. (This is not as severe as noted with arteriography.) Inform the patient that occasionally, mild degrees of nausea, vomiting, or skin itching can also occur.

After

- Continue appropriate hydration of the patient to prevent dehydration caused by the diuretic action of the dye.
- Observe the puncture site for infection, cellulitis, or bleeding.
- Assess the patient's vital signs for signs of bacteremia (e.g., high temperature, tachycardia, chills, fever).
- Evaluate the patient for signs of allergic reaction (e.g., rash, chills, fever, irritability). Treat with antihistamines or steroids.

Abnormal findings

Obstructed venous systems caused by thrombosis, tumor, or inflammation
Acute deep vein thrombosis

Notes

V

ventriculography (Ventriculogram)

Type of test X-ray

Normal findings No ventricular abnormalities

Test explanation and related physiology

For ventriculography, serial x-ray examinations are taken of the skull after air or contrast material in injected *directly* into the ventricles through burr holes in the skull. The size, shape, and filling of the ventricles are observed. Lesions (e.g., brain tumors), cerebral anomalies, and the patency of the ventricular system are identified. This procedure should *not* be performed when less invasive procedures, such as computed tomography (CT) or magnetic resonance imaging (MRI) scans, would suffice for diagnosis.

Contraindications

- Patients with increased intracranial pressure
- Patients with infection near the insertion site
  Meningitis can result from contamination.

Potential complications

- Severe headache caused by loss of cerebrospinal fluid (CSF)
- Brainstem compression from shifts in intracranial pressure

Procedure and patient care

Before

- Explain the procedure to the patient.
- Ensure that the physician has obtained informed and written consent for ventriculography and craniotomy before premedicating the patient. Craniotomy may be necessary to prevent brainstem compression.
- Prepare the patient using the normal preoperative routine.

During

- Note the following procedural steps:
  1. A specified area (e.g., top, back, side) of the head

must be shaved according to the neurosurgeon's orders.

2. The patient is prepared as for brain surgery because if brain displacement occurs, an immediate craniotomy must be performed.
3. The fasting patient is taken to the operating room and placed in a special chair.
4. Using either general or local anesthesia for the patient, the neurosurgeon makes burr holes through scalp incisions and then punctures the ventricles with a special needle or catheter.
5. After removing some CSF, either air or contrast material is injected into the ventricles.
6. The patient is repositioned during the x-ray study that follows to ensure adequate visualization of the ventricular structures.
7. If the test results are normal, the needle is removed and the skin over the burr holes is sutured closed.
8. The scalp wounds are covered with a sterile dressing.

- Note that this procedure is performed by a neurosurgeon in approximately 30 minutes.
- Remember that immediate surgery (craniotomy) may be necessary if an intracranial tumor is detected or if the procedure itself caused dangerous intracranial pressure shifts.
- Tell the patient that no discomfort occurs during this test because it is done with him or her under anesthesia.

After

- Monitor the patient's vital signs and neurologic signs frequently for the first 12 to 24 hours.
- Elevate the head of the patient's bed 10 to 15 degrees for the first 24 hours and then elevate as tolerated.
- Check the patient's scalp dressing for drainage and reinforce as necessary.
- When the patient is alert and oriented, encourage fluids to replace the CSF lost during the procedure.
- Since most patients have a headache that will last for about 24 to 48 hours, use an ice bag to help relieve the pain.
- If ordered, administer analgesics to relieve severe patient discomfort.

- Tell the patient that the scalp sutures are usually removed in 4 to 5 days.

Abnormal findings

Brain tumors
Cerebral anomalies
Abnormal patency of ventricular system

Notes

waxy casts

Type of test Urine

Normal findings No casts present

Test explanation and related physiology

Casts are clumps of material or cells. They are formed in the renal collecting tubule and have the shape of the tubule, thus the term *cast*. Waxy casts may be cell casts, hyaline casts, or renal failure casts. Waxy casts are found especially in patients with chronic renal diseases and are associated with chronic renal failure. They also occur in patients with diabetic nephropathy, malignant hypertension, and glomerulonephritis.

Procedure and patient care

Before

- Explain the procedure to the patient.

During

- Collect a freshly voided specimen in a urine container.
- If the specimen is contaminated by vaginal discharge or bleeding, collect a "clean-catch" or "midstream" specimen. This requires meticulous cleansing of the urinary meatus with an iodine preparation to reduce contamination of the specimen by external organisms. Then the cleansing agent must be completely removed, or it will contaminate the specimen. The midstream collection is obtained by:

  1. Having the patient begin to urinate in a bedpan, urinal, or toilet and then stop urinating (This washes the urine out of the distal urethra.)
  2. Correctly positioning a sterile urine container, into which the patient voids 3 to 4 ounces of urine
  3. Capping the container
  4. Allowing the patient to finish voiding

After

- Send the urine specimen immediately to the laboratory.
- Do *not* allow the specimen to sit, since the casts will break up.

W

Abnormal findings

Chronic renal diseases
Chronic renal failure
Diabetic nephropathy
Malignant hypertension
Glomerulonephritis
Renal transplant rejection
Nephrotic syndrome

Notes

white blood cell count and differential count (WBC and differential, Leukocyte count, Neutrophil count, Lymphocyte count, Monocyte count, Eosinophil count, Basophil count)

Type of test Blood

Normal findings

Total WBCs
Adult/child over 2 years: 5000-10,000/mm^3
Child 2 years and younger: 6200-17,000/mm^3
Newborn: 9000-30,000/mm^3
Differential count
Neutrophils: 55%-70%
Lymphocytes: 20%-40%
Monocytes: 2%-8%
Eosinophils: 1%-4%
Basophils: 0.5%-1%

Possible critical values WBCs <2500 or >30,000/mm^3

Test explanation and related physiology

The WBC count has two components. One is a count of the total number of WBCs (leukocytes) in 1 mm^3 of peripheral venous blood. The other component, the differential count, measures the percentage of each type of leukocyte present in the same specimen. An increase in the percentage of one type of leukocyte means a decrease in the percentage of another type. Neutrophils and lymphocytes make up 75% to 90% of the total leukocytes. These leukocyte types can be identified easily by their morphology on a venous blood smear. The total leukocyte count has a wide range of normal values, but many diseases can induce abnormal values. An increased total WBC count (leukocytosis) usually indicates infection, inflammation, tissue necrosis, or leukemic neoplasia. Trauma or stress, either emotional or physical, can increase the WBC count. Leukopenia (i.e., a decreased WBC count) occurs in many forms of bone marrow failure (e.g., following antineoplastic chemotherapy or radiation therapy or in agranulocytosis), overwhelming infections, dietary deficiencies, and autoimmune diseases.

The major function of the WBCs is to fight infection and

W

react against foreign bodies or tissues. Five types of WBCs can easily be identified on a routine blood smear. These cells, in order of frequency, include neutrophils, lymphocytes, monocytes, eosinophils, and basophils. All these WBCs arise from the same "pluripotent" stem cell within the bone marrow as the red blood cell (RBC) does. Beyond this origin, however, each cell line differentiates separately. Most mature WBCs are then deposited into the circulating blood.

Polymorphonuclear (PMN) *neutrophils* are produced in 7 to 14 days and exist in the circulation for only 6 hours. The primary function of the neutrophil is phagocytosis (killing and digestion of bacterial microorganisms). Acute bacterial infections and trauma stimulate neutrophil production, resulting in an increased WBC count. Often, when neutrophil production is stimulated, early immature forms of neutrophils enter the circulation. These immature forms are called *band* or *stab cells*. This process, referred to as a "shift to the left" in WBC production, is indicative of an ongoing acute bacterial infection.

Lymphocytes are divided into two types: T cells and B cells. T cells are primarily involved with cellular-type immune reactions, whereas B cells participate in humoral immunity (antibody production). The primary function of the lymphocytes is fighting chronic bacterial infection and acute viral infections. The differential count does not separate the T and B cells, but rather counts the combination of the two.

Monocytes are phagocytic cells capable of fighting bacteria in a way very similar to that of the neutrophil. However, monocytes can be produced more rapidly and can spend a longer time in the circulation than the neutrophils.

Basophils, and especially *eosinophils,* are involved in the allergic reaction. Parasitic infestations also are capable of stimulating the production of these cells.

The WBC and differential count are routinely measured as part of the complete blood count (CBC, see p. 212). Serial WBCs and differential counts have both diagnostic and prognostic value. For example, a persistent increase in the WBC count may indicate a worsening of an infectious process (e.g., appendicitis). A dramatic decrease in the WBC count may indicate marrow failure and delay further chemotherapy in patients undergoing cancer treatment.

Interfering factors

- Eating, physical activity, and stress may cause an increase in WBC and differential values.
- Pregnancy (final month) and labor may cause increased WBC levels.
- Drugs that may cause increased WBC levels include adrenalin, allopurinol, aspirin, chloroform, epinephrine, heparin, quinine, steroids, and triamterene (Dyrenium).
- Drugs that may cause decreased WBC levels include antibiotics, anticonvulsants, antihistamines, antimetabolites, antithyroid drugs, arsenicals, barbiturates, chemotherapeutic agents, diuretics, and sulfonamides.
- Patients who have had a splenectomy have a persistent mild elevation of WBC counts.

Procedure and patient care

Before

- Explain the procedure to the patient.
- Tell the patient that no fasting is required.

During

- Collect approximately 5 to 7 ml of venous blood in a lavender-top tube.

After

- Apply pressure or a pressure dressing to the venipuncture site.
- Check the venipuncture site for bleeding.

Abnormal findings

Increased WBC count (leukocytosis)	Decreased WBC count (leukopenia)
Infection	Drug toxicity (e.g., chloramphenicol)
Leukemic neoplasia	Bone marrow failure
Trauma	Overwhelming infections
Stress	Dietary deficiency
Tissue necrosis	Autoimmune disease
Inflammation	Bone marrow infiltration (e.g., myelofibrosis)

W

Increased/decreased differential count

See Table 13.

TABLE 13 Causes for abnormalities in the WBC differential count

Type of WBC	Elevated	Decreased
Neutrophils	*Neutrophilia* Physical or emotional stress Acute suppurative infection Myelocytic leukemia Trauma Cushing's syndrome Inflammatory disorders (e.g., rheumatic fever, thyroiditis, rheumatoid arthritis) Metabolic disorders (e.g., ketoacidosis, gout, eclampsia)	*Neutropenia* Aplastic anemia Dietary deficiency Overwhelming bacterial infection (especially in the elderly) Viral infections (e.g., hepatitis, influenza, measles) Radiation therapy Addison's disease Drug therapy: myelotoxic drugs (as in chemotherapy)
Lymphocytes	*Lymphocytosis* Chronic bacterial infection Viral infection (e.g., mumps, rubella) Lymphocytic leukemia Multiple myeloma Infectious mononucleosis Radiation Infectious hepatitis	*Lymphocytopenia* Leukemia Sepsis Immunodeficiency diseases Lupus erythematosus Later stages of human immunodeficiency virus (HIV) infection Drug therapy: adrenocorticosteroids, antineoplastics Radiation therapy

TABLE 13 Causes for abnormalities in the WBC differential count—cont'd

Type of WBC	Elevated	Decreased
Monocytes	*Monocytosis* Chronic inflammatory disorders Viral infections (e.g., infectious mononucleosis) Tuberculosis Chronic ulcerative colitis Parasites (e.g., malaria)	*Monocytopenia* Drug therapy: prednisone
Eosinophils	*Eosinophilia* Parasitic infections Allergic reactions Eczema Leukemia Autoimmune diseases	*Eosinopenia* Increased adrenosteroid production
Basophils	*Basophilia* Myeloproliferative disease (e.g., myelofibrosis, polycythemia rubra vera) Leukemia	*Basopenia* Acute allergic reactions Hyperthyroidism Stress reactions

Notes

W

white blood cells and casts

Type of test Urine

Normal findings
WBCs: 0-4/low-power field
WBC casts: negative

Test explanation and related physiology

Normally, few white blood cells (WBCs) are found in the urine sediment on microscopic examination. The presence of five or more WBCs in the urine indicates a urinary tract infection. A clean-catch urine culture should be done for further evaluation.

Casts are clumps of material or cells. They are formed in the renal collecting tubule and have the shape of the tubule, thus the term *cast*. On microscopic examination of the urine sediment, WBC casts are most frequently found in patients with acute pyelonephritis. WBC casts are also seen in patients with glomerulonephritis and lupus nephritis.

Interfering factors

- Vaginal discharge can contaminate the urine specimen.

Procedure and patient care

Before

- Explain the procedure to the patient.

During

- Collect a freshly voided specimen in a urine container.
- If the specimen is contaminated by vaginal discharge or bleeding, collect a "clean-catch" or "midstream" specimen. This requires meticulous cleansing of the urinary meatus with an iodine preparation to reduce contamination of the specimen by external organisms. Then the cleansing agent must be completely removed, or it will contaminate the specimen. The midstream collection is obtained by:

  1. Having the patient begin to urinate in a bedpan, urinal, or toilet and then stop urinating (This washes the urine out of the distal urethra.)

2. Correctly positioning a sterile urine container, into which the patient voids 3 to 4 ounces of urine
3. Capping the container
4. Allowing the patient to finish voiding

After

- Send the specimen immediately to the laboratory or refrigerate.
- Note that urine should be checked for casts when it is fresh.

Abnormal findings
Increased WBCs

Bacterial infection in urinary tracts

Increased WBC casts

Acute pyelonephritis
Glomerulonephritis
Lupus nephritis

Notes

W

wound culture and sensitivity (C&S)

Type of test Microscopic examination

Normal findings Negative

Test explanation and related physiology

Wound cultures are obtained to determine the presence of pathogens in patients with suspected wound infections. Wound infections are most often caused by pus-forming organisms.

All cultures should be performed before antibiotic therapy is initiated. Otherwise the antibiotic may interrupt the growth of the organism in the laboratory. More often than not, however, the physician will want to institute antibiotic therapy before the culture results are reported. In these instances a *Gram stain* of the specimen smeared on a slide is most helpful and can be reported in less than 10 minutes. All forms of bacteria are grossly classified as gram positive (blue staining) or gram negative (red staining). Knowledge of the shape of the organism (e.g., spheric, rod shaped) can also be very helpful in the tentative identification of the infecting organism. With knowledge of the Gram stain results, the physician can institute a reasonable antibiotic regimen based on past experience as to the organism's possible identity. Most organisms require about 24 hours to grow in the laboratory, and a preliminary report can be given at that time. Occasionally, 48 to 72 hours are required for growth and identification of the organism. Cultures may be repeated after appropriate antibiotic therapy to assess for complete resolution of the infection.

Interfering factors

- Drugs that may alter test results include antibiotics.

Procedure and patient care

Before

- Explain the procedure to the patient.

During

- Aseptically place a sterile cotton swab into the pus of the patient's wound and then place the swab into a sterile, covered test tube. (Culturing specimens from the skin edge are much less accurate than culturing the suppurative material.)

- If an anaerobic organism is suspected, obtain an anaerobic culture tube from the microbiology laboratory.
- If wound cultures are to be obtained on a patient requiring wound irrigation, obtain the culture *before* the wound is irrigated.
- If any antibiotic ointment or solution has been previously applied, remove it with sterile water or saline before obtaining the culture.
- Handle all specimens as though they were capable of transmitting disease.
- Indicate on the laboratory slip any medications the patient may be taking that could affect test results.

After

- Transport the specimen to the laboratory immediately after testing (at least within 30 minutes).
- Notify the physician of any positive results so that appropriate antibiotic therapy can be initiated.

Abnormal finding

Wound infection

Notes

W

D-**xylose absorption test** (Xylose tolerance test)

Type of test Blood; urine

Normal findings

Adult/elderly: blood levels equal to 25-40 mg/dl 2 hours after ingestion
80%-95% excreted in urine 5 hours after ingestion.

Child: blood levels equal to 30 mg/dl 1 hour after ingestion
16%-33% excreted in urine 5 hours after ingestion

Test explanation and related physiology

D-Xylose is a monosaccharide that is easily absorbed by the normal intestine. In patients who have malabsorption, intestinal D-xylose absorption is diminished and, as a result, blood levels and urine excretion will be reduced. D-Xylose is the monosaccharide chosen for the test because it is not metabolized by the body. Its serum levels directly reflect intestinal absorption.

Also, this monosaccharide is used because absorption does not require pancreatic or biliary exocrine function. Its absorption is directly determined by the small intestine. This test is used to separate patients with diarrhea caused by maldigestion (pancreatic/biliary dysfunction) from those with diarrhea caused by malabsorption (sprue, Whipple's disease, Crohn's disease).

In this test the patient is asked to drink a fluid containing a prescribed amount of D-xylose. Blood and urine levels are subsequently evaluated. Excellent gastrointestinal absorption would be documented by high blood levels and good urine secretion of D-xylose. Poor intestinal absorption would be marked by decreased blood levels and urine excretion.

Contraindications

- Patients with abnormal kidney function
- Patients who are dehydrated

Interfering factors

- Drugs that may affect test results include aspirin, atropine, and indomethacin.

Procedure and patient care

Before

- Explain the procedure to the patient.
- Instruct the adult patient to fast for 8 hours before testing.
- Tell the pediatric patient or the parents that the patient should fast for at least 4 hours before testing.

During

- Collect approximately 7 ml of venous blood in a red-top tube before the patient ingests the D-xylose.
- Collect a first-voided morning urine specimen and send it to the laboratory.
- Ask the patient to drink 25 g of D-xylose dissolved in 8 ounces of water. Record the time of ingestion.
- Calibrate pediatric doses according to the patient's body weight.
- Repeat venipunctures to obtain blood in exactly 2 hours for an adult and 1 hour for a child.
- Collect urine for a designated time, usually 5 hours. Refrigerate the urine during the collection period.
- Observe the patient for nausea, vomiting, and diarrhea, which may occur as side effects to D-xylose.
- Instruct the patient to remain in a restful position. Intense physical activity can alter the digestive process and affect the test results.

After

- Observe the venipuncture site for bleeding.
- Provide the patient with food or drink and inform the patient that normal activity can be resumed after completion of the study.

Abnormal findings

Decreased levels

Malabsorption caused by:
  Sprue
  Lymphatic obstruction

X

Enteropathy (e.g., radiation)
Crohn's disease
Whipple's disease
Small intestine bacterial overgrowth
Hookworm
Viral gastroenteritis
Giardia lamblia infestation

Notes

Appendix: Typical Abbreviations and Units of Measurement

$<$	Less than
$\leq$	Less than or equal to
$>$	Greater than
$\geq$	Greater than or equal to
C	Celsius
cc	Cubic centimeter
cg	Centigram
cm	Centimeter
cm H_2O	Centimeter of water
cu	Cubic
dl	Deciliter (100 ml)
g	Gram
hr	Hour
IU	International unit
ImU	International milliunit
IμU	International microunit
K	Kilo
kg	Kilogram
L	Liter
m	Meter
m^2	Square meter
m^3	Cubic meter
mEq	Milliequivalent
mEq/L	Milliequivalent per liter
mg	Milligram
min	Minute
ml	Milliliter
mm	Millimeter
mm^3	Cubic millimeter
mM	Millimole
mm Hg	Millimeter of mercury
mm H_2O	Millimeter of water

mol	Mole
mmol	Millimole
mOsm	Milliosmole
mμ	Millimicron
mU	Milliunit
mV	Millivolt
ng	Nanogram
nmol	Nanomole
Pa	Pascal
pg	Picogram (or micromicrogram)
pl	Picoliter
pm	Picomole
S	Second (SI)
sec	Second
SI units	International System of Units
μ	Micron
μ^3	Cubic micron
μg	Microgram
μIU	Microinternational unit
μmol	Micromole
μU	Microunit
U	Unit
yr	Year

Bibliography

Behrman, RE, Vaughan VC, Nelson WE, editors: *Nelson textbook of pediatrics,* ed 13, Philadelphia, 1987, WB Saunders.

Bertagnolli ME, and others: Use of endoscopic ultrasound in patients with motility disorders, *Gastroenterol Nurs* 12(2):98-99, 1989.

Bordow RA, Moser KM: *Manual of clinical problems in pulmonary medicine,* Boston, 1985, Little, Brown.

Breslau PJ: *Ultrasonic duplex scanning in the evaluation of carotid artery disease,* Voerendaal, Holland, 1981, Heerlen.

Christman C, Bennett J: Diabetes: new names, new test, new diet, *Nursing '87* 17(1):34-41, 1987.

Comella CL, Bleck TP: The technique of lumbar procedure, *J Crit Illness* 3(9):61-66, 1988.

Comella CL, Bleck TP: Selecting the right neurologic test for the critically ill patients, *J Crit Illness* 3(9):47-59, 1988.

Conway J: The aging kidney, *J Urol Nurs* 8(3):704-707, 1989.

Croft JE, Grodzicki RL, Steere AC: Antibody response in Lyme disease: evaluation of diagnostic tests, *J Infect Dis* 149(5):789-795, 1984.

D'Ambrosia RD, editor: *Musculoskeletal disorders: regional examination and differential diagnosis,* ed 2, Philadelphia, 1986, JB Lippincott.

Doershuk CF, Boat TF: Cystic fibrosis. In Behrman RE, Vaughan VC, Nelson WE, editors: *Nelson textbook of pediatrics,* ed 13, Philadelphia, 1987, WB Saunders.

Dowling JJ: *Musculoskeletal disease: staged for rapid comprehension,* St Louis, 1985, Mosby–Year Book.

Easton EJ: *Musculoskeletal magnetic resonance imaging,* Thorofare, NJ, 1986, Slack.

Felig P, and others: *Endocrinology and metabolism,* ed 2, New York, 1987, McGraw-Hill.

Fishman AP: *Pulmonary diseases and disorders,* ed 2, New York, 1987, McGraw-Hill.

Fritz M: Noninvasive bladder volume measurement, *Urol Nurs* 9(1):8-9, 1988.

Glenn J and others: Evaluation of the utility of a radioimmunoassay for serum CA 19-9 levels in patients before and after treatment of carcinoma of the pancreas, *J Clin Oncol* 6(3):462-468, 1988.

Halila H, and others: Ovarian cancer antigen CA 125 levels in pelvic inflammatory disease and pregnancy, *Cancer* 57(7):1327-1329, 1986.

Hudson MA, and others: Clinical use of prostate specific antigen in patients with prostate cancer, *J Urol* 142(10):1011-1017, 1989.

Jacobs DS, and others: *Laboratory test handbook,* St Louis, 1988, Mosby–Year Book.

Johnson JB: Laboratory tests: clinical, financial, and professional implications, *Emerg Nurs Rep* 2(10):1-8, 1988.

Kee JL, Hayes ER: Assessment of patient laboratory data in the acutely ill, *Nurs Clin North Am* 25(4):751-759, 1990.

Kisslo J, Adams DB, Belkin RN: *Doppler color flow imaging,* New York, 1988, Churchill Livingstone.

Knight CG: Assessing the preoperative adult, *Nurse Pract* 13(1):6, 8, 13+, 1988.

Knoben JE, Anderson PO: *Handbook of clinical drug data,* ed 6, Hamilton, Ill, 1988, Drug Intelligence.

Lam J, and others: Safety and diagnostic accuracy of dipyridamole-thallium imaging in the elderly, *J Am Coll Cardiol* 11:585-589, 1988.

Lange PH, Brawer MK: Serum prostate-specific antigen: its use in diagnosis and management of prostate cancer, *Urology* 33(6)(suppl):13-17, 1989.

Lopez E: Prenatal diagnosis by ultrasound, *J Perinat Neonat Nurs* 2(4):34-42, 1989.

McBride EV, Distefano K: Explaining diagnostic tests for M.S., *Nursing '88* 18(2):68-72, 1988.

Pagana KD, Pagana TJ: *Diagnostic testing and nursing implications: a case study approach,* ed 3, St Louis, 1990, Mosby–Year Book.

Peddecord KM, Janon EA, Robins JM: Use of MR imaging in an outpatient MR center, *AJR* 148:809-812, 1987.

Pope CE: Diseases of the esophagus. In Wyngaardenn JB, Smith LH, editors: *Cecil textbook of medicine,* ed 17, Philadelphia, 1985, WB Saunders.

Rainwater LM, and others: Prostate-specific antigen testing in untreated and treated prostatic adenocarcinoma, *Mayo Clin Proc* 65(8):1118-1126, 1990.

Rakel RE: *Conn's current therapy 1990,* Philadelphia, 1991, WB Saunders.

Rudolphi DM: Duplex scanning, *Am J Nurs* 90(4):123-124, 1990.

Sabiston DC, editor: *Textbook of surgery,* ed 13, Philadelphia, 1986, WB Saunders.

Sakahara H, and others: Serum 19-9 concentrations and computed tomography findings in patients with pancreatic carcinoma, *Cancer* 57(7):1324-1326, 1986.

Serologic testing for antibody to human immunodeficiency virus (update), *MMWR* 36(52):833-840, 1988.

Sher PP: Drug interferences with clinical laboratory tests, *Drugs* 24:25-63, 1982.

Thompson S: Ultrasonography: intraoperative diagnosis of choledocholithiasis, *AORN J* 51(4):983-985, 1990.

Van Dyke JA, and others: Pancreatic imaging, *Ann Intern Med* 102:212, 1985.

Wallach J: *Interpretation of diagnostic tests,* ed 4, Boston, 1986, Little, Brown.

Wilson JD, and others: *Harrison's principles of internal medicine,* ed 12, New York, 1991, McGraw-Hill.

Williford ME, and others: Computed tomography of pleural disease, *Am J Roentgenol* 140:909, 1983.

Wong CA: Preoperative patient preparation, *J Post Anesth Nurs* 5(3):149-156, 1990.

Index of Tests by Body System

Cancer studies
acid phosphatase, 3-4
Bence Jones protein, 90-91
bone scan, 120-122
CA 15-3 tumor marker, 136-137
CA 19-9 tumor marker, 138-139
CA-125 tumor marker, 134-135
carcinoembryonic antigen, 151-152
gallium scan, 360-361
lymphangiography, 497-499
mammography, 504-506
Papanicolaou smear, 539-541
prostate-specific antigen, 590-591
sputum cytology, 685-686
thermography, 704-705

Cardiovascular system
aldosterone assay, blood, 22-25
antistreptolysin O titer, 60-61
arteriography of lower extremities, 65-68
aspartate aminotransferase, 78-80
cardiac catheterization, 153-159
cardiac nuclear scanning, 160-163
carotid duplex scanning, 164-165
catecholamines, 775-778
chest x-ray, 174-176
cholesterol, 190-191
computed tomography of chest, 223-225

Cardiovascular system—cont'd
creatinine phosphokinase, 248-250
cryoglubulin, 251-252
digital subtraction angiography, 272-274
Doppler studies, 278-280
echocardiography, 281-283
electrocardiography, 284-287
electrophysiologic study, 300-302
exercise stress testing, 333-335
Holter monitoring, 414-416
lactic dehydrogenase, 450-452
lipoproteins, 464-466
myoglobin, 518-519
pericardiocentesis, 555-557
plethysmography
arterial, 566-567
venous, 568-569
positron emission tomography, 575-577
renin assay
plasma, 638-640
renal vein, 641-643
triglycerides, 736-737
vanillylmandelic acid, 775-778
venography of lower extremities, 779-781

Endocrine system
adrenal angiography, 5-7
adrenal venography, 8-10
adrenocorticotropic hormone, 11-12
stimulation test, 13-14
aldosterone assay, blood, 22-25

Tests in this list are grouped by the following body systems: cancer, cardiovascular, endocrine, gastrointestinal, hematologic, hepatobiliary, immunologic, miscellaneous studies, nervous, pulmonary, reproductive, skeletal, and urologic.

Endocrine system—cont'd
antidiuretic hormone, 51-53
antithyroglobulin antibody,
62-63
antithyroid microsomal
antibody, 64
blood glucose, 379-381
calcium
blood, 140-142
urine, 143-144
catecholamines, 775-778
computed tomography of
adrenals, 217-219
cortisol
blood, 237-238
urine, 239-240
cortisone administration test,
241-242
dexamethasone suppression
test, 268-271
estriol excretion, 325-327
gastrin, 372-373
glucose tolerance test,
388-390
glycosylated hemoglobin,
391-392
17-hydroxycorticosteroids,
419-421
insulin assay, 430-431
ketones, 441-442
17-ketosteroids, 443-445
long-acting thyroid stimulator,
474-475
luteinizing hormone assay,
493-494
metyrapone, 509-510
osmolality, blood, 533-534
parathyroid hormone,
542-543
phosphorus, 561-562
postprandial glucose, 382-383
radioactive iodine uptake,
612-614
renin assay
plasma, 638-640
renal vein, 641-643
sella turcica x-ray, 658
thyroid scanning, 713-715
thyroid ultrasound, 720-721

Endocrine system—cont'd
thyroid-stimulating hormone,
716-717
stimulation test, 718-719
thyrotropin-releasing hormone
test, 722-723
thyroxine, 724-726
free, index of, 727-728
triiodothyronine, 738-739
uptake test, 740-741
tubular phosphate
reabsorption, 744-745
urine glucose, 384-385
vanillylmandelic acid, 775-778
Gastrointestinal system
barium enema, 81-84
barium swallow, 85-87
carcinoembryonic antigen,
151-152
clostridial toxin assay,
197-198
colonoscopy, 205-207
computed tomography of
abdomen, 213-216
esophageal function studies,
317-320
esophagogastroduodenoscopy,
321-324
fecal fat, 340-342
gastric analysis, 364-367
gastric cytology, 368-369
gastric emptying scan,
370-371
gastrin, 372-373
gastroesophageal reflux scan,
374-375
gastrointestinal bleeding scan,
376-378
5-hydroxyindoleacetic acid,
422-423
lactose tolerance test, 453-454
laparoscopy, 455-457
obstruction series, 527-529
protein, blood, 592-594
Schilling test, 653-655
sialography, 661-662
sigmoidoscopy, 665-667
small bowel follow-through,
672-675
stool culture, 687-688

Gastrointestinal system—cont'd
  stool for occult blood testing,
    689-691
  upper gastrointestinal x-ray
    study, 746-748
  urea nitrogen blood test,
    749-751
  D-xylose absorption test,
    796-798
Hematologic system
  bleeding time, 98-100
  blood smear, 109-111
  blood typing, 112-114
  bone marrow biopsy, 115-119
  clot retraction test, 199-201
  coagulating factors
    concentration, 202-204
  complete blood count and
    differential count, 212
  Coombs' test
    direct, 233-234
    indirect, 235-236
  delta-aminolevulinic acid,
    266-267
  disseminated intravascular
    coagulation screening,
    275-277
  euglobulin lysis time, 328-329
  ferritin, 343-344
  fibrin degradation products,
    349-350
  folic acid, 354-355
  glucose-6-phosphate
    dehydrogenase, 386-387
  haptoglobin, 398-399
  hematocrit, 400-401
  hemoglobin, 402-403
    electrophoresis, 404-406
  iron level and total
    iron-binding capacity,
    437-440
  partial thromboplastin time,
    activated, 544-546
  platelet count, 563-565
  porphyrins and
    porphobilinogens,
    573-574
  prothrombin time, 600-603
  red blood cell count, 617-619

Hematologic system—cont'd
  red blood cell indices,
    620-623
  red blood cell survival study,
    624-626
  red blood cells and casts,
    615-616
  reticulocyte count, 644-645
  sickle cell test, 663-664
  white blood cell count and
    differential count,
    787-791
Hepatobiliary system
  alanine aminotransferase,
    18-19
  aldolase, 20-21
  alkaline phosphatase, 26-27
  alpha-fetoprotein, 30-31
  ammonia level, 32-33
  amylase
    blood, 43-44
    urine, 45-46
  aspartate aminotransferase,
    78-80
  bilirubin
    blood, 92-94
    urine, 95-97
  CA 19-9 tumor marker,
    138-139
  cholangiography, 183-185
  cholecystography, 186-189
  cholesterol, 190-191
  computed tomography of
    abdomen, 213-216
  endoscopic retrograde
    cholangiopancreatography,
    305-308
  Epstein-Barr virus, 311-313
  fecal fat, 340-342
  gallbladder scanning, 358-359
  gamma-glutamyl
    transpeptidase, 362-363
  hepatitis virus studies,
    407-409
  lactic dehydrogenase, 450-452
  leucine aminopeptidase,
    458-459
  lipase, 462-463

Hepatobiliary system—cont'd
liver and pancreatobiliary
system ultrasonography,
470-471
liver biopsy, 467-469
liver scanning, 472-473
5'-nucleotidase, 522-523
obstruction series, 527-529
percutaneous transhepatic
cholangiography,
551-554
protein, blood, 592-594
secretin-pancreozymin,
656-657
sweat electrolytes test,
692-694
T-tube and operative
cholangiogram, 697-699
Immunologic system
AIDS serology, 15-17
aldolase, 20-21
antimitochondrial antibody
test, 54-55
antinuclear antibody test,
56-57
anti–smooth muscle antibody
test, 54-55
complement assay, 210-211
cryoglubulin, 251-252
Epstein-Barr virus, 311-313
febrile/cold agglutinins,
338-339
HLA-B27 antigen, 412-413
immunoglobulin
electrophoresis, 427-429
lupus erythematosus test,
491-492
Lyme disease test, 495-496
mononucleosis spot test,
511-512
protein electrophoresis,
597-599
rheumatoid factor, 649-650
Miscellaneous tests
blood culture and sensitivity,
101-103
blood glucose, 379-381
carbon dioxide content,
147-148
carboxyhemoglobin, 149-150
chloride

Miscellaneous tests—cont'd
chloride—cont'd
blood, 179-180
urine, 181-182
erythrocyte sedimentation
rate, 314-316
positron emission
tomography, 575-577
potassium
blood, 578-580
urine, 581-582
protein, blood, 592-594
sialography, 661-662
sodium
blood, 676-678
urine, 679-680
therapeutic drug monitoring,
700-703
throat culture and sensitivity,
711-712
toxicology screening, 730-733
urine culture and sensitivity,
764-766
urine glucose, 384-385
wound culture and sensitivity,
794-795
Nervous system
brain scan, 123-125
caloric study, 145-146
cerebral angiography, 166-168
cisternal puncture, 194-196
computed tomography of
brain, 220-222
digital subtraction
angiography, 272-274
electroencephalography,
288-291
electromyography, 292-294
electroneurography, 295-297
electronystagmography,
298-299
evoked potential studies,
330-332
lumbar puncture and
cerebrospinal fluid
examination, 478-484
magnetic resonance imaging,
500-503
myelography, 513-517
oculoplethysmography,
530-532

Nervous system—cont'd
positron emission
tomography, 575-577
skull x-ray, 670-671
spinal x-rays, 681-682
ventriculography, 782-784
Pulmonary system
acid-fast bacilli, 1-2
alpha$_1$-antitrypsin, 28-29
angiotensin-converting
enzyme, 47-48
blood gases, 104-108
bronchography, 126-128
bronchoscopy, 129-133
carbon dioxide content,
147-148
carboxyhemoglobin, 149-150
chest tomography, 172-173
chest x-ray, 174-176
computed tomography of
chest, 223-225
lung biopsy, 485-487
lung scan, 488-490
mediastinoscopy, 507-508
oximetry, 537-538
pleural biopsy, 570-572
pulmonary angiography,
604-606
pulmonary function tests,
607-611
sputum culture and sensitivity,
683-684
sputum cytology, 685-686
thoracentesis and pleural fluid
analysis, 706-710
tuberculin test, 742-743
urine pH, 771-772
Reproductive system
alpha-fetoprotein, 30-31
amniocentesis, 34-40
amnioscopy, 41-42
antispermatozoal antibody,
58-59
Barr body analysis, 88-89
CA 15-3 tumor marker,
136-137
CA-125 tumor marker,
134-135
cervical mucus test, 169-171
chlamydial smear, 177-178

Reproductive system—cont'd
chorionic villus sampling,
192-193
colposcopy, 208-209
contraction stress test,
229-232
culdoscopy, 254-255
cytomegalovirus, 265
endometrial biopsy, 303-304
estriol excretion, 325-327
fetal scalp blood pH, 345-346
fetoscopy, 347-348
galactose-1-phosphate uridyl
transferase, 356-357
gonorrhea culture, 393-395
herpes genitalis, 410-411
human placental lactogen, 416
hysterosalpingography,
424-426
laparoscopy, 455-457
luteinizing hormone assay,
493-494
mammography, 504-506
nonstress test, 520-521
obstetric ultrasonography,
524-526
Papanicolaou smear, 539-541
pelvimetry, 549-550
phenylketonuria test, 558-560
pregnancy tests, 583-585
pregnanediol, 586-587
progesterone assay, 588-589
rubella antibody test, 651-652
semen analysis, 659-660
Sims-Huhner test, 668-669
syphilis detection test,
695-696
thermography, 704-705
TORCH test, 729
toxoplasmosis antibody titer,
734-735
Skeletal system
aldolase, 20-21
alkaline phosphatase, 26-27
arthrocentesis with synovial
fluid analysis, 69-72
arthrography, 73-74
arthroscopy, 75-77
bone scan, 120-122
electromyography, 292-294

Skeletal system—cont'd
  HLA-B27 antigen, 412-413
  lactic dehydrogenase, 450-452
  long bones x-ray, 476-477
  magnetic resonance imaging,
      500-503
  myoglobin, 518-519
  rheumatoid factor, 649-650
  spinal x-rays, 681-682
  uric acid
      blood, 754-756
      urine, 757-758
Urologic system
  acid phosphatase, 3-4
  aldosterone assay, 22-25
  antegrade pyelography, 49-50
  antidiuretic hormone, 51-53
  antistreptolysin O titer, 60-61
  bilirubin, urine, 95-97
  carbon dioxide content,
      147-148
  catecholamines, 775-778
  chloride
      blood, 179-180
      urine, 181-182
  computed tomography of
      kidney, 226-228
  creatinine, blood, 243-244
  creatinine clearance, 245-247
  crystals, 253
  cystography, 256-257
  cystometry, 258-260
  cystoscopy, 261-264
  epithelial casts, 309-310
  fatty casts, 336-337
  granular casts, 396-397
  hyaline casts, 417-418
  intravenous pyelogram,
      432-436
  ketones, 441-442
  kidney, ureter, and bladder
      x-ray study, 448-449
  kidney sonogram, 446-447
  leukocyte esterase, 460-461

Urologic system—cont'd
  osmolality
      blood, 533-534
      urine, 535-536
  pelvic floor sphincter
      electromyography,
      547-548
  potassium
      blood, 578-580
      urine, 581-582
  prostate-specific antigen,
      590-591
  protein, urine, 595-596
  renal angiography, 627-630
  renal biopsy, 631-633
  renal scanning, 634-637
  renin assay
      plasma, 638-640
      renal vein, 641-643
  retrograde pyelography,
      646-648
  sodium
      blood, 676-678
      urine, 679-680
  urea nitrogen blood test,
      749-751
  urethral pressure profile,
      752-753
  uric acid
      blood, 754-756
      urine, 757-758
  urinalysis, 759
  urine appearance and color,
      760-763
  urine culture and sensitivity,
      764-766
  urine flow studies, 767-768
  urine odor, 769-770
  urine pH, 771-772
  urine specific gravity, 773-774
  vanillylmandelic acid, 775-778
  waxy casts, 785-786
  white blood cells and casts,
      792-793

Index of Tests by Type

Blood tests
  acid phosphatase, 3-4
  adrenocorticotropic hormone,
    11-12
    stimulation test, 13-14
  AIDS serology, 15-17
  alanine aminotransferase,
    18-19
  aldolase, 20-21
  aldosterone assay, 22-25
  alkaline phosphatase, 26-27
  alpha$_1$-antitrypsin, 28-29
  alpha-fetoprotein, 30-31
  ammonia level, 32-33
  amylase, 43-44
  angiotensin-converting
    enzyme, 47-48
  antidiuretic hormone, 51-53
  antimitochondrial antibody
    and anti–smooth muscle
    tests, 54-55
  antinuclear antibody test,
    56-57
  antispermatozoal antibody,
    58-59
  antistreptolysin O titer, 60-61
  antithyroglobulin antibody,
    62-63
  antithyroid microsomal
    antibody, 64
  aspartate aminotransferase,
    78-80
  bilirubin, 92-94
  bleeding time, 98-100
  blood culture and sensitivity,
    101-103
  blood gases, 104-108

Blood tests—cont'd
  blood smear, 109-111
  blood typing, 112-114
  CA-125 tumor marker,
    134-135
  CA-15-3 tumor marker,
    136-137
  CA-19-9 tumor marker,
    138-139
  calcium, 140-142
  carbon dioxide content,
    147-148
  carboxyhemoglobin, 149-150
  carcinoembryonic antigen,
    151-152
  chloride, 179-180
  cholesterol, 190-191
  clot retraction test, 199-201
  coagulating factors
    concentration, 202-204
  complement assay, 210-211
  complete blood count and
    differential count, 212
  Coombs' test
    direct, 233-234
    indirect, 235-236
  cortisol, 237-238
  cortisone administration test,
    241-242
  creatinine, 243-244
  creatinine clearance, 245-247
  creatinine phosphokinase,
    248-250
  cryoglobulin, 251-252
  cytomegalovirus, 265
  dexamethasone suppression
    test, 268-271

index of tests by type

Tests in this list are grouped by the following types of test: blood, electrodiagnostic, endoscopy, fluid analysis, manometric, microscopic examination, nuclear scan, other studies, sputum, stool, ultrasound, urine, and x-ray.

Blood tests—cont'd
  disseminated intravascular
    coagulation screening,
    275-277
  Epstein-Barr virus titer,
    311-313
  erythrocyte sedimentation
    rate, 314-316
  estriol excretion, 325-327
  euglobulin lysis time, 328-329
  febril/cold agglutinins,
    338-339
  ferritin, 343-344
  fetal scalp blood pH, 345-346
  fibrin degradation products,
    349-350
  folic acid, 354-355
  galactose-1-phosphate uridyl
    transferase, 356-357
  gamma-glutamyl
    transpeptidase, 362-363
  gastrin, 372-373
  glucose, 379-381
    postprandial, 382-383
  glucose tolerance test,
    388-390
  glucose-6-phosphate
    dehydrogenase, 386-387
  glycosylated hemoglobin,
    391-392
  haptoglobulin, 398-399
  hematocrit, 400-401
  hemoglobulin, 402-403
    electrophoresis, 404-406
  hepatitis virus studies,
    407-409
  HLA-B27 antigen, 412-413
  human placental lactogen, 416
  immunoglobulin
    electrophoresis, 427-429
  insulin assay, 430-431
  iron level and total
    iron-binding capacity,
    437-440
  lactic dehydrogenase, 450-452
  lactose tolerance test, 453-454
  leucine aminopeptidase,
    458-459
  lipase, 462-463
  lipoproteins, 464-466
  long-acting thyroid stimulator,
    474-475

Blood tests—cont'd
  lupus erythematosus test,
    491-492
  luteinizing hormone assay,
    493-494
  Lyme disease test, 495-496
  metyrapone, 509-510
  mononucleosis spot test,
    511-512
  myoglobin, 518-519
  5′-nucleotidase, 522-523
  osmolality, 533-534
  parathyroid hormone,
    542-543
  partial thromboplastin time,
    activated, 544-546
  phenylketonuria test, 558-560
  phosphorus, 561-562
  platelet count, 563-565
  potassium, 578-580
  pregnancy, 583-585
  progesterone assay, 588-589
  prostate-specific antigen,
    590-591
  protein, 592-594
    electrophoresis, 597-599
  prothrombin time, 600-603
  red blood cell count, 617-619
  red blood cell indices,
    620-623
  renin assay
    plasma, 638-640
    renal vein, 641-643
  reticulocyte count, 644-645
  rheumatoid factor, 649-650
  rubella antibody test, 651-652
  sickle cell test, 663-664
  sodium, 676-678
  syphilis detection test,
    695-696
  therapeutic drug monitoring,
    700-703
  thyroid-stimulating hormone,
    716-719
    stimulation test, 718-719
  thyrotropin-releasing hormone
    test, 722-723
  thyroxine, 724-726
    free, index of, 727-728
  toxicology screening, 730-733

Blood tests—cont'd
  toxoplasmosis antibody titer, 734-735
  triglycerides, 736-737
  triiodothyronine, 738-739
    uptake test, 740-741
  tubular phosphate reabsorption, 744-745
  urea nitrogen blood test, 749-751
  uric acid, 754-756
  white blood cell count and differential count, 787-791
  D-xylose absorption test, 796-798
Electrodiagnostic tests
  caloric study, 145-146
  electrocardiography, 284-287
  electroencephalography, 288-291
  electromyography, 292-294
  electroneurography, 295-297
  electronystagmography, 298-299
  electrophysiologic study, 300-302
  evoked potential studies, 330-332
  exercise stress testing, 333-335
  Holter monitoring, 414-416
  pelvic floor sphincter electromyography, 547-548
Endoscopy
  amnioscopy, 41-42
  arthroscopy, 75-77
  bronchoscopy, 129-133
  colonoscopy, 205-207
  culdoscopy, 254-255
  cystoscopy, 261-264
  endoscopic retrograde cholangiopancreatography, 305-308
  esophagogastroduodenoscopy, 321-324
  fetoscopy, 347-348
  laparoscopy, 455-457
  mediastinoscopy, 507-508

Endoscopy—cont'd
  sigmoidoscopy, 665-667
Fluid analysis
  amniocentesis, 34-40
  antispermatozoal antibody, 58-59
  arthrocentesis with synovial fluid analysis, 69-72
  cervical mucus test, 169-171
  cisternal puncture, 194-196
  gastric analysis, 364-367
  lumbar puncture and cerebrospinal fluid examination, 478-484
  pericardiocentesis, 555-557
  secretin-pancreozymin, 656-657
  semen analysis, 659-660
  Sims-Huhner test, 668-669
  sweat electrolytes test, 692-694
  thoracentesis and pleural fluid analysis, 706-710
Manometric tests
  contraction stress test, 229-232
  cystometry, 258-260
  esophageal function studies, 317-320
  oculoplethysmography, 530-532
  plethysmography
    arterial, 566-567
    venous, 568-569
  urethral pressure profile, 752-753
Microscopic examinations
  Barr body analysis, 88-89
  bone marrow biopsy, 115-119
  chlamydial smear, 177-178
  endometrial biopsy, 303-304
  gastric cytology, 368-369
  gonorrhea culture, 393-395
  herpes genitalis, 410-411
  liver biopsy, 467-469
  lung biopsy, 485-487
  Papanicolaou smear, 539-541
  pleural biopsy, 570-572
  renal biopsy, 631-633
  throat culture and sensitivity, 711-712

Microscopic examinations—
  cont'd
  wound culture and sensitivity,
    794-795
Nuclear scans
  bone scan, 120-122
  brain scan, 123-125
  cardiac nuclear scanning,
    160-163
  fibrinogen uptake test with
    125I, 351-353
  gallbladder scanning, 358-359
  gallium scan, 360-361
  gastric emptying scan,
    370-371
  gastroesophageal reflux scan,
    374-375
  gastrointestinal bleeding scan,
    376-378
  liver scanning, 472-473
  lung scan, 488-490
  positron-emission
    tomography, 575-577
  radioactive iodine uptake,
    612-614
  red blood cell survival study,
    624-626
  renal scanning, 634-637
  thyroid scanning, 713-715
Other studies
  chorionic villus sampling,
    192-193
  colposcopy, 208-209
  magnetic resonance imaging,
    500-503
  nonstress test, 520-521
  oximetry, 537-538
  pulmonary function tests,
    607-611
  tuberculin test, 742-743
Sputum tests
  acid-fast bacilli, 1-2
  culture and sensitivity,
    683-684
  cytology, 685-686
Stool tests
  clostridial toxin assay,
    197-198
  culture, 687-688
  fecal fat, 340-342

Stool tests—cont'd
  for occult blood testing,
    689-691
Ultrasound tests
  carotid duplex scanning,
    164-165
  Doppler studies, 278-280
  echocardiography, 281-283
  kidney sonogram, 446-447
  liver and pancreatobiliary
    system ultrasonography,
    470-471
  obstetric ultrasonography,
    524-526
  thyroid ultrasound, 720-721
Urine tests
  aldosterone assay, 22-25
  amylase, 45-46
  appearance and color,
    760-763
  Bence Jones protein, 90-91
  bilirubin, 95-97
  calcium, 143-144
  chloride, 181-182
  cortisol, 239-240
  creatinine clearance, 245-247
  crystals, 253
  culture and sensitivity,
    764-766
  delta-aminolevulinic acid,
    266-267
  dexamethasone suppression
    test, 268-271
  epithelial tests, 309-310
  estriol excretion, 325-327
  fatty casts, 336-337
  flow of, studies, 767-768
  glucose, 384-385
  glucose tolerance test,
    388-390
  granular casts, 396-397
  hyaline casts, 417-418
  17-hydroxycorticosteroids,
    419-421
  5-hydroxyindoleacetic acid,
    422-423
  ketones, 441-442
  17-ketosteroids, 443-445
  leucine aminopeptidase,
    458-459

Urine tests—cont'd
  leukocyte esterase, 460-461
  metyrapone, 509-510
  odor, 769-770
  osmolality, 535-536
  pH, 771-772
  phenylketonuria test, 558-560
  porphyrins and
      porphobilinogens,
      573-574
  potassium, 581-582
  pregnancy, 583-585
  pregnanediol, 586-587
  protein, 595-596
  red blood cells and casts,
      615-616
  Schilling test, 653-655
  sodium, 679-680
  specific gravity, 773-774
  toxicology screening, 730-733
  tubular phosphate
      reabsorption, 744-745
  uric acid, 757-758
  urinalysis, 759
  vanillylmandelic acid and
      catecholamines, 775-778
  waxy casts, 785-786
  white blood cells and casts,
      792-793
  D-xylose absorption test,
      796-798
X-ray examinations
  adrenal angiography, 5-7
  adrenal venography, 8-10
  antegrade pyelography, 49-50
  arteriography of lower
      extremities, 65-68
  arthrography, 73-74
  barium enema, 81-84
  barium swallow, 85-87
  bronchography, 126-128
  cardiac catheterization, 153-159
  cerebral angiography, 166-168
  chest tomography, 172-173
  chest x-ray, 174-176
  cholangiography, 183-185
  cholecystography, 186-189

X-ray examinations—cont'd
  computed tomography
    of abdomen, 213-216
    of adrenals, 217-219
    of brain, 220-222
    of chest, 223-225
    of kidney, 226-228
  cystography, 256-257
  digital subtraction
      angiography, 272-274
  hysterosalpingography,
      424-426
  intravenous pyelogram,
      432-436
  kidney, ureter, and bladder
      x-ray study, 448-449
  long bones x-ray, 476-477
  lymphangiography, 497-499
  magnetic resonance imaging,
      500-503
  mammography, 504-506
  myelography, 513-517
  obstruction series, 527-529
  pelvimetry, 549-550
  percutaneous transhepatic
      cholangiography,
      551-554
  positron-emission
      tomography, 575-577
  pulmonary angiography,
      604-606
  renal angiography, 627-630
  retrograde pyelography,
      646-648
  sella turcica x-ray, 658
  sialography, 661-662
  skull x-ray, 670-671
  small bowel follow-through,
      672-675
  spinal x-rays, 681-682
  thermography, 704-705
  T-tube and operative
      cholangiogram, 697-699
  upper gastrointestinal x-ray
      study, 746-748
  venography of lower
      extremities, 779-781
  ventriculography, 782-784

Comprehensive Index

A

Abdomen
  computed tomography of, 213-216
  plain film of, 527-529
Abdominal abscess, 527
Abdominal aorta
  on computed tomography of abdomen, 213
  calcification of, 528
Abdominal scintigraphy, 376-378
ABO typing, 113
Abortion, threatened, 416
Abruptio placentae, 524
Abscess, pancreatic and hepatic, 470
Accelerated erythrocyte hemolysis, 93
Acetaminophen
  therapeutic, monitoring of, 702t
  in toxicology screening, 732t
Acetones, urine, 441-442
Achalasia, 317
Acid clearing, 318
Acid phosphatase, 3-4
Acid reflux with pH probe, 317-318
Acid-base balance, 181, 533, 578
Acidemia, 771
Acid-fast bacilli, 1-2
Acid-fast stains for tubercle bacilli on synovial fluid, 70
Acidosis, 581
  metabolic, 105, 106t, 107t
  respiratory, 105, 106t, 107t
Acquired immunodeficiency serology, 15-17

Acquired immunohemolytic anemia, 109
ACTA suppression test, 268-271
ACTH, 11-12, 22, 268, 419, 658
  stimulation of, 13-14, 237, 239
Activated partial thromboplastin time (APTT), 544-546
Acute demyelinating polyneuropathy, 478
Addison's disease, 6, 11, 13, 217, 237, 419, 443
Adrenal adenoma, 269, 509
Adrenal angiography, 5-7
Adrenal arteriography, 5-7
Adrenal cortex, tumor of, 22
Adrenal gland
  computed tomography of, 217-219
  hyperfunction of, 268, 419
  tumors of, 5, 13
Adrenal hyperplasia, 5, 8, 13, 22, 419, 509
Adrenal insufficiency, 6, 11, 13, 217, 237, 419, 443
Adrenal suppression, 419
Adrenal venography, 8-10
Adrenocortical dysfunction, 443
AFP, 30-31, 37
Agglutination of red blood cells, 233
Agglutination inhibition test (AIT), 583
Agglutinins, cold and febrile, 338-339
Agranulocytosis, 115
AIDS
  high risk for, 15
  serology, 15-17

Page numbers designated *i* refer to illustrations; those designated *t* refer to tables.

Air-contrast barium enema, 81
Air-contrast myelography, 514
ALA, 266-267
Alanine aminotransferase (ALT), 18-19
Albumin, 597
  blood, 592-594
  urine, 595-596
Alcohol
  detection of ingestion of, 362
  in toxicology screening, 732t
Alcoholic, nutritional status of, 354
Alcoholic cirrhosis, 47, 78
Aldolase, 20-21
Aldosterone, 578, 676
  assay of, 22-25
Aldosteronism, primary, 22
Alkalemia, 771
Alkaline phosphatase (ALP), 26-27
Alkalosis, 581
  metabolic, 105, 106t, 107t
  respiratory, 105, 106t, 107t
Allen test, 107
Alpha globulins, 597
Alpha₁ antitrypsin test (A1AT, ATT), 28-29
Alpha-fetoprotein (AFP), 30-31, 37
ALT, 18-196
Ambulatory electrocardiography, 414-416
Ambulatory monitoring, 414-416
Amenorrhea, 88
Amikacin, therapeutic, monitoring of, 702t
Aminolevulinic acid (ALA), 266-267
Aminophylline, therapeutic, monitoring of, 702t
Amitriptyline, therapeutic, monitoring of, 702t
Ammonia level, 32-33
Amniocentesis, 34-40, 39i
  timing of, 37
Amnioscopy, 41-42
Amniotic fluid, 113
  analysis of, 34-40

Amniotic fluid—cont'd
  embolism of, 275
  meconium staining of, 34, 41
Amobarbital in toxicology screening, 732t
Amphetamine in toxicology screening, 731t
Amylase
  blood, 43-44
  pleural fluid, 707
  urine, 45-46
Amylase/creatinine clearance ratio, 45
Amyloidosis, 90-91, 467, 472
ANA, 56-57
  in pleural fluid, 708
Anemia, 109, 199, 343, 354
  aplastic, 116
  hemolytic, 79, 110, 113, 115, 233, 276, 343, 354, 405, 624
  hemorrhagic, 115
  iron deficiency, 115, 437-438
  megaloblastic, 110, 343, 354
  and red blood cell indexes, 621t
  sickle cell, 109, 404-405, 663, 664
    maternal, 416
Anencephaly, 30, 34
Aneurysm
  arterial, 65
  cerebral, 166
  ventricular, 153
Angina, 78
Angiocardiography, 153-159
Angiography, 65-68
  adrenal, 5-7
  bronchial, 604-606
  cerebral, 166-168
  coronary, 153-159
  digital subtraction, 272-274
  pulmonary, 604-606
  renal, 627-630
Angioplasty
  balloon, 153, 156
  transluminal coronary, 156
Angiotensin-converting enzyme (ACE), 47-48
Anisocytosis, 109

Ankylosing spondylitis, 412
Anomalous venous return, 153
Anoscopy, 665-667
Antegrade pyelography, 49-50
Antibiotic-associated colitis
  assay, 197-198
Antibody(ies), 592
  antimitochondrial, 54-55
  antinuclear, 56-57
    in pleural fluid, 708
  antismooth muscle, 54-55
  antispermatozoal, 58-59
  antithyroglobulin, 62-63
  antithyroid microsomal, 64
  blood typing, 112
  circulating, 427
  hepatitis, 407-408
  to human immunodeficiency
    virus, 15
  rubella, 651-652
  toxoplasmosis, 734-735
  to *Treponema pallidum,* 695
Antideoxyribonuclease B
    (antiDNase B), 60
Antidiuretic hormone (ADH),
    51-53, 676
Antigen(s)
  blood typing, 112
  carcinoembryonic, 151-152
    in pleural fluid, 707
  Epstein-Barr nuclear, 311
  hepatitis, 407-409
  HLA-B27, 412-413
  prostate-specific, 590-591
Antigen-antibody complexes,
    210
Antihemophilic factor, 202
Antiinflammatory drugs, 98
Antimicrosomal antibody, 64
Antimitochondrial antibody
    (AMA) test, 54-55
Antinuclear antibody (ANA),
    56-57
  in pleural fluid, 708
Antismooth muscle antibody
    (ASMA) test, 54-55
Antisperm antibodies, 58-59
Antispermatozoal antibody,
    58-59

Antistreptolysin O titer (ASO
    titer), 60-61
Antithyroglobulin antibody,
    62-63
Antithyroid microsomal
    antibody, 64
Aortic artery pressure, 154*t*
Aplastic anemia, 116
Appearance
  pleural fluid, 706
  urine, 760-761, 762*t*-763*t*
Appendicitis, 81, 527
Arborization of cervical mucus,
    169
Argentaffin (enteroendocrine)
    cells, 422
Arrhythmias, cardiac, 285, 300,
    414
Arterial blood gases, 104-108
Arterial Doppler studies, 278
Arterial oxygen saturation
    (SaO$_2$), 537
Arterial plethysmography,
    566-567
Arterial trauma, 65
Arteriography
  adrenal, 5-7
  cerebral, 166-168
  coronary, 156
  of gastric bleeding site, 376
  of lower extremities, 65-68
  pulmonary, 604-606
  renal, 627-630
Arteriosclerotic heart disease,
    464
  cholesterol in, 190
Arteriosclerotic occlusive disease,
    65, 278
Arteriovenous (AV)
    malformation, 123-124,
    166, 205, 220
Arthritis, 120, 476, 495
  crystal-induced, 69
  rheumatoid, 26, 70, 251, 649
  septic, 69
Arthrocentesis with synovial
    fluid analysis, 69-72
Arthrogram, 73-74
Arthrography, 73-74
Arthroscopy, 75-77

Ascaris, 687
Aspartate aminotransferase
    (AST), 78-80
Aspermia, 659
Aspiration scan, 374-375
AST, 78-80
Atelectasis, 35
Atherosclerosis, renal artery, 245
Atherosclerotic occlusive
    coronary artery disease,
    153
Atherosclerotic thrombi, 65
Auditory brainstem evoked
    potentials (ABEPs),
    330-331
Australia antigen, 407-409
Autoantibodies against red
    blood cells, 233
Autoimmune diseases, 56, 210,
    427
    of central nervous system, 478
    inflammatory, 314

B

Bacilli, acid-fast, 1-2
Bacteremia, 101
Bacteria in stool, 687
Bacterial endocarditis, 60
Bacterial infectious arthritis, 70
Bacteroides, 687
Balloon angioplasty, 153, 156
Band cells, 788
Barium, 746
Barium enema (BE), 81-84
Barium swallow, 85-87
Barr body analysis, 88-89
Basophil count, 787-791
    causes of abnormalities in,
    791*t*
Basophilic stippling, 110
Bence Jones protein, 90-91
Beriberi, 79
Bernstein test, 318
Beta globulins, 597
Beutler fluorometric test, 356
Bilateral adrenal hyperplasia, 5,
    8, 13, 22, 269
Bile duct(s)
    autoimmune disease of, 54
    obstruction of, 305, 340

Bile duct(s)—cont'd
    patency of, 183
Biliary and pancreatic ducts,
    ERCP of, 305-308
Biliary calculi, 186
Biliary ducts, 551
Biliary tract radionuclide scan,
    358-359
Bilirubin
    amniotic fluid, 36
    blood, 92-94
    and fetal hemoglobin, 34
    urine, 95-97
Biologic pregnancy tests, 583
Biopsy
    bone marrow, 115-119
    colonoscopy, 205
    cone, 208
    endometrial, 303-304
    fetal skin, 347
    liver, 467-469
    lung, 485-487
    percutaneous liver, 467
    pleural, 570-572
    renal, 631-633
Bladder
    function of, 258
    on x-ray films, 256
Bleeding scan, gastrointestinal,
    376-378
Bleeding time, 98-100
Bleeding ulcer, 110
Blocked efferent ducts in testes,
    58
Blood in cerebrospinal fluid,
    479
Blood amylase, 43-44
Blood antibody screening,
    235-236
Blood bilirubin, 92-94
Blood calcium, 140-142
Blood cell abnormalities, 79
Blood chloride, 179-180
Blood clotting factors, 202-204
Blood components in fibrin
    production, 200*t*
Blood cortisol, 237-238
Blood creatinine, 243-244
Blood culture and sensitivity,
    101-103

Blood gases, 104-108
Blood groups, 112*t*
Blood indices, 620-623
Blood smear, 109-111
Blood sugar, 379-381
Blood transfusion
  hepatitis from, 409
  reaction to, 233, 235, 275
Blood typing, 112-114
Blood urea nitrogen, 749-751
Blood-brain barrier, disruption
  of, 123
Bone
  alkaline phosphatase in, 26
  necrosis of, 120
  tumor metastases to, 90, 542
Bone marrow
  aspiration of, 115-119
  biopsy of, 115-119
  examination of, 115-119
  failure of, 563
Bone scan, 120-122
Bordetella pertussis, 711
Bowel
  on computed tomography of
    abdomen, 213
  perforation of, 43, 45
Brachial artery in cardiac
  catheterization, 156
Brachial vein in cardiac
  catheterization, 156
Brain
  computed tomography of,
    220-222
  electrical activity of, 288
  neoplasm of, 478
Brain potentials, evoked,
  330-332
Brain scan, 123-125
Brainstem, abnormalities of, 145
Breakdown, fibrin, products of,
  349-350
Breast
  cancer of, 504, 704
    CA 15-3 tumor marker in,
      136
    carcinoembryonic antigen
      in, 151
  fibrocystic disease of, 704
  mammography of, 504-506

Breast—cont'd
  thermography of, 704-705
Breast stimulation technique,
  232
Bronchi, obstruction in, 126
Bronchial angiography, 604-606
Bronchial washings, collection
  of, 130
Bronchitis, chronic, 28
Bronchogram, 126-128
Bronchography, 126-128
Bronchoscopy, 129-133
  insertion of bronchoscope in,
    132*i*
Bruits, cardiac, 530
Buerger's disease, 65
Bulbocavernous reflex, 547
BUN, 749-751
Burkitt's lymphoma, 511
Burns, 79, 275
Butabarbital in toxicology
  screening, 732*t*

C

Ca^{++}, 140-142
CA 15-3 tumor marker,
  136-137
CA 19-9 tumor marker,
  138-139
CA-125 tumor marker, 134-135
Calcium
  blood, 140-142
  urine, 143-144
Calculi; *see also* Gallstones
  biliary, 186
  renal or pelvic, 446
    and hyperuricosuria, 757
Caloric study, 145-146
Campylobacter, 687
Cancer
  breast, 504, 704
    CA 15-3 tumor marker in,
      136
    carcinoembryonic antigen
      in, 151
    epithelial ovarian, 134
    metastatic, 343
    prostatic, 590
Candida albicans, 687

Carbamazepine, therapeutic, monitoring of, 702t
Carbon dioxide content, 147-148
Carbon monoxide, 149-150
  in toxicology screening, 732t
Carboxyhemoglobin, 149-150
  in toxicology screening, 732t
Carcinoembryonic antigen (CEA), 151-152
  in pleural fluid, 707
Carcinoid syndrome, 422
Carcinoid tumors, 422
Carcinoma, 507
  adrenal, 509
  carcinoembryonic antigen in, 151
  cervical, 539
  hepatic, 266
  in situ, 208
  intestinal, 52
  lung, 52, 485
  pancreas, 52
  urologic tract, 52
Cardiac bruits, 530
Cardiac catheterization, 153-159
Cardiac echo and heart sonogram, 281-283
Cardiac index (CI), 155t
Cardiac mapping, 300-302
Cardiac muscle function, 153
Cardiac nuclear scanning, 160-163
Cardiac output (CO), 155t
Cardiac scan, 160-163
Cardiac tamponade, 555
Carotid duplex scanning, 164-165
Carotid endarterectomy, 288
Casts
  epithelial, 309-310
  fatty, 336-337
  granular, 396-397
  hyaline, 417-418
  and red blood cells, 615-616
  waxy, 785-786
  and white blood cells, 792-793
CAT scan; *see also* CT scan
  of abdomen, 213-216

Catecholamines, 8
  and vanillylmandelic acid, 775-778
Catheterization, cardiac, 153-159
CEA, 151-152
  pleural fluid, 707
Celiac disease, 354
Cell counts in pleural fluid, 706
Cells
  in cerebrospinal fluid, 479
  cervical, classification of, 539
Central nervous system, autoimmune diseases involving, 478
Central venous pressure (CVP), 154t
Cephalopelvic disproportion (CPD), 549
Cerebellum, abnormalities of, 145
Cerebral angiography, 166-168, 272
Cerebral arteriography, 166-168
Cerebral blood flow, 123-125
Cerebral hemorrhage, 478
Cerebral infarction, 123
Cerebrospinal fluid (CSF), 124
  analysis of, 478-484
Cerebrovascular accident (CVA), 123
Cervical carcinoma, 539
Cervical culture, 177
  gonorrhea, 393
Cervical intraepithelial neoplasia (CIN), 539-540
Cervical mucus, 169-171, 668
  sperm penetration test, 668-669
Cervical x-rays, 681-682
Chalasia, 317
Chemotherapy, 115
Chest
  computed tomography of, 223-225
  radiography of, 174-176
  tomography of, 172-173
  x-ray of, 174-176
Chest leads, EKG, 284, 285 286-287

Chlamydial smear, 177-178
Chloramphenicol, therapeutic, monitoring of, 702*t*
Chloride
 blood, 179-180
 cerebrospinal fluid, 480
 urine, 181-182
Cholangiogram, T-tube and operative, 697-699
Cholangiography, 183-185
 percutaneous transhepatic, 551-554, 552*i*
Cholangiopancreatography, endoscopic retrograde, 305-308
Cholecystitis, 358
Cholecystography, 186-189
Cholescintigraphy, 358-359
Cholestasis, 362, 458, 522
Cholesterol, 190-191, 464
 in pleural fluid, 708
Choriocarcinoma of uterus, testes, or ovaries, 584
Chorionic somatomammotropin, human, 416
Chorionic villus biopsy (CVB), 192-193
Chorionic villus sampling (CVS), 192-193
Christmas factor, 202
Chromatin-positive body, 88-89
Chromosomal aberrations, 34
Chronic hepatitis, 20
Chronic lymphocytic leukemia, 90
Chronic myeloid leukemia, 116
Chylomicrons, 464
CIN, 539-540
Circulating antibodies, 427
Cirrhosis, 20, 26, 54, 151, 251, 275, 472
 alcoholic, 47, 78
  CA 19-9 tumor marker in, 138
Cisternal puncture, 194-196
Cisternal scan, 123-125
Clearance, creatinine, 245-247
Closed technique lung biopsy, 485
Clostridial enterocolitis, 197

Clostridial toxin assay, 197-198
Clostridium, 687
Clostridium difficile, 197-198
Clot retraction test, 199-200
Clotting factors, 544, 600-603
Cloudy urine, 760
CMV, 265, 729
CO_2 combining content, 147-148
CO_2 content, 147-148
Coagulating factors, 202-204
 concentration of, 202-204
 conditions resulting in, 204*t*
 in fibrin production, 200*t*
Coagulopathy, consumptive, 544
Coccygeal x-rays, 681-682
Coefficient, fat retention, 341
COHb, 149-150
Cold agglutinins, 338-339
Colitis
 pseudomembranous, 197
 ulcerative, 151
Collagen vascular disease, 98, 593
Colon cancer, 135
Colonoscopy, 205-207
Color
 cerebrospinal fluid, 479
 urine, 760-761, 762*t*-763*t*
Color Doppler echocardiography, 281-282
Colorectal cancer, 151
Colposcopy, 208-209
Coma, 533
 hepatic, 32
Combined one-stage and two-stage Schilling test, 654-655
Complement assay, 210-211
Complete blood count, 212
Computed tomography
 of abdomen, 213-216
 of adrenals, 217-219
 of brain, 220-222
 of chest, 223-225
 of kidney, 226-228
 single-photon emission, 162

Computerized axial transverse tomography (CATT), 220-222
Conduction defects, 285
Conduction velocity, 295
Cone biopsy, 208
Congenital adrenal hyperplasia, 443
Congenital enzyme deficiency, 419
Congenital heart defects, 153
Congenital herpes infection, 410
Congenital infections, cytomegalovirus, 265
Congenital toxoplasmosis, 734
Conjugated bilirubin, 92, 95
Conn's syndrome, 22
Consumptive coagulopathy, 544
Contraction stress test (CST), 229-232
Contrast material in myelography, 513
Coombs' test
  direct, 233-234
  indirect, 235-236
Coronary angiography, 153-159
Coronary arteriogram, 156
Coronary artery disease, atherosclerotic occlusive, 153
Corticotropin, 11-12
Cortisol
  blood, 237-238
  metabolites of, 419
  plasma, 268
  precursors of, 509
  suppression test, 268-271
  urine, 239-240
Cortisone administration test, 241-242
Corynebacterium diphtheriae, 711
Cosyntropin test, 13-14
Coumarin ingestion, 601
Cranial nerve, eighth, 145
Creatinine
  amniotic fluid, 36
  blood, 243-244
  clearance of, 245-247
Creatinine kinase (CK), 248-250

Creatinine phosphokinase (CPK, CP), 248-250
Crohn's disease, 81, 340
Cross-matching blood, 113
Cryoglobulin, 251-252
Crystal-induced arthritis, 69
Crystals, urinary, 253
C&S
  blood, 101-103
  cerebrospinal fluid, 479
  handling of specimens for, 101
  sputum, 683-684
  stool, 687-688
  throat, 711-712
  urine, 764-766
  wound, 794-795
CT scan
  of abdomen, 213-216
  of adrenals, 217-219
  of brain, 220-222
  of chest, 223-225
  of kidney, 226-228
Cuff pressure test, 568-569
Culdoscopy, 254-255
Culture
  chlamydial, 177
  gonorrhea, 393-395
  of pleural fluid, 707
Culture and sensitivity
  blood, 101-103
  cerebrospinal fluid, 479
  handling of specimens for, 101
  sputum, 683-684
  stool, 687-688
  throat, 711-712
  urine, 764-766
  wound, 794-795
Cushing's syndrome, 8, 11, 98, 237, 239, 268, 419, 509, 658
CVA, 123
CVP, 154*t*
CXR, 174-176
Cystic fibrosis, 34, 340, 692
  CA 19-9 tumor marker in, 138
Cystography, 256-257
Cystometrogram (CMG), 258-260

Cystometry, 258-260
Cystoscopy, 261-264
Cystourethrography, 256-257
Cysts, renal, 446
Cytologic test for cancer, 539-541
Cytology
  amniotic fluid, 36
  cerebrospinal fluid, 480-481
  gastric, 368-369
  pleural fluid, 707
  seminal, 659-660
  sputum, 685-686
Cytomegalovirus (CMV), 265, 729
Cytotoxic antibody, anti-HLA-B27, 412

D

Dane particle, 407-408
Dead space, 609*i*
Decubitus view chest x-ray, 174
Deep vein thrombophlebitis (DVT), 351
Deep vein thrombosis, 568
Degenerative bone changes, 120
Degenerative brain disease, 478
Degradation products, fibrin, 349-350
Dehydration, 535
Delta-aminolevulinic acid (delta-ALA), 266-267
Demyelinating disorders, 478
Dent test, 241-242
Depression, 722
Dermatomyositis, 20
Desipramine, therapeutic, monitoring of, 702*t*
Dexamethasone suppression test (DST), 268-271
Dextroamphetamine, in toxicology screening, 731*t*
Diabetes, 391, 430
  gestational, 388
  insipidus, 51, 535
  juvenile, 430
  ketoacidosis in, 441
  maternal, 416
  mellitus, 379, 382, 384

Diabetic control index, 391-392
Diabetic ketoacidosis, 79
Diabetic nephropathy, 785
Diagnex Blue test, 364-367
Diaphragm, air under, 527
Diaphragmatic hernia, 174
Dicumarol, 601
Diethylenetriamine pentaacetic acid, 488
Diethylstibestrol (DES), in utero exposure to, 208
Differential count, 212
  causes of abnormalities in, 790*t*-791*t*
  and white blood cell count, 787-791
Diffusing capacity of lung, 610-611
Digital radiography, 272-274
Digital subtraction angiography (DSA), 272-274
Digital venous subtraction angiography (DVSA), 272-274
Digitoxin, therapeutic, monitoring of, 702*t*
Digoxin, therapeutic, monitoring of, 702*t*
Dilantin in toxicology screening, 733*t*
Dipyridamole-thallium scan, 160-163
Direct antiglobulin test, 233-234
Direct Coombs' test, 233-234
DISIDA scanning, 358-359
Disopyramide, therapeutic, monitoring of, 702*t*
Disseminated intravascular coagulation (DIC), 98, 328, 349, 564
  pathophysiology of, 276*i*
  screening for, 275-277
Diverticula, 81
  esophageal, 85
Diverticulitis, 151
DMSA renal scan, 634-637
Doppler studies, 278-280
Down's syndrome, 34

Drugs
  affecting urine color,
    762t-763t
  therapeutic, monitoring of,
    700-701, 702t-703t
DSA, 272-274
DTPA renal scan, 634-637
Duodenum
  on esophagogastroduode-
    noscopy, 321
  fiberoptic scope in, 307i
Duplex scanning, carotid,
  164-165
DVSA, 272-274
Dysgenesis, ovarian, 88
Dysplasia, cellular, 208
Dysrhythmias, cardiac, 285,
  300, 414

E

Ear oximetry, 537-538
Early antigen diffuse component
  (EAD), 312
Early antigen restricted
  component (EAR), 312
EBNA, 311
EBV, 311-313, 511
Echocardiography, 281-283
Echogram
  of liver, biliary tree,
    gallbladder, and pancreas,
    470-471
  obstetric, 524-526
  thyroid, 720-721
Ectopic pregnancy, 45, 254
Effusion, pleural, 706
Eighth cranial nerve, 145
Ejection fraction (EF), 155t
Electrocardiogram (ECG,
  EKG), 284-287
  in stress test, 333
Electrocardiograph (EKG) stress
  testing, 333-335
Electrocardiography, 284-287
Electroencephalogram (EEG),
  288-291
Electroencephalography,
  288-291
Electrolyte balance, 535

Electrolytes, sweat, test of,
  692-694
Electromyography (EMG),
  292-294
  pelvic floor sphincter,
    547-548
Electromyoneurography, 292,
  295
Electroneurography (ENG),
  295-297
Electronystagmography,
  298-299
Electrophoresis
  hemoglobin, 404-406
  immunoglobulin, 427-429
  protein, 597-599
Electrophysiologic study (EPS),
  300-302
ELISA test
  for HIV and antibody, 15-17
  for Lyme disease, 495
  sensitivity and specificity of,
    16
Elliptocytes, 109
Embolic occlusions, 65
Embolism
  amniotic fluid, 275
  pulmonary, 47, 488, 604
Emphysema, 28
Encephalitis, 478, 480
Encephalopathy, hepatic, 32
End diastolic left ventricular
  pressure, 154t
End diastolic volume (EDV),
  155t
End systolic volume (ESV),
  155t
Endarterectomy, carotid, 288
Endocarditis, 101, 251
  bacterial, 60
    subacute, 649
Endometrial biopsy, 303-304
Endometrial carcinoma, 539
Endometriosis, 455
Endoscopic retrograde
  cholangiopancreatography
    (ERCP), 305-308
Endotracheal lesions, laser
  therapy for, 129
Endourology, 261-264

Enema
   barium, 81-84
   small bowel, 672, 674
Enteritis, regional, 81
Enterobius, 688
Enterococcus, 687
Enterocolitis, clostridial, 197
Enteroendocrine cells, 422
Enteroscopy, 321
Enzyme deficiency, congenital,
      419
Enyzme-linked immunosorbent
      assay (ELISA)
   for HIV and antibody, 15-17
   for Lyme disease, 495
   sensitivity and specificity of,
      16
Enzymes
   liver, 467
   pancreatic, 656-657
Eosinophils, 787-791
   causes of abnormalities in,
      791*t*
EP studies, 330-332
Epiphrenic diverticula, 85
Epithelial casts, 309-310
Epithelial ovarian cancer, 134
Epstein-Barr nuclear antigen
      (EBNA), 311
Epstein-Barr virus (EBV), 511
   titer of, 311-313
Erythema chronicum migrans
      (ECM), 495
Erythrocyte count, 617-619
Erythrocyte indices, 620-623
Erythrocyte sedimentation rate
      (ESR), 314-316
Erythroid hypoplasia, 115
Escherichia coli, 687
Esophageal function studies,
      317-320
Esophageal manometry,
      317-320
Esophageal motility studies,
      317-320
Esophageal reflux, 85
Esophagogastroduodenoscopy
      (UGD), 321-324
Esophagus
   on computed tomography of
      chest, 223

Esophagus—cont'd
   on esophagogastroduode-
      noscopy, 321
ESR, 314-316
Estriol excretion, 325-327
Estrogen fractions, 325-327
Estrogen-secreting tumors, 443
Ethosuximide, therapeutic,
      monitoring of, 702*t*
Euglobulin clot lysis, 328-329
Euglobulin lysis time, 328-329
Evoked brain potentials,
      330-332
Evoked potential studies,
      330-332
Evoked responses, 330-332
Excretory function of kidneys,
      634
Excretory urography (EUG),
      432-436
Exercise stress testing, 333-335
   with thallium scanning, 161
Exophthalmos, malignant, 474
Expiratory reserve volume
      (ERV), 609*i*
Extraadrenal
      pheochromocytoma, 8
Extracorporeal heart bypass, 275
Extraesophageal tumors, 85
Exudates in pleural fluid, 707

F

Factor
   clotting, 600-603
   rheumatoid, 649-650
Factor assay, 202-204
Fasting blood sugar (FBS),
      379-381
Fat absorption, 340-342
Fat retention coefficient, 341
Fatty casts, 336-337
Febrile/cold agglutinins,
      338-339
Fecal fat, 340-342
Femoral vein in cardiac
      catheterization, 156
Fern test, 169-171
Ferning of cervical mucus, 169
Ferritin, 343-344
Fertility workup, 659

Fetal activity determination, 520-521
Fetal distress, 34, 416
Fetal heart rate (FHR), 229, 520
Fetal hypoxia, 41, 345
Fetal infections, intrauterine, 427
Fetal lung maturity, 35
Fetal maturity, test of, 34
Fetal scalp blood pH, 345-346
Fetal skin biopsy, 347
Fetal well-being, index of, 325
α_1-Fetoprotein, 30-31
Fetoscopy, 347-348
Fetus
  hemoglobin in, 404
  human placental lactogen and, 416
Fiberoptic bronchoscope, 129, 570
Fiberoptic scope in duodenum, 307*i*
Fibrin breakdown products, 349-350
Fibrin clots, intravascular formation of, 275
Fibrin degradation products (FDPs), 276, 349-350
Fibrin production, coagulation factors in, 200*t*
Fibrin split products (FSPs), 349-350
Fibrinogen, 202, 600
Fibrinogen uptake test (FUT), 351-353
  with ^{125}I, 351-353
Fibrinolysis, 203*i*
  primary, 328
Fibrinolysis/euglobulin lysis, 328-329
Fibroadenoma, 504
Fibrocystic breast disease, 504, 704
Fibromuscular dysplasia, 65
Fibrosis, marrow, 98
Flat plate of abdomen, 527-529
Flat plate x-ray film, 448
Flexible fiberoptic bronchoscope, 129

Flipped LDH, 451
Flow studies, urine, 767-768
Fluoescent treponemal antibody absorption test (FTA-ABS), 695
Fluorescent treponemal antibody test, 695-696
Foam stability test, 35
Folate, 354-355
Folic acid, 354-355
  deficiency of, 109
Follow-through, small bowel, 672-675
Forced expiratory reserve volume in 1 second (FEV$_1$), 608, 609*i*
Forced vital capacity (FVC), 608, 609*i*
Foreign bodies
  bronchial, removal of, 129
  ingestion of, 527
Fracture(s), 26, 120
  healing of, 476
  skull, 670
  stress, of vertebrae, 681
FT$_4$ index, 727-728
FTA, 695-696
FTI, 727-728
Functional residual volume (FRV), 609*i*
Fungus, culture of pleural fluid for, 706, 707

G

Galactose-1-phosphate uridyl transferase (Gal-1-PUT), 356-357
Galactosemia, 34
  screening for, 356-357
Gallbladder scanning, 358-359
Gallbladder series, 186-189
Gallium scam, 360-361
Gallstones, 93, 183, 186, 470, 551, 697
  CA 19-9 tumor marker in, 138
Gammaglobulins, 597
  electrophoresis of, 427-429
Gamma-glutamyl transferase (GGT), 362-363

Gamma-glutamyl transpeptidase (GGTP, γ-GTP), 362-363
Gangrene, 20
Gases, arterial blood, 104-108
Gastric analysis, 364-367
Gastric cytology, 368-369
Gastric emptying scan, 370-371
Gastric ulcer, 364
Gastrin, 372-373
Gastroesophageal reflux scan, 374-375
Gastrogafin, 746
Gastrointestinal bleeding scan, 376-378
Gastrointestinal cancer, carcinoembryonic antigen in, 151
Gastrointestinal x-ray study, upper, 746-748
Gastroscopy, 321-324
Gated pool ejection fraction (GPEF), 160-161
Gated pool imaging, 160-161
Gaucher's disease, 47
GB series, 186-189
G-cell hyperplasia, 372
GE reflux scan, 374-375
Genetic aberrations, 34
Genetic typing, 28
Gentamicin, therapeutic, monitoring of, 702t
German measles test, 651-652
Gestational diabetes, 388
GI scintigraphy, 376-378
Giardia, 687
Globulin(s), 597
  thyroid-binding, 740
Glomerular filtration rate (GFR), 245
Glomerulonephritis, 60, 245, 251, 309, 432, 595, 711, 786, 792
Glucose
  blood, 379-381
  cerebrospinal fluid, 480
  pleural fluid, 707
  postprandial, 382-383
  urine, 384-385

Glucose tolerance test (GTT), 388-390
Glucose-6-phosphate dehydrogenase (G-6-PD screen), 386-387
Glutamine in cerebrospinal fluid, 481
Glutethimide in toxicology screening, 733t
Glycohemoglobin (Hb A$_{1c}$), 391-392
Glycosuria, 384
Glycosylated hemoglobin (GHb, GHB), 391-392
Goiter, 713
Gonadal insufficiency, 493
Gonorrhea culture, 393-395
Gout, 253, 757
  and pseudogout, 70
Graded exercise testing, 333-335
Gram stain, 101
  pleural fluid, 707
  sputum, 683-684
  with throat culture, 711
  urine, 764
  wound, 794
Granular casts, 396-397
Granuloma, lung, 485
Granulomatous infections, 507
Graves' disease, 474, 713
Guthrie test, 558-560
Gynecologic laparoscopy, 455-457

H

Hageman factor, 202
HAI, 651-652
Haptoglobin, 398-399
Hashimoto's thyroiditis, 62, 64
HCO$_3$−, 105, 106t
Headache, 123
Healing of fracture, 476
Heart scan, 160-163
Heart sonogram and cardiac echo, 281-283
Heinz bodies, 110
Hemagglutination inhibition test, 651-652
Hematocrit (Hct), 400-401
Heme synthesis, 266

Hemochromatosis, 343
Hemoglobin (Hb, Hgb), 402-403, 620
    electrophoresis, 404-406
    fetal, and bilirubin, 34
    glycosylated, 391-392
Hemoglobin C disease, 405
Hemoglobin H disease, 405
Hemoglobinopathies, 110, 404
Hemolysis of red blood cells, 398
    accelerated, 93
Hemolytic anemia, 79, 110, 113, 115, 233, 276, 343, 354, 405, 624
Hemophilia, 34, 544
Hemoptysis, 126
Hemorrhage
    cerebral, 478
    colonic, 205
    on computed tomography of adrenals, 217
    gastrointestinal, 321
    intracranial, 220
    spontaneous, 563
Hemorrhagic anemia, 115
Hemosiderosis, 343
Hemostasis, 203i
Henoch-Schönlein syndrome, 98
Heparin, 544
Hepatic abscess, 470
Hepatic coma, 32
Hepatic encephalopathy, 32
Hepatitis, 20, 54, 78, 93, 266, 467, 649
    viral, 251
Hepatitis A virus (HAV), 407
Hepatitis B virus (HBV), 407
Hepatitis C, 409
Hepatitis virus studies, 407-409
Hepatitis-associated antigen (HAA), 407-409
Hepatobiliary cancer, CA 19-9 tumor marker in, 138
Hepatobiliary imaging, 358-359
Hepatobiliary scintigraphy, 358-359
Hepatocellular cancer, 30
Hepatocellular liver disease, 600
Hepatocyte function, 593

Hepatoma, 26, 54
Hepatomegaly, 467
Hereditary elliptocytosis, 109
Hereditary metabolic disorders, 34
Hereditary spherocytosis, 109
Hernia, diaphragmatic, 174
Herpes, 729
Herpes genitalis, 410-411
Herpes simplex type 2 (HSV 2), 410-411
Herpesvirus type 2, 410-411
Heterophil antibody test, 511-512
Hgb S test, 663-664
Hiatal hernia, 85
HIDA scanning, 358-359
High-density lipoprotein (HDL), 190, 464-466
Histamine challenge test, 611
Histoplasmosis, 47
HIV antibody test, 15-17
HLA-B27 antigen, 412-413
Hodgkin's disease, 30, 47, 116
Holter monitoring, 414-416
Hookworm, 687
Hormone
    thyroid-stimulating, 716-717
        stimulation test of, 718-719
    thyrotropin-releasing, test of, 722-723
Howell-Jolly bodies, 110
Human chorionic gonadotropin (HCG), 583
Human chorionic somatomammotropin (HCS), 416
Human immunodeficiency virus (HIV), 15
Human lymphocyte antigen B27, 412-413
Human placental lactogen (HPL), 416
Hyaline casts, 417-418
Hydatidiform mole, 524, 584
Hydrocephalus, 124
Hydrocortisone
    blood, 237-238
    urine, 239-240
Hydronephrosis, 49, 432, 446

17-Hydroxycorticosteroids (17-OCHS), 419-421
5-Hydroxyindoleacetic acid (5-HIAA), 422-423
Hyperaldosteronism, 638
Hyperbilirubinemia, 93, 95
Hypercalcemia, 140, 241, 542
Hyperchloremia, 179
Hyperchromasia, 110
Hyperglycemia, 379
Hyperkalemia, 578-579
Hypernatremia, 676
Hyperparathyroidism, 140, 143, 241, 253, 542, 744
Hypersensitivity, 116, 427
Hypersplenism, 98, 563
  secondary, 116
Hypertension, 638, 641
  malignant, 786
  portal, 116
Hyperthyroidism, 612, 713, 722, 724, 727, 738
Hyperuricemia, 754
Hyperuricosuria, 757
Hyperventilation in electroencephalography, 290
Hypochloremia, 179
Hypoglycemia, 379
Hypogonadism, male, 88
Hypokalemia, 578-579
Hyponatremia, 679
Hypoparathyroidism, 143, 542
Hypophosphatemia, 561
Hypopituitarism, 13, 419
Hypothyroidism, 612, 722, 724, 727, 738
  primary and secondary, 716, 718
Hypoxemia, 110
Hypoxia, fetal, 41, 345
Hysterogram, 424-426
Hysterosalpingography, 424-426

I

131I uptake test, 612-614
IDA gallbladder scanning, 358-359
Idiopathic hemolytic anemia, 233

Idiopathic pulmonary fibrosis, 47
Ileus, 672
Imipramine, therapeutic, monitoring of, 702t
Immune complexes, 649
Immune deficiency, 427
Immunoglobulin
  electrophoresis, 427-429
  thyroid-stimulating, 474-475
Immunoglobulin G, cerebrospinal fluid level of, 480
Immunologic pregnancy tests, 583
Incontinence, 258
Indirect Coombs' test, 235-236
Infarction
  cerebral, 123, 220
  myocardial, 78, 153, 285, 450, 518
  renal, 45
Infection, 69
  chronic, 427
Infectious hepatitis, 407
Infectious mononucleosis, 54, 78, 251, 311, 649
Infertility, 455
  evaluation of, 58-59, 254
Inhalation tests, 611
Inspiratory capacity (IC), 609i
Inspiratory reserve volume (IRV), 608, 609i
Insulin assay, 430-431
Intestinal motility, diminished, 672
Intestine, carcinoma of, 52
Intraglandular lymph nodes, 495
Intrauterine device (IUD), 455
Intrauterine fetal infections, 427
Intrauterine growth retardation, 416
Intravascular clots, 276
Intravenous cholangiogram (IVC), 183-185
Intravenous glucose tolerance test (IV-GTT), 388-389
Intravenous pyelography (IVP), 49, 432-436

Intravenous urography (IUG, IVU), 432-436
Intussusception, nonstrangulated ileocolic, 81
Iodine uptake test, 612-614
Iodine-125 fibrinogen uptake test, 351
Ionized calcium, blood, 140
Iontophoretic sweat test, 692-694
Iron deficiency anemia, 115, 437-438
Iron level and total iron-binding capacity (Fe and TIBC), 437-440
Iron storage, 343
Ischemia
  cerebral, 288
  myocardial, 161
Isoenzymes
  of alkaline phosphatase, 26
  of bone origin (ALP$_2$), 26
  creatinine phosphokinse, 248-249
  of liver origin (ALP$_1$), 26
IUD, 455
IVP, 49, 432-436
Ivy bleeding time, 98-100
Ixodes dammini, 495

J

Jaundice, 92, 95, 305, 467
  obstructive, 20, 54
  physiologic, of newborn, 92-93, 95
Joint aspiration, 69-72
Juvenile diabetes, 427

K

Kanamycin, therapeutic, monitoring of, 703t
Kernicterus, 93, 95
Ketoacidosis, 441
  diabetic, 79
Ketones, 441-442
17-Ketosteroids (17-KS), 443-445
Kidney(s)
  biopsy of, 631-633
  computed tomography of, 226-228

Kidney(s)—cont'd
  on computed tomography of abdomen, 213
  on intravenous pyelography, 432, 433
Kidney, ureter, and bladder x-ray study (KUB), 448-449
Kidney scan, 634-637
Kidney sonogram, 446-447
Kidney stones, 527
Klinefelter's syndrome, 88
Kupffer cells, 26

L

Lactic dehydrogenase, 450-452
  in cerebrospinal fluid, 480
  in pleural fluid, 707
Lactogen, human placental, 416
Lactose tolerance test, 453-454
Laparoscopy, 455-457
Laryngography, 126-128
Laser therapy for endotracheal lesions, 129
Latency, 330
Lateral view chest x-ray, 174
Latex fixation test, 649-650
Lead poisoning, 110, 266
Lead in toxicology screening, 733t
Lecithin/sphingomyelin (L/S ratio), 35-36
Leprosy, 47
Leptocytes, 110
Leucine aminopeptidase (LAP), 458-459
Leukemia, 52, 98, 110, 115, 116, 251, 511, 564
  chronic lymphocytic, 90
Leukemoid drug reactions, 113
Leukocyte count, 787-791
Leukocyte esterase, 460-461
Lidocaine, therapeutic, monitoring of, 703t
Limb leads, EKG, 284, 285, 286-287
Lipase, 462-463
Lipid and cholesterol count in pleural fluid, 708
Lipoproteins, 464-466
  high- and low-density, 190

Liquid-emptying study, 370
Lithium
  therapeutic, monitoring of,
      703*t*
  in toxicology screening, 733*t*
Liver
  on computed tomography of
      abdomen, 213
  and pancreatobiliary system
      ultrasonography, 470-471
Liver autoimmune disease, 54
Liver biopsy, 467-469
Liver cell dysfunction, 362
Liver congestion, 78
Liver disease, 18, 110, 533
  cholesterol in, 190
  chronic, 593
Liver scanning, 472-473
Liver tumors, primary, 26
Long bones x-ray, 476-477
Long-acting thyroid stimulator
      (LATS), 474-475
Lordotic view chest x-ray, 174
Low-density lipoprotein (LDL),
      190, 464-466
Lower esophageal sphincter
      (LES) pressure, 317
Lower extremities
  arteriography of, 65-68
  venography of, 779-781
Lower GI series, 81-84
Lumbar puncture
  and cerebrospinal fluid
      examination (LP and
      CSF examination),
      478-484
  patient position for, 482*i*
Lumbar x-rays, 681-682
Lung
  carcinoma of, 52, 269
  diffusing capacity of, 610-611
Lung biopsy, 485-487
Lung scan, 488-490
Lupus erythematosus, 210
Lupus erythematosus test (LE
      cell prep), 491-492
Lupus nephritis, 792
Luteinizing hormone assay (LH
      assay), 493-494
Lyme disease test, 495-496

Lymphangiogram, 497-499
Lymphangiography, 497-499
Lymphocyte count, 787-791
Lymphocytes, causes of
      abnormalities in, 790*t*
Lymphocytic leukemia, 116
Lymphography, 497-499
Lymphoma(s), 30, 116, 343,
      497
  concentrating gallium, 360
  thymus, 52

M

Macroamylasemia, 45
Macrocytes, 109
Macrocytic normochromic
      anemia, 621*t*
Macroglobulinemia, 251
  Waldenström's, 199
Magnetic resonance imaging
      (MRI), 500-503
Malabsorption, 253, 340, 354,
      672
Maldigestion, 340
Male hypogonadism, 88
Malignant exophthalmos, 474
Malignant hypertension, 786
Malnutrition, 354
  cholesterol in, 190
Mammogram, 504-506
Mammography, 504-506
Mammothermography, 704-705
Marrow infiltrative diseases, 116
Master's two-step test, 333
Mastitis, 504
Maximal heart rate, 333
Maximal midexpiratory flow
      (MMF), 608, 609*i*
Maximal volume ventilation
      (MVV), 608, 609*i*
MCH, 620-623
MCHC, 620-623
MCV, 620-623
M/E ratio, 116
Mean corpuscular hemoglobin
      (MCH), 620-623
Mean corpuscular hemoglobin
      concentration (MCHC),
      620-623

Mean corpuscular volume (MCV), 620-623
Meconium staining of amniotic fluid, 34, 41
Medianoscopy, 507-508
Mediastinal structures on computed tomography of chest, 223
Mediterranean G-6-PD deficiency, 386
Megakaryocytes, 115-116
Megaloblastic anemia, 110, 343, 354
Meningitis, 478, 480
  recurrent, 124
Meprobamate in toxicology screening, 733*t*
Metabolic acidosis, 105, 106*t*, 107*t*
Metabolic alkalosis, 105, 106*t*, 107*t*
Metabolic disorders, hereditary, 34
Metapyrone, 509-510
Metastasis, 98, 113, 116, 120, 343, 507
Methacholine challenge test, 611
Methamphetamine in toxicology screening, 731*t*
Methotrexate, therapeutic, monitoring of, 703*t*
Methyprylon in toxicology screening, 733*t*
Metrizamide, 513-514
Microcytes, 109
Microcytic hypochromic anemia, 621*t*
Microcytic normochromic anemia, 621*t*
Microsomal antibody, 64
Milk-alkali syndrome, 542
Minimal hemostatic levels of coagulation factors, 200*t*, 202
Minute ventilation, 609*i*
Minute volume (MV), 609*i*
M-mode echocardiography, 281
Monitoring
  Holter, 414-416
  therapeutic drug, 700-701, 702*t*-703*t*

Monospot test, 511-512
Monocyte count, 787-791
Monocytes, causes of abnormalities in, 791*t*
Mononuclear heterophil test, 511-512
Mononucleosis, 116
Mononucleosis spot test, 511-512
Motility, esophageal, 317
Mucin clot test, 69-70
Mucosal inflammation, colonic, 205
Mucus, cervical, 169-171, 668
Multiple myeloma, 90, 116, 251, 427
Multiple pregnancy, 524-526
Multiple sclerosis, 20, 330, 478
Mumps, 43, 45
Murphy-Pattee test, 724
Muscle injury, myocardial, 248
Muscle mass and creatinine, 243
Muscular dystrophy, 20
Muscular trauma, 20
Musculoskeletal trauma, 79
Myasthenia gravis, 20
Mycobacterium tuberculosis, 1, 479, 683, 706
Mycoplasma pneumoniae, 338
Myelitis, 480
Myelofibrosis, 113
  drug-induced or idiopathic, 116
Myelogram, 513-517
Myelography, 513-517
Myeloma, 47, 110
Myelomeningocele, 30, 34
Myocardial infarction (MI), 78, 153, 285, 450, 518
Myocardial muscle injury, 248
Myocardial scan, 160-163
Myoglobin, 518-519

N

Natiuretic hormone, 676
Necrosis, bone, 120
Neisseria gonorrhea, 393
Neoplasia, 69, 275
  colonic, 205
  intracranial, 220
  metastatic, 113

Nephritis, lupus, 792
Nephropathy, diabetic, 786
Nephrotic syndrome, 336, 595
Nephrotomography, 433
Nerve conduction studies,
    295-297
Neural tube defects (NTDs), 30,
    34, 347
Neurologic bladder dysfunction,
    258
Neurologic disorders, 330
Neuropathies, 295
Neurosyphilis, 478
Neutrophil count, 787-791
Neutrophils, causes of
    abnormalities in, 790*t*
Newborn
    cytomegalovirus in, 265
    physiologic jaundice of,
        92-93, 95
Nipple stimulation technique,
    232
Nitrogen, blood urea, 749-751
Nodules, thyroid, 713
    cystic and solid, 720
Non-A, non-B hepatitis, 409
Nonstrangulated ileocolic
    intussusception, 81
Nonstress test (NST), 520-521
Normocytic normochromic
    anemia, 621*t*
Nortriptyline, therapeutic,
    monitoring of, 703*t*
Nuclear cardiac scanning,
    160-163
Nuclear imaging of kidney,
    634-637
Nuclear magnetic resonance
    (NMR), 500-503
5-Nucleotidase, 522-523
Nutrition, 593
Nystagmus, 298
    rotary, 145

O

O₂ saturation, 107
OB, stool for, 689-691
Oblique view chest x-ray,
    174
Obstetric echography, 524-526

Obstetric ultrasonography,
    524-526
Obstruction series, 448,
    527-529
Obstructive biliary disease, 26,
    600
Obstructive jaundice, 20, 54
Obstructive pulmonary disease,
    607
Occlusion cuff, 568
Occult blood testing, stool for,
    689-691
Oculoplethysmography (OMG),
    530-532
Oculovestibular reflex, 298
    study of, 145-146
Odor, urine, 769-770
Oil-based contrast material,
    513
Oligoclonal gammaglobulin
    bands, 480
Oligospermia, 659
O&P, stool test for, 687, 688
Opacification of nasal sinuses,
    670
Open method lung biopsy, 485,
    487
Open pleural biopsy, 570
Operative cholangiogram,
    697-699
Ophthalmic artery, blood flow
    in, 530
Oral cholecystogram, 186-189
Oral glucose tolerance test
    (OGTT), 388-390
Oropharyngeal culture,
    gonorrhea, 394
Osmolality
    blood, 533-534
    urine, 535-536
Osteodystrophy, 120
Osteomyelitis, 120, 476
Ova and parasites, stool test for,
    687-688
Ovarian cancer, 134
Ovarian dysgenesis, 88
Ovarian enlargement, 524
Ovaries and laparoscopy, 455
Overnight dexamethasone
    suppression test, 270

Ovulation, 493, 586, 588
  detection of, 169
Oximetry, 537-538
Oxygen, fetal, 229
Oxygen content of blood, 105,
    106t, 107
Oxygen saturation, 537-538
  arterial (SaO₂), 537
Oxytocin challenge test (OCT),
    229-232

P

P wave, 285
Packed cell volume (PCV),
    400-401
Packed red cell volume, 400-401
Paget's disease, 26, 120
Paigen assay, 356
Panacinar emphysema, 28
Pancreas
  carcinoma of, 43, 45, 52
    CA 19-9 tumor marker in,
    138
  on computed tomography of
    abdomen, 213
Pancreatic abscess, 470
Pancreatic ducts, 656-657
  obstruction of, 340
Pancreatic enzymes, 656-657
Pancreatitis, 43, 45, 79, 462,
    470
    CA 19-9 tumor marker in,
    138
Pancreatobiliary system
    ultrasonography, 470-471
Pantopaque, 513
Pap smear, 539-541
Pap test, 539-541
Papanicolaou smear, 539-541
Paralytic ileus, 527
Paraneoplastic syndrome ectopic
    ADH production, 51-52
Parasites, stool test for, 687-688
Parathormone, 542-543
Parathyroid function, 140
Parathyroid hormone (PTH),
    542-543
Parenchymal liver disease,
    600-601
Parkinson's disease, 330

Parotiditis, 43, 45
Partial thromboplastin time
    (PTT), 544-546
Patent ductus arteriosus, 153
Patient position for lumbar
    puncture, 482i
Peak drug level, 700
Pelvic endoscopy, 455-457
Pelvic floor sphincter
    electromyography
    (EMG), 547-548
Pelvic ultrasonography on
    pregnancy, 524-526
Pelvimetry, 549-550
Pelvis on computed tomography
    of abdomen, 213
Penetrating peptic ulcer, 43, 45
Peptic ulcer, 364, 372
  penetrating, 43, 45
Percutaneous liver biopsy, 467
Percutaneous needle biopsy,
    lung, 486
Percutaneous transhepatic
    cholangiography (PTC,
    PTHC), 551-554, 552i
Perforated viscus, 527
Perfusion
  of kidneys, 634
  pulmonary, 488
Pericardiocentesis, 555-557
Pericarditis, 78
Peripheral blood smear, 109-111
Peripheral vascular disease, 464
Peripheral vascular occlusion,
    566
Pernicious anemia, 354, 653
PFT, 607-611
pH
  blood, 104-105, 106t
    fetal scalp, 345-346
  pleural fluid, 707-708
  urine, 771-772
Pharyngitis, streptococcal, 711
Phenmetrazine in toxicology
    screening, 731t
Phenobarbital
  therapeutic, monitoring of,
    703t
  in toxicology screening, 733t

Phenylalanine screening, 558-560
Phenylketonuria (PKU) test, 558-560
Pheochromocytoma, 5, 8
Phlebography, 779-781
Phorphorus (P), 561-562
Phosphate (PO$_4$), 561-562
  tubular reabsorption of, 744-745
Photostimulation in electroencephalography, 290
Physiologic jaundice of newborn, 92-93, 95
Phytonadione, 601
Pilocarpine iontophoresis, 692
Pineal glands, 670
Pinworms, 688
Pituitary gland, 658, 722
  ACTH-producing tumor of, 11
Placenta previa, 524
Placental blood flow, 229
Placental function, 325
Placental lactogen, human, 416
Plain film, 448
  of abdomen, 527-529
Plasma cortisol level, 8
Plasma estriol determination, 325-326
Plasma renin assay, 638-640
Plasma thromboplastin antecedent, 202
Platelet count, 563-565
Platelet precursors, 115-116
Plethysmography
  arterial, 566-567
  venous, 568-569
Pleura, fluid accumulation in, 174
Pleural biopsy, 570-572
Pleural effusion, 706
Pleural fluid analysis, 706-710
Pleural tap, 706-710
Pleuroscopy, 570
Plummer's disease, 713
Pneumonia, localized, 126
Poikilocytosis, 109
Poliomyelitis, 20

Polycythemia vera, 115, 116, 564
Polymyositis, 20
Polyneuropathy, acute demyelinating, 478
Polyps, 81
  colonic, 205
Porphobilinogens and porphyrins, 573-574
Porphyria, 266
Porphyrins and porphobilinogens, 573-574
Portal hypertension, 116
Positron-emission tomography (PET), 575-577
Postcoital cervical mucus test, 668-669
Postcoital test, 668-669
Posteroanterior view chest x-ray, 174
Postmaturity, fetal, 416
Postprandial glucose, 382-383
Postsplenectomy syndromes, 564
Poststreptococcal disease, 60
Potassium
  blood (K$^+$), 578-580
  urine (K$^+$), 581-582
P-R interval, 285
PRA, 638-640
Prealbumin, thyroid-binding, 740
Pregnancy, 79, 354
  blood typing in, 112
  ectopic, 45, 254, 455
  hemoglobin in, 402
  herpes infection in, 411
  high-risk, 229
  human placental lactogen in, 416
  iron in, 438
  multiple, 416, 524-526
  pelvic ultrasonography in, 524-526
  Rh-sensitized, 34
  rubella antibody test in, 651
  syphilis detection test in, 695
  tests for, 583-585
  thyroid status in, 727

Pregnancy—cont'd
toxoplasmosis in, 734
tuberculin test in, 742
uterus ultrasonography in, 524-526
Pregnanediol, 586-587
Pressure(s)
in cardiac monitoring, 154*t*
cerebrospinal fluid, 478-479
urethral, 752-753
Primary aldosteronism, 22
Primidone, therapeutic, monitoring of, 703*t*
Proaccelerin, 202
Procainamide, therapeutic, monitoring of, 703*t*
Proconvertin stable factor, 202
Proctoscopy, 665-667
Progesterone assay, 588-589
Progesterone supplementation, 586
Proliferative endometrium, 303
Prolonged dexamethasone suppression test (DSP), 268-271
Propranolol, therapeutic, monitoring of, 703*t*
Prostate gland, 3
Prostate-specific antigen (PSA), 590-591
Prostatic acid phosphatase (PAP), 3-4
Prostatic carcinoma, 3, 590
Prosthetic heart valves, 563
Protein(s)
Bence Jones, 90-91
blood, 592-594
cerebrospinal fluid, 479
electrophoresis, 597-599
free hemoglobin–binding, 398
pleural fluid, 706-707
urine, 595-596
Proteinuria, 417, 595
and edema, 595
Proteus, 687
Prothrombin, 202
Prothrombin time, 600-603
Pro-time, 600-603
Protozoans, 687

P_{CO_2}, 105, 106*t*
P_{O_2}, 105, 106*t*, 107
Pseudocyst, pancreatic, 470
Pseudogout, 70
Pseudomembranous colitis, 197
Pseudomembranous colitis toxic assay, 197-198
Pseudomonas, 687, 760
PT, 600-603
Pulmonary angiography, 604-606
Pulmonary arteriography, 604-606
Pulmonary artery pressure, 153, 154*t*
Pulmonary diseases, 52
Pulmonary embolism, 47, 488, 604
Pulmonary function tests, 607-611
Pulmonary scintiphotography, 488-490
Pulmonary toilet, 130
Pulmonary wedge pressure, 153, 154*t*
Pulse oximetry, 537-538
Pulse wave, arterial, 566
Purified protein derivative, 742
Purpura, Henoch-Schönlein, 98
Pyelography
antegrade, 49-50
retrograde, 646-648
Pyelonephritis, 792

Q
QRS complex, 285
Quantitative calcium, 143-144
Quantitative fibrinogen, 200*t*, 202
Quantitative stool fat determination, 340-342
Queckenstedt-Stookey test, 479, 483
Quinidine, therapeutic, monitoring of, 703*t*

R
Radiation therapy, 115
Radioactive fibrinogen scanning, 351-353

Radioactive iodine uptake, 612-614
Radiographic pelvimetry, 549-550
Radioimmunoassay (RIA) for pregnancy, 583-584
Radioisotope liver scanning, 472-473
Radionuclide renal imaging, 634-637
Radioreceptor (RRA) for pregnancy, 584
Radiorenography, 634-637
RAIU, 612-614
Rape, 3
Rapid dexamethasone suppression test (DSP), 268-271
Rapid plasma reagin, 695-696
Rapid surfactant test, 35
Raynaud's phenomenon, 251
RBC count, 617-619
RBC indexes, 620-623
RBC intracellular structure, 110
RBC shape, variations in, 109
RBC size, variations in, 109
RBC smear, 109-111
RBC survival study, 624-626
RBCs and casts, 615-616
Reabsorption, tubular phosphate, 744-745
Recording cuff, 568
Rectal culture, gonorrhea, 393
Rectal EMG procedure, 547-548
Red blood cell count, 617-619
Red blood cell indices, 620-623
Red blood cell morphology, 109-111
Red blood cell survival study, 624-626
Red blood cells and casts, 615-616
Reflux scan, gastroesophageal, 374-375
Regional enteritis, 81
Reiter's syndrome, 412
Renal angiography, 627-630
Renal arteriography, 627-630
Renal biopsy, 631-633

Renal calculi, 446, 771
and hyperuricosuria, 757
Renal cell cancer, 30
Renal failure, 535
Renal function studies, 243, 750
Renal infarction, 45
Renal scanning, 634-637
Renal stone formation, 253
Renal tubular casts, 309-310
Renal ultrasonography, 446-447
Renal vein renin assay, 641-643
Renin assay
plasma, 638-640
renal vein, 641-643
Renin-angiotensin system, 22
Renogram, 634
Renography, 634-637
Residual blood level, 700
Residual volume (RV), 609*i*
Resin triiodothyronine uptake test, 740-741
Respiratory acidosis 105, 106*t*, 107*t*
Respiratory alkalosis, 105, 106*t*, 107*t*
Respiratory distress syndrome (RDS), 35
Restrictive pulmonary disease, 607
Retention of dead fetus, 275
Retic count, 644-645
Reticulocyte count, 644-645
Reticulocyte index, 644
Reticulocytosis, 109, 110
Retrograde pyelography, 49, 646-649
Retroperitoneal lymph nodes on computed tomography of abdomen, 213
Reye's syndrome, 481
RF, 649-650
Rh isoimmunization, 34
Rh sensitization, 416
Rh typing, 113
Rheumatic carditis, 78
Rheumatic disease, 56
Rheumatic fever, 60, 116, 711
Rheumatoid arthritis, 26, 70, 251, 649

Rheumatoid factor, 649-650
RhoGAM, 113
Right femoral artery in cardiac
    catheterization, 156
Rigid bronchoscope, 129
Rotary nystagmus, 145
RPR, 695-696
RT₃U, 740-741
Rubella, 729
Rubella antibody test, 651-652

S

Sacral x-rays, 681-682
Salicylate
    therapeutic, monitoring of,
        703t
    in toxicology screening, 733t
Salivary ducts, 661
Salmonella, 687
Salpingitis, 455
Sarcoidosis, 47, 241, 467, 472,
        507, 542
    lung, 485
SBF, 672-675
Scalp blood, fetal, pH of,
        345-346
Scanning
    renal, 634-637
    thyroid, 713-715
Scarlet fever, 60
Schilling test, 653-655
Scintigraphy, hepatobiliary,
        358-359
Scintiphotography, pulmonary,
        488-490
Scintiscan, thyroid, 713-715
Scleroderma, 47
Scout film, 448
    of abdomen, 527-529
Secretin-pancreozymin, 656-657
Secretory endometrium, 303
Sed rate test, 314-316
Seizures, 123, 533
Sella turcica x-ray, 658
Semen analysis, 659-660
Semen examination, 659-660
Seminal cytology, 659-660
Seminal fluid, 3
Septal defects, cardiac, 153
Septic arthritis, 70

Septicemia, 275
Sequestration, splenic, study of,
        624-626
Serologic test for syphilis,
        695-696
    of cerebrospinal fluid, 481
Serum agglutination and
        inhibition, 58-59
Serum albumin, 592-594
Serum angiotensin-converting
        enzyme (SACE), 47-48
Serum calcium, 140-142
Serum cortisol, 237-238
Serum creatinine, 243-244
Serum globulin, 592-594
Serum glutamic-oxaloacetic
        transaminase (SGOT),
        78-80
Serum glutamic-pyruvic
        transaminase (SGPT),
        18-19
Serum hepatitis, 407
Serum osmolality, 533-534
Serum sickness, 210
Serum urea nitrogen, 749-751
Sex chromatin body, 88-89
Sex of fetus, 34
Sexually transmitted diseases,
        393, 410
SGOT, 78-80
SGPT, 18-19
Shake test, 35
Shatzski's rings, 85
Sheep cell agglutination test,
        649-650
Shigella, 687
Short gut syndrome, 340
Sialography, 661-662
Sickle cell anemia, 109,
        404-405, 663, 664
    maternal, 416
Sickle cell preparation, 663-664
Sickle cell test, 663-664
Sickle cell trait, 405
Sickledex, 663-664
Sigmoidoscopy, 665-667
Sims-Huhner test, 668-669
Single-photon emission
        computed tomography
        (SPECT), 162

Sinuses, opacification of, 670
Skeletal muscle and creatinine phosphokinse, 249
Skull x-ray, 670-671
SLE, 56, 70, 251, 491, 511, 649, 708
Sleep electroencephalography, 290
Small bowel enema, 672-675
Small bowel follow-through, 672-675
Smear
 blood, 109-111
 chlamydial, 177-178
Sodium (Na^+)
 blood, 676-678
 reabsorption of, 578
 urine, 679-680
Solid-emptying study, 370
Somatomammotropin, human chorionic, 416
Somatosensory evoked responses (SERs), 331
Sonogram
 heart, and cardiac echo, 281-283
 kidney, 446-447, 446-447
 thyroid, 720-721
Specific gravity of urine, 773-774
Sperm
 examination of, 659-660
 penetration of cervical mucus, test of, 668-669
Sperm antibodies, 58-59
Sperm count, 659-660
Spherocytosis, hereditary, 109
Spina bifida, 34
Spinal canal, myelography of, 513
Spinal cord injuries, 331
Spinal cord neoplasm, 478
Spinal puncture, 478-484
Spinal tap, 478-484
Spinal x-rays, 681-682
Spinnbarkheit of cervical mucus, 169, 170i
Spleen on computed tomography of abdomen, 213

Splenic sequestration study, 624-626
Split fibrin, products of, 349-350
Spondylolisthesis, 681
Spondylosis, 681
Sprue, 354
Sputum
 culture and sensitivity of, 683-684
 cytology of, 685-686
ST segment, 285
Stab cells, 788
Staphylococcus, 687
Staphylococcus aureus, 687
Stationary bicycle stress test, 333
Steatorrhea, 340
Stenosis of renal artery, 627
Stomach
 emptying ability of, 370
 on esophagogastroduodenoscopy, 321
Stool culture, 687-688
Stool for occult blood testing, 689-691
Streptococcal pharyngitis, 711
Streptokinase, administration of, 153
Streptolysin O, 60
Stress fracture of vertebrae, 681
Stress test, 333-335
 contraction, 229-232
 thallium, 161
Stroke, 123
Stroke volume (SV), 155t
Strongyloides, 687
STS, 695-696
Stuart factor, 202
Subacute bacterial endocarditis, 649
Subclavian vein in cardiac catheterization, 156
Survival study, red blood cell, 624-626
Swallow, barium, 85-87
Swallowing pattern, 317
Sweat electrolytes test, 692-694
Syndrome of inappropriate antidiuretic hormone secretion (SIADH), 51, 535

Synovial fluid analysis, 69-72
Synovial fluid glucose value, 70
Synovitis, 69
Syphilis, serology for, 695-696
  of cerebrospinal fluid, 481
Systemic lupus erythematosus
    (SLE), 56, 70, 251, 491,
    511, 649, 708
Systolic left ventricular pressure,
    154t

T

T wave, 285
T₃ by RAI, 738-739
T₃ radioimmunoassay, 738-739
T₃ resin uptake test, 740-741
T₃ᵣᵤ, 740-741
T₄, 724-726
Tap, pleural, 706-710
Tape test for pinworms, 688
Tapeworm, 687
Technetium-99m, 160
Technetium (Tc) sulfur, 472
Testes, blocked efferent ducts in,
    58
Testicular cancer, 30
Testosterone-secreting tumors,
    443
TGs, 736-737
Thalassemia, 109, 110
Thalassemia major, 405
Thalassemia minor, 405
Thallium scan, 160-163
Thallium stress testing, 161
Thallium-201, 160
Theophylline, therapeutic,
    monitoring of, 703t
Therapeutic drug monitoring,
    700-701, 702t-703t
Thermography, 704-705
Thoracentesis and pleural fluid
    analysis, 706-710
Thoracic x-rays, 681-682
Throat culture
  gonorrhea, 393
  and sensitivity, 711-712
Thrombasthenia, 199
Thrombi, atherosclerotic, 65
Thrombocyte count, 563-565

Thrombocytopenia, 98, 199,
    563
Thrombocytosis, 563, 564
Thromboembolic disease, 601
Thromboembolism, 545
Thrombolytic therapy, 248
Thrombophlebitis, 101
  deep vein, 351
Thrombosis
  deep vein, 568
  vascular, 563
  venous, 779
Thymus lymphoma, 52
Thyroglobulin antibody, 62-63
Thyroid, inflammation of, 62
Thyroid antimicrosomal
    antibody, 64
Thyroid antithyroglobulin
    antibody, 62-63
Thyroid autoantibody, 62-63,
    64
Thyroid scanning, 713-715
Thyroid ultrasound, 720-721
Thyroid-binding globulin, 740
Thyroid-binding prealbumin,
    740
Thyroid-stimulating hormone,
    716-717
  stimulation test, 718-719
Thyroid-stimulating
    immunoglobulin (TSIG),
    474-475
Thyrotoxicosis, 738
Thyrotropin, 716-717
Thyrotropin-releasing factor test,
    722-723
Thyrotropin-releasing hormone
    test, 722-723
Thyroxine, 724-726
  free, index of, 727-728
Thyroxine screen, 724-726
TIA, 530
Tidal volume (TV, VT), 608,
    609i
Tobramycin, therapeutic,
    monitoring of, 703t
Tolerance test, glucose, 388-390
Tomogram, 172-173
Tomography of lungs, 172-173
TORCH test, 729

Total iron-binding capacity (TIBC), 437-440
Total lung capacity (TLC), 609i
Total protein, 592-594
Total/ionized calcium, 140-142
Toxemia, 416
Toxicology screening, 730-731t, 732t-733t
Toxin, clostridial, assay of, 197-198
Toxoplasma gondii, 734
Toxoplasmosis, 729
Toxoplasmosis antibody titer, 734-735
TPR, 744-745
Tracheobronchial malformation, 126
Trachoma, 177
Trait, sickle cell, 663, 664
Transbronchial lung biopsy, 485, 486
Transbronchial needle aspiration, 485, 486
Transcatheter bronchial brushing, 485, 486
Transferrin saturation, 437-440
Transfusion, blood
  hepatitis from, 409
  reaction to, 233, 235, 275
Transient ischemic attacks (TIAs), 530
Transluminal coronary angioplasty, 156
Transposition of great vessels, 153
Transudates in pleural fluid, 707
Trauma
  muscular, 20
  nerve, 295
Treadmill test, 333
Treponema pallidum, antibodies to, 695
TRF test, 722-723
TRH test, 722-723
Trichinosis, 20
Triglycerides, 464, 736-737
Triiodothyronine, 738-739
  uptake test, 740-741
Triple renal study, 634
Trough blood level, 700

TRP, 744-745
TSH, 716-717
  stimulation test, 718-719
T-tube and operative cholangiogram, 697-699
Tubal ligation, 455
Tube gastric analysis, 364-367
Tubeless gastric analysis, 364-367
Tuberculin test, 742-743
Tuberculosis, 1, 47, 649
Tubular necrosis, 245
Tubular phosphate reabsorption, 744-745
Tumor(s)
  in adrenal hyperfunction, 419
  associated with SIADH, 52
  bone marrow, 98
  carcinoid, 422
  cardiac, 282
  on computed tomography of adrenals, 217
  concentrating gallium, 360
  extraesophageal, 85
  intestine, 81
  liver, 467
  lung, 174
  metastatic, 78, 90, 116
  pancreatic, 470
  renal, 432
  skull, 670
  testosterone- or estrogen-secreting, 443
  uterus, testes, or ovaries, 584
Tumor marker
  CA 15-3, 136-137
  CA 19-9, 138-139
  CA-125, 134-135
Turner's syndrome, 88
Two-dimensional echocardiography, 281
Two-hour postprandial blood sugar, 382-383
Two-hour postprandial glucose (2-hour PPG), 382-383
Two-stage Schilling test, 654
Type A G-6-PD deficiency, 386
Typing, blood, 112-114

U

UGI, 746-748
Ulcer, 364
Ulceration, colonic, 205
Ulcerative colitis, 151
Ultrasonography
  liver and pancreatobiliary
    system, 470-471
  obstetric, 524-526
  renal, 446-447
Unconjugated bilirubin, 92, 95
UPP, 752-753
Upper gastrointestinal cancer,
    135
Upper gastrointestinal (UGI)
    endoscopy, 321-324
Upper gastrointestinal x-ray
    study, 746-748
Upper GI series, 746-748
Uptake
  fibrinogen, 351
  triiodothyronine, test of,
    740-741
Urea nitrogen blood test,
    749-751
Uremia, 98, 110
Ureters, obstruction of, 49, 646
Urethral culture, 177, 178
  gonorrhea, 393
Urethral pressure measurements,
    752-753
Urethral pressure profile,
    752-753
Uric acid
  blood, 754-756
  urine, 757-758
Urinalysis, 759
Urinary crystals, 253
Urinary tract infection, 460
Urine amylase, 45-46
Urine appearance and color,
    760-761, 762t-763t
Urine bilirubin, 95-97
Urine calcium, 143-144
Urine chloride, 181-182
Urine cortisol, 239-240
Urine culture and sensitivity,
    764-766
Urine flow studies, 767-768
Urine glucose, 384-385

Urine ketones, 441-442
Urine odor, 769-770
Urine osmolality, 535-536
Urine pH, 771-772
Urine specific gravity, 773-774
Urine sugar, 384-385
Urochrome, 760
Urodynamic studies, 767-768
Uroflowmetry, 767-768
Urography, excretory, 432-436
Urologic tract, carcinoma of, 52
Uterine enlargement, 524
Uterosalpingography, 424-426
Uterotubography, 424-426

V

Valproic acid, therapeutic,
    monitoring of, 703t
Valves, prosthetic, of heart, 563
Valvular defects, cardiac, 153
Vanillylmandelic acid and
    catecholamines, 775-778
Varices, esophageal, 85
Vascular structures on computed
    tomography of chest, 223
Vascular thrombosis, 563
Vasopressin, 51-53
VDRL, 695-696
Venereal Disease Research
    Laboratory test, 695-696
Venogram, 779-781
Venography
  adrenal, 8-10
  of lower extremities, 779-781
Venous patency, 278
Venous plethysmography,
    568-569
Venous thrombosis, 779
Ventilation/perfusion scanning
    (VPS), 488-490
Ventricular aneurysms, 153
Ventricular hypertrophy, 285
Ventriculogram, 782-784
Ventriculography, 153-159,
    782-784
Vertebrae, stress fracture of, 681
Very low-density lipoprotein
    (VLDL), 464-466
Vestibular portion of eighth
    cranial nerve, 145

Viral capsid antigen (VCA), 312
Viral hepatitis, 78, 251
Virus
  Epstein-Barr, 311-313
  hepatitis, 407-409
Visual evoked responses
      (VERs), 330
Vital capacity (VC), 609*i*
Vitamin B$_{12}$ absorption test,
      653-655
Vitamin B$_{12}$ deficiency, 109
Vitamin D intoxication, 542
Vitamin K, 600-601
Voiding cystography, 256-257
Voiding cystourethrography,
      256-257
Volumes in cardiac monitoring,
      154*t*
von Willebrand's disease, 98

W

Waldenström's
      macroglobulinemia, 199
Warfarin, 601
Water-soluble contrast material,
      513
Waxy casts, 785-786
WBC and differential, 787-791
WBC esterase, 460-461

Western blot test for HIV and
      antibody, 15-17
Whipple's disease, 340
White blood cell count and
      differential count,
      787-791
  causes of abnormalities in,
      790*t*-791*t*
White blood cells and casts,
      792-793
Whole blood clot retraction test,
      199-201
Wound culture and sensitivity,
      794-795

X

Xeromammogram, 505
X-ray, chest, 174-176
D-Xylose absorption test,
      796-798
Xylose tolerance test, 796-798

Y

Yersinia, 687

Z

Zenker's diverticula, 85
Zollinger-Ellison (ZE)
      syndrome, 364, 372

I

Ig	Immunoglobulin
IVC	Intravenous cholangiography
IV-GTT	Intravenous glucose tolerance test
IVP	Intravenous pyelography
IVU, IUG	Intravenous urography

K

K	Potassium
KS	Ketosteroid
KUB	Kidney, ureters, and bladder x-ray study

L

LAP	Leucine aminopeptidase
LATS	Long-acting thyroid stimulator
LDH	Lactic dehydrogenase
LDL	Low-density lipoprotein
LE	Lupus erythematosus
LES	Lower esophageal sphincter
LFT	Liver function tests
LH	Luteinizing hormone
LP	Lumbar puncture
L/S ratio	Lecithin/sphingomyelin ratio
LS spine	Lumbosacral spine

M

MCH	Mean corpuscular hemoglobin
MCHC	Mean corpuscular hemoglobin concentration
MCV	Mean corpuscular volume
MRI	Magnetic resonance imaging

N

Na	Sodium
NMR	Nuclear magnetic resonance
NST	Nonstress test

O

O&P	Ova and parasites
OB	Occult blood
OCT	Oxytocin challenge test
OGTT	Oral glucose tolerance test
17-OHCS	17-hydroxycorticosteroids
OPG	Oculoplethysmography

P

PAP	Prostatic acid phosphatase
PET	Positron-emission tomography
PFT	Pulmonary function tests
pH	Hydrogen ion concentration
PKU	Phenylketonuria
PO_2	Partial pressure of oxygen
PPBS	Postprandial blood sugar
PPD	Purified protein derivative
PPG	Postprandial glucose
PRA	Plasma renin assay